Mental Health and the Built Environment

Mental Health and the Built Environment
More than Bricks and Mortar?

David Halpern

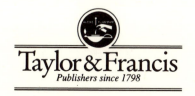

Taylor & Francis
Publishers since 1798

UK	Taylor & Francis Ltd, 4 John St., London WC1N 2ET
USA	Taylor & Francis Inc., 1900 Frost Road, Suite 101, Bristol, PA 19007

First published 1995

A Catalogue Record for this book is available from the British Library

ISBN 0 7484 0235 7
ISBN 0 7484 0236 5 pbk

Library of Congress Cataloging-in-Publication Data are available on request

Typeset in 10/12 pt ITC Garamond
by Solidus (Bristol) Limited

Printed in Great Britain by SRP, Ltd., Exeter

Contents

Contents

Preface and Acknowledgments

This book is about whether the environment can affect mental health. About eight years ago I was working in an architectural practice in anticipation of taking a second degree in urban planning and design. However, there was a question that bothered me: what made us so sure that what we were building was any 'better' than that which it replaced? The dominant perspective within architecture and design emphasised aesthetics, and while architectural students learned to produce beautiful collages and dramatic pastel drawings, they learned little or nothing of the potential social or behavioural consequences of design. Perhaps the over-confidence of planners in the fifties and sixties had made the next generation cautious, or perhaps the social and behavioural consequences of design were too small to matter and it was a mistake to think that the criteria for design should be anything other than aesthetic. Certainly, this was the position taken by many within the design professions.

I found it difficult to be entirely at ease with this conception of the world. Was it really true that we, as designers, only had to concern ourselves with aesthetics? It seemed like a wonderful freedom, but what if we were wrong? What of the people who had to live in our designs? Was it really so arbitrary if the building was for ten people or a thousand, if the road went straight or around, or if the city was built in one way or another? Was it really true that the built environment did not affect our social behaviour and well-bring? I tried to answer these questions by reference to architectural, planning and psychology texts, but with little success. There were plenty of assertions (in both directions) about how the environment affected mental health and well-bring, but very little evidence.

This book explores some of these questions. It is partly based on research conducted for my doctoral thesis at the Faculty of Social and Political Sciences, the University of Cambridge between 1988 and 1992, and partly on work conducted since then. I have tried to make the book accessible without compromising the detail and comprehensiveness of the analysis. The chapters are intended to be relatively self-contained such that the reader can jump between them or go straight to the sections of particular interest. I believe that the data and reviews that are drawn together in this book make significant progress towards answering the questions I started with.

There are many people who helped with the research behind this book. Before the research even began, there were frank discussions with architects, planners and designers. I am grateful to those who encouraged me to think that the project was worth pursuing such as David Good (who was to become my supervisor), Raymond Cochrane (Professor of Psychology at Birmingham University), and Ray Jobling (St. John's College, Cambridge). Other figures who were helpful sources of guidance and encouragement included Frazer Watts (MRC Applied Psychology Unit, Cambridge), John Parker (Greater London Consultants), Eugene Pakel (Department of Psychiatry, Cambridge), Tirril Harris (Royal Holloway and Bedford College, London) and Hugh Freeman (University of Manchester and British Journal of Psychiatry). I am also indebted to the large number of people who gave practical help and assistance including: with identifying suitable data for secondary analysis (parts of chapters 2, 3 and 4), to the staff of the ESRC data archive for help with identifying suitable data; with the Southgate study (chapter 6), to John Reid (Consultant in Public Health, Halton Health Authority), the doctors of the Brookvale and Weavervale practices and especially Drs Frood, Murphy, Zurek, and Richards, the practice administrators, Hugh Owen (Merseyside Improved Housing), Paul Sturgen and the Halton General Hospital Community Psychiatric Nurses, the Research and Intelligence Unit of Cheshire County Council, Margaret Davies and the representatives of the Southgate Residents' Association, and the staff of the local library; and with the Eastlake study (chapter 7), to Chris Wilkinson (City Council), John Barker (Architectural liaison officer, Police Headquarters), Joan Tibbs, Alan Pearson and the other staff at the local housing office, the County Council research unit, and most of all, to the many residents who gave of their time to make the study possible.

I am also very grateful to St. John's College for awarding me the Benefactors' Studentship which financed most of the research presented here, and to the Policy Studies Institute, London, and Nuffield College, Oxford, for allowing me the time to write up the research into the present book. Thanks also to the crew at Taylor and Francis who helped turn the manuscript into something presentable, notably Comfort Jegede, Anthony Levings and Carol Saumarez; and to those who gave permission for plates to be reproduced including Herbert Gans and Oscar Newman.

Finally, I wish to thank my family, friends and colleagues who made the whole process a pleasure rather than a burden, and especially Dave Good, William Watson, David Smith, Avner Offer, and – of course – Jennifer Rubin. Occasionally it is tempting to wonder what answers I would have found if I had stuck with building buildings instead of regressions, but I hope that the present book makes some sense of the decision.

DSH
August 1995

List of Figures and Tables

Figures

Tables

Chapter 1

Introduction and Background

'What a dreadful room you have, Rodya, just like a coffin,' said Pulkeria Alexandrovna, breaking the oppressive silence. 'I'm sure it is responsible for at least half your depression.'

'Room?' said he absently. 'Yes, the room has made a big contribution . . . I've thought of that too . . .' (*Crime and Punishment*, Dostoevsky, 1865: 222.)

Introduction

There is a widespread lay belief that the environment around us affects our mental health and well-being. In everyday speech, people often describe environments in terms of the moods that they evoke: 'It's such a relaxing environment'. 'What a cheerful room' or more negatively, 'I do not like that building, it's so depressing.' In this book we shall be exploring whether this belief – that the environment can affect our mental health and well-being – is literally true. It is certainly true that people have strong views about the environment, and people will pay substantial amounts of money in order to live in pleasant surroundings. But is it also true that some environments are literally depressing while others are not? Can the design of a house, the length of a street or the form of a development affect our mental health? These are the types of questions that this book will try to answer.

What is Meant by 'The Built Environment'?

The research presented in the following chapters focuses on the effects of certain aspects of the environment. When psychologists use the term *environment*, they are often referring to a very wide range of phenomena including the child's early experience and socialization, family dynamics, and life events, to name but a few, but here the term will be used more narrowly. The *built environment* refers to those aspects of the environment that urban planners, architects and urban geographers study. The built environment includes, but is not limited to the physical form of specific dwellings, developments, streets and cities. The term *planned environment* is sometimes used to indicate the broader, more social aspects of the built environment, but here the terms will be used interchangeably.

Physical and social planning are unavoidably enmeshed. Environments are typically constructed for social reasons, designs lead to social consequences whether intended or not, and even the humblest construction inevitably acquires a socially ascribed meaning. Consider, for example, the development of public housing projects or of suburbs; they have both a physical and a social manifestation. The public housing and private suburban housing tend to have distinctive physical forms, and the spatial divisions between these housing types has reflected and emphasized the spatial division between the social groups who live in them. The focus in this book is on the overlap between those aspects of the physical and social environment that have concerned urban planners, geographers and architects and those that may be linked to mental health.

Four Possible Channels of Influence

A broad reading of the psychological and planning literatures suggests that if the planned environment has any influence on mental health, then it is likely to be through four inter-related channels of influence. These potential channels of influence of the environment over mental health are:

- as a source of stress;
- as an influence over social networks and support;
- through symbolic effects and social labelling;
- through the action of the planning process itself.

The evidence on the first of these issues – the role of the environment as a source of stress – is explored in Chapters 2 and 3. These chapters explore the influence on mental health of pollution, the weather, noise, crowding and environmentally related fear of crime. The influence of the environment on social networks, patterns of friendship, neighbouring behaviour and social support is examined in Chapter 4. Chapter 5 examines the effects of symbolic and social labelling aspects of the environment on mental health, and Chapter 6 examines the effect of the planning process itself on mental health. Finally, Chapter 7 presents a detailed case study to explore whether mental health can be improved through altering the environment.

However, before beginning on these detailed reviews, it is wise to ask ourselves, 'what is mental health and mental illness?' Also, it is helpful to contextualize the later chapters with a brief review of how earlier researchers have approached the topic of mental health and the environment and to draw out the major recurrent methodological difficulties that face researchers working on the topic.

What is Mental Illness?

The term *mental illness* refers to a range of chronic, subjectively unpleasant psychological conditions, which may range from a cluster of mild symptoms such as listlessness, bodily symptoms without organic causes, and feelings of depressed or anxious mood, to gross pathology, such as hearing voices that are not there, feeling that one's thoughts are being broadcast, or showing grossly disordered thought. In this book, the focus will be on the types of mild psychopathology and symptoms that are common in the community, though where the evidence is available, reference will be made to the occurrence of more severe disorders. The term *mental health* will be understood as referring to the condition of being free of psychiatric symptoms and having a subjective feeling of well-being.

American early community surveys suggested that as many 70 to 80 per cent of general population reported at least one psychiatric symptom (Srole *et al.*, 1962; Leighton, *et al.*, 1963). More recent estimates using stricter clinically grounded criteria have been substantially lower (Robins and Regier, 1991). Clearly, estimates vary according to the severity of the cut-off point used and to the time period covered, but most researchers report that, over a month, around 1 in 3 to 1 in 5 people suffer from some form of mental illness. A recent survey of 10,000 people in private households in the United Kingdom found that about 1 in 7 adults aged 16 to 64 had some sort of mental health problem in the week prior to interview (Meltzer *et al.*, 1994). However, many more people were found to be suffering from just one of the symptoms such as fatigue (27%), sleep problems (25%) or irritability (22%). Most of the symptoms reported are relatively mild, for example, headaches, sleeplessness, irritability, or feeling under strain, and less than a fifth (17 per cent) of these people go to see their doctor about the symptom (*General Household Survey*, 1980). These very common conditions, sometimes described as *sub-clinical* (Taylor and Chave, 1964) or *undifferentiated neuroses* (Gelder, Gath and Mayou, 1983) constitute the vast bulk of mental illness.

It is found that, to a very large extent, the different kinds of symptom cited above co-vary, that is, an individual who reports one kind of symptom is very likely to report another. Those people who report physical symptoms (headaches, stomach-aches, nausea) are very likely to report mood disturbance (feeling sad, hopeless, lonely). The covariance between physical and mental symptoms allowed early researchers to disguise questionnaires about mental health as questionnaires about physical health (Langner, 1962; Goldberg, 1972). This was done because researchers were afraid that survey respondents would not be prepared to answer questions about feelings as these were thought to be too personal. More recent scales have tended to exclude physical symptoms on the basis that these items could lead to the misclassification of genuine physical complaints as mental illness (especially in the elderly), but still, very similar estimates of prevalence (rates of occurrence) continue to be reported.

Most researchers agree that certain psychological symptoms tend to occur together, and this is the main basis of psychiatric nosologies (Kendall, 1975; Kaplan and Saddock, 1988). The significance of a cluster of simultaneously occurring symptoms is that they constitute a *syndrome*. The two most common clusters of symptoms in community surveys justify a distinction between depression and anxiety. The cluster of symptoms identified with depression include feelings of sadness, failure, low spirits, that things never turn out, and wishing you were dead. Physical symptoms found to co-vary include loss of appetite, trouble concentrating, trouble sleeping, reduced talking, and lethargy. Symptoms identified with anxiety include feeling tense, worried, afraid, irritable, and anxious. Physical symptoms found to co-vary include shortness of breath, dizziness, heart palpitations, cold sweats, and trembling hands. However, a number of studies have shown that all the various measures of mental illness and clusters of symptoms, including anxiety and depression, are statistically closely related (Mirowsky and Ross, 1989), and for most purposes they can be taken as interchangeable indicators of *non-specific psycho-logical distress* (Dohrenwend, *et al.*, 1980) or *demoralization* (Frank, 1973). More extreme disorders, both in the sense of their low prevalence and in the sense of how debilitating they are to the individual, tend to be relatively discrete, but even these co-vary to a surprisingly large extent.

What is this distress from which so many appear to suffer? Is mental illness the opposite of happiness? How does psychological distress relate to clinical disorder? Is the pattern of mental illness random, or does it have identifiable causes? These are some of the questions that we should briefly consider before beginning our exploration of the relationship between the environment and mental health.

Everyday Psychopathology and Clinical Disorder

The most common way of estimating the level of mental illness in the community is by establishing a clinically validated cut-off score above which respondents are classified as *cases*. If a number of questions are asked of samples identified by clinicians as without pathology and another sample identified as psychiatric cases, then two things can be established. First, the questions that discriminated best between the two samples can be identified (this technique was used, for example, in the selection of items in the Langer–22 scale used by Srole *et al.*, 1962). Second, it can be established how well any given symptom score divides between those identified as cases or not by the clinicians. In principal, a cut-off point can be established above which 70, 80, 90 or whatever per cent of individuals could be expected to be classified as cases by clinicians – in other words – those who would be thought to need formal psychiatric care of some kind.

This technique gives rise to the figure of a point prevalence rate for all psychiatric illness in the general population of around 1 in 5 to 1 in 10 (Goldberg and Huxley, 1980). Similar proportions have been reported in Britain (Ingham, Rawsley and Hughes, 1972; Goldberg, 1972); Germany (Dilling, 1980); North America (Weissman *et al.*, 1978); Australia (Finlay-Jones and Burvill, 1977) and Africa (Orley and Wing, 1979).[1] However, it is important to note that no sharp dichotomy exists between cases and non-cases. Most researchers use a cut-off point at which the probability of being able to assign a diagnosis exceeds at least 0.5, but then many also use a category of *borderline, threshold,* or *sub-clinical disturbance* (Brown and Harris, 1978; Goldberg and Huxley, 1980).

The absence of a clear dichotomy between cases and non-cases has led to two types of critique. The first is that more sophisticated techniques should be used in the identification of cases. Epidemiologists have stressed the importance of establishing separate cut-off points for different groups in the population, such as the elderly, and for men and women. Some have emphasized the importance of using more sophisticated psychometric techniques, and especially the more critical use of Receiver Operating Characteristics (ROC) analysis depending upon the consequences of incorrect classifications and the distributions of scale scores among normal individuals and cases (Fombonne, 1991). This is a relatively conservative critique. The second kind of critique is more radical. Some have argued that the absence of a clear dichotomy between cases and non-cases means that attempts to impose a cut-off point are artificial and result in the loss of a large amount of important information.

> Diagnosis throws away information about the similarity of some cases and the dissimilarity of others . . . As an assessment becomes broader, it becomes less sensitive to meaningful changes or differences, and the ratio of information to random noise declines. When a full range of symptoms is split into only two categories, such as: enough symptoms for a diagnosis of depression; and not enough symptoms for a diagnosis of depression, most of the information is lost, but all of the random error remains. (Mirowsky and Ross, 1989: 30–1)

A similar critique can be made of many of the distinctions employed by psychiatrists; even in the most sophisticated psychiatric nosologies, many cases do not fit within a set of tidy and mutually exclusive categories. The evolution of diagnostic frameworks has therefore coincided with a massive proliferation of diagnostic categories to soak up the cases that are not clear-cut, such as *schizoaffective disorder, schizophreniform disorder,* or *depressive disorder not otherwise specified.*

Which of the two perspectives is most valid depends largely on what you want out of the data. If you are a clinician and must make judgments as to the appropriateness of treatment for a given individual, then the first perspective or critique is most valid: you need some kind of cut-off point, albeit one as sophisticated as possible. However, if you are a researcher investigating the causes of disorder then the use of cut-offs is generally unnecessary and obscures important information.

It is very likely that research into the aetiology (or causes) of mental illness would miss many significant associations if only categorical variables were used. The position taken here is that *mental illness* is a phenomena ranging from relatively mild everyday psychopathologies through to extremely severe and debilitating types of disorder as manifested in psychotic psychiatric patients, with the divisions between categories of severity being relatively arbitrary.

The Relationship between Mental Illness, Misery and Happiness

Psychological distress and happiness

A number of writers have argued that contrary to popular understanding, psycho-logical distress (manifested as misery or symptoms) is not the opposite of happiness (Argyle, 1987; 1992). Bradburn (1969) asked subjects which of a number of feelings had they felt over the past few weeks. Some of the items were positive, and some were negative. Bradburn found that there was no relationship between the reporting of positive and negative items; individuals who reported feeling bored were just as likely as others to report, for example, feeling pleased at having accomplished something. Further evidence for the independence of happiness and distress are findings that suggest that slightly different factors influence the two (Headey, Holmstorm and Wearing, 1984; Argyle, 1987). Also, it is clearly possible to think of certain disorders, such as in the manic phase of manic-depression, during which the person can appear to be extremely happy (though such phases tend to be limited). Similarly, a person suffering from schizophrenia may often appear to show inappropriate affect rather than unhappiness *per se*. Argyle (1992) has argued that if distress, or at least depression, really was the opposite of happiness then this would imply that to make normal people happier we would just have to give them 'the same treatment that is used for depressives' – electric shocks, anti-depressives and so on' (p. 284).

However, electric shocks and anti-depressives are not normally given for the types of mild disorder found in the community, and the argument suggesting that happiness and distress are not opposites has probably been somewhat overstated. Similarly, disorders such as mania are relatively rare (lifetime prevalence rates certainly being less than 1 per cent) and the vast majority of people identified by community surveys as suffering from mental illness are suffering from *neuroses* such as anxiety or depression. When subjects are asked how they feel at a particular time as opposed to over a period of weeks, positive and negative feelings are strongly negatively associated (Kammann and Flett, 1983; Diener, 1984; Fordyce, 1985). Typical correlations between scales of happiness and scales of psychological distress are around –.4 to –.7. Of these subjective well-being measures, the scales developed by Fordyce are particularly well respected (Larsen, Diener and Emmons, 1985). Fordyce (1985) reports strong negative correlations (in the range –.5 to –.8) between all forms of the Psychap Inventory (the happiness scale); and anxiety, depression, and hostility on the MAACL (Multiple Affect Adjective Check-list); tension, depression, and confusion on the POMS (Profile of Mood States); depression on the DACL (Depression Adjective Check-list); and depression, anxiety, psychopathy, psychasthenia, and schizophrenia subscales on the MMPI (Minnesota Multiphasic Personality Inventory). In terms of psychometrics these correlations are very high and strongly suggest that, at least to a large extent, psychological distress and happiness *are* opposites. Once account is taken of random measurement error, the degree of independence between global measures of distress and happiness must be quite small. Being unhappy is clearly a central, though not necessarily sufficient, aspect of the psychological distress as measured by psychometric scales.

Mental illness and misery

Suffering from the type of mental illness that is common in the community typically involves being unhappy or miserable, but if a person is unhappy, are they necessarily suffering from mental illness? It is certainly true that according to psychiatric definitions, being unhappy – even if profoundly so – is not enough to automatically lead to a diagnostic label. If a person's spouse dies, then provided that the bereavement occurred within the previous two years, the diagnostic label of clinical depression is not normally applied, even though the symptoms may be identical. More straightforwardly, being unhappy or in a bad mood is not considered, in itself, enough to constitute mental illness. Periodic negative affective states are normal: if your car gets scratched by vandals or if you miss your train you feel irritated or annoyed, and if nothing ever happens you feel bored. Emotions are part of being alive, and we do not describe someone as suffering from mental illness every time they experience a bad mood. So what distinguishes mental illness from normal unhappiness?

Part of the answer is to do with the length of time involved – if a person's bad

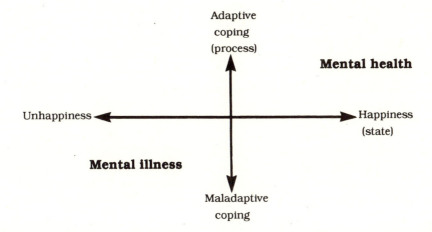

Figure 1.1: *Diagram showing the relationship between psychological distress and well-being*

or depressed mood lasts for a period of months or even years, then we are more likely to describe this as mental illness rather than just unhappiness. However, mental illness is constituted not only by negative affect but also by characteristic mental processes. An individual who suffers from depression is not just feeling down, he or she also exhibits social, behavioural and cognitive patterns which act to reinforce and propagate the subjective experience of the negative mood. The depressed person is passive and withdrawn, reducing the possibility of positive experiences that might induce a more positive mood. His or her style of thought is characterized by negative, generalized and internally directed attributions which act to exaggerate the negative impact of any event; his or her affect and manner can make them less pleasant to be with and reduces the likelihood of positive social interaction. The central difference between unhappiness and mental illness lies in the distinction between *state* and *process*. The mental state which characterizes psychological distress can be fairly described as unhappiness, even misery, and as the opposite of happiness. The pathological coping mechanisms or process that act to maintain the state are what distinguish mental illness from normal unhappiness. These relationships are depicted in the diagram above, where the horizontal axis represents the mental state and the vertical axis represents the style of coping.

Satisfaction

A further concept widely used in the literature is *satisfaction*. Satisfaction is more specific than happiness and refers to the positive appraisal of something or someone rather than a global internal state. It is possible to be satisfied with some aspects of life or a situation while simultaneously dissatisfied with others. A person can be happy in general but dissatisfied about something specific, and can be miserable in general but simultaneously satisfied about something specific. Clearly, the more important something is to a person, the more likely it is that dissatisfaction with that object or aspect of their life will lead to overall dissatisfaction and unhappiness. Campbell, Converse and Rogers (1976) attempted to predict overall ratings of satisfaction with life from a range of specific domains. Overall satisfaction was most closely related to satisfaction with family life (r=.41); followed by marriage (r=.36); financial situation (r=.33); housing (r=.30); work (r=.27); friendship (r=.26); health (r=.22); and leisure activities (r=.21) [figures in brackets are correlations].

Both theoretical and empirical work shows that overall moods are not simple summations of satisfactions and dissatisfactions. Studies such as that of Campbell, *et al.*, show that some kind of weighting operates to determine overall levels of satisfaction. Detailed studies of more specific appraisals show that these involve complex combinations and the simplification of enormous numbers of micro-satisfactions and dissatisfactions. To take a simple example, Morton-Williams, *et al.* (1978) found that residents would often say that they were not bothered by road noise. Nonetheless, these same residents would often then go on to say, in response to more specific questions, that they were very bothered by *certain* road noises (for example, by motor bikes). Minsky (1987) has illustrated this kind of phenomenon with computational models which point to how overall subjective appraisals of satisfaction can conceal an enormous cognitive complexity and a large number of specific appraisals.

In summary, the presence of a negative internal state (the absence of happiness) is a necessary but not sufficient condition of most forms of mental illness, but mental illness also implies maladaptive patterns of coping. Specific satisfactions and dissatisfactions are important determinants of happiness and unhappiness, but the relative importance of any particular source of satisfaction and dissatisfaction varies. Sources of satisfaction and dissatisfaction have a correspondingly less direct impact on mental health and illness.

The Causes of Mental Illness

A very large number of factors have been implicated in the aetiology of mental illness. Classical debates revolve around the relative importance of broadly *environmental* as opposed to *genetic* factors in the onset and course of mental illness, with both proving important. A multitude of environmental factors (in the broader sense) and genetic predispositions weave in and out to form complex, intertwined aetiologies, often difficult to untangle across a population, let alone within an individual patient. Even in schizophrenia, a disorder in which genetic factors have been strongly implicated, the concordance rate of MZ (genetically identical) twins is far from 100 per cent (50 to 60 per cent), emphasizing that generally, both environmental and genetic factors are involved in its aetiology (Gottesman and Shields, 1982).

Most forms of mental illness, including the minor neuroses and psychological distress common in the community, are strongly associated with a number of social variables including low socio-economic status, unemployment, and impoverished social networks. Psychological distress has also been found to be associated with certain dimensions of personality such as neuroticism and *low hardiness* (see later chapters for further details). However, it has become clear that many of the social variables associated with psychologically distressed individuals, such as poverty and poor social networks, are at least as much the result of mental illness as the cause. As in debates over the relative importance of genetic and environmental factors, debates over the relative importance of *selection* over *causation* have led to strong evidence for the occurrence of *both* processes (Antunes *et al.*, 1974; Cochrane, 1983; Mirowsky and Ross, 1989; Halpern, 1993). The relationship between personality types and mental illness is a very strong one, but is greatly confused by the similarity of the items used in the scales to assess them and by the problematic distinction between the concept of the trait and the chronic mood state.

Nonetheless, a wide consensus exists that at least some non-constitutional factors causally relate to the occurrence of mental illness. For example, following the work of Holmes and Rahe (1967) and others, a large literature has developed on the association between *life-events* – significant occurrences in individuals' lives – and mental illness. A number of studies have shown that major life events increase the probability that an individual will develop depression or some other neurosis, and that they can (at least) trigger the occurrence of psychotic episodes (Brown and Harris, 1978; Paykel and Dowlatshahi, 1988). It has also been shown that life events increase the probability of physical illness and reduce the effectiveness of the immune system (Kennedy, Kiecolt-Glaser and Glaser, 1990). However, despite their significance, life events explain only a small part of the variance in the occurrence of mental illness. For example, Brown and Harris (1978) showed that in only 1 out of 5 women did a major life event or chronic stress lead to an episode of depression. Other risk factors included having several young children, the absence or failure of a close confiding relationship, and low self-esteem. Brown and Harris suggested that a further set of *symptom formation factors* influenced the form and severity of any subsequent disorder, including age and the experience of the early death of the individual's mother. Recent work has shown that daily hassles also predict levels of psychological symptoms, and sometimes do so better than major life events: the more hassles, the worse mood and the more symptoms (Kanner, *et al.*, 1981; Caspi, Bolger and Eckenrode, 1987).

Space is too restricted here for an exploration of the state of knowledge about the aetiologies of specific disorders, and this information can be found in standard texts (Gelder, *et al.*, 1983; Meyer and Salmon, 1984; Kaplan and Sadock, 1990). It will serve my purpose sufficiently just to emphasize a number of general points. First, non-constitutional (environmental) variables are implicated in the occurrence of all forms of mental illness, though to varying extents. Second, the clinical divisions that are made between disorders to facilitate and guide treatment do not exclude the possibility that many of the same factors are aetiologically relevant in these disorders. In fact, it is already known that many of the same factors do operate in differing disorders (for example, life events and the absence of supportive relationships), though their relative importance may differ. Secondary sets of factors (including constitutional, social and cultural variables) operate to determine the form and severity that the illness takes, and these variables are not necessarily the same as the initial causal agents. Third, aetiologies and various causal agents are not exclusive in their occurrence or effects. Although academic debates tend to juxtapose one possible aetiological route against another, there is little evidence to suggest that this juxtaposition reflects the actual relationships between causal routes. Many social and constitutional variables are relevant in the complex and various aetiologies of mental illness. This book is an exploration of the aetiological relevance of one particular, relatively narrow group of factors referred to as the *the planned* or *built environment*. Whatever is decided about the relevance of these factors, it should be clearly understood that these factors are being explored as *complementary* rather than as *alternative* explanations of mental illness and psychological distress. The book explores the possibility that the planned environment may be able to soak up some of the sizeable amount of variability in who suffers from mental illness left unexplained by other, more conventional explanations.

In the chapters that follow, a wide range of literatures will be examined. Not all researchers have used the same terms or outcome measures, and terms such as *emotional disturbance, dissatisfaction, unhappiness* and *annoyance* have often been used interchangeably with the term *mental illness.* Where possible, I have tried to maintain a distinction between mental illness and other forms of distress (such as annoyance and dissatisfaction). In retrospect, perhaps a better way of describing this range of phenomenon would be through a term such as *mental ill-health* or *psychological distress.* It may be that the term mental *ill*ness is too medical in that it raises images of organic pathogens, bacteria and the like, and this distracts from the more social and environmental causes that are implicated in the aetiology of most psychological distress. Perhaps the best that we can do for now is to highlight the definitional problems in the literature and to try to avoid the use of terms that pre-judge the aetiology of phenomena under consideration. I can only hope that the current work will enable later scholars to be more precise.

Mental Illness and the Environment: Early Studies

In the mid-nineteenth century, the idea forcefully emerged that poor quality environments were a major cause of the high levels of physical sickness and frequent epidemics that were common among the poor. Friedrich Engels in *The Condition of the Working Class in England* (1844–1845) was one of the first to state the link clearly:

> There is ample proof that the dwellings of the workers who live in the slums, combined with other adverse factors, give rise to many illness. (p. 111) ...
> The middle classes ... have no grounds for complaint if I accuse them of social murder (p. 123).

On both sides of the Atlantic, continuing outbreaks of disease associated with the poor housing conditions of many working-class families eventually led to the development of reformist based slum clearance programmes, the enforcement of systems of health regulations and planning law, and other efforts to improve the quality of the housing stock (Jacobs and Stevenson, 1981). Through improvements to the housing stock, water supplies, sanitation, and the reduction of pollution, enormous reductions in the occurrence of many diseases have been achieved. The link between today's poor housing and physical health is much weaker, as even the poorest quality of housing tends to be of a much higher physical standard than that of poor housing in the previous century, though some links persist (Byrne, *et al.,* 1986; Lowry, 1991). For example, Martin (1990) was able to demonstrate that damp found in poor housing led to significant increases in the ill-health of children residents. The assessments of housing conditions were made separately and a few days after the interview to assess health. Controls were also made for smoking, mothers' mental health (using the *General Health Questionnaire*; (Goldberg, 1972), unemployment and other socio-demographic variables.

The formal recognition of the influence of housing on health gave planners and politicians a mandate to clear substandard housing and unhealthy slums, and to replace them with modern and healthy alternatives. The success that planners achieved initially brought them considerable powers, not least being the power to order the demolition of large areas and organize their rebuilding. Ironically, the success of planners in reducing the link between housing and health in recent decades may have somewhat undermined the planners' *raison d'etre*. Today the argument is frequently advanced that, whereas the main goal of the planner was once the creation of designs that were good for physical health, today the main aim of the planner is the creation of designs that are good for mental health (Parker, 1985). As one design textbook explains:

> Most official housing standards, which originated in the nineteenth-century public health laws, emphasise physical health and safety and ignore both individual and community *mental* health ... But we have also learned that the design of environments affects people in a multitude of ways and that, in terms of their well-being, it matters deeply. (Cooper-Marcus and Sarkissian, 1986: 5–9, authors' italics.)

However, despite their claims, almost no references are made by planners to psychological literatures to support the assertion that mental health is affected by the planned environment. Sceptics might argue that the reason for the absence of these references is that very little evidence for a link between the built environment and mental health actually exists.

Psychiatric Geographies

In 1939 Faris and Dunham published a study of the geographical distribution of the home addresses of persons admitted for psychiatric disorders in Chicago. They discovered that the pattern of psychiatric admissions across the city was far from even: the psychiatric admission rate was lowest in the outer suburbs and became steadily higher towards the inner-city core. Faris and Dunham argued that the isolation and disorganization of the inner-city rooming-house areas led to a social and mental disorganization of the individuals who lived in those areas, and hence to elevated levels of psychiatric disorder, and in particular, schizophrenia, (though not for mania which showed a more random pattern).

Later researchers have successfully replicated Faris and Dunham's findings in a number of places including Chicago (Levy and Rowitz, 1973) and a number of cities within Britain (Giggs, 1973; Taylor 1975; Dean and James, 1984). However, Faris and Dunham's original interpretation – that the disorganization and isolation of the environment *caused* the elevated rates of psychiatric admissions – has been strongly contested. An alternative explanation which is now widely accepted is that the dramatic maps of psychiatric admissions plotted by Faris and Dunham were the result of *social drift* rather than social causation (Cochrane, 1983). Theories of social drift

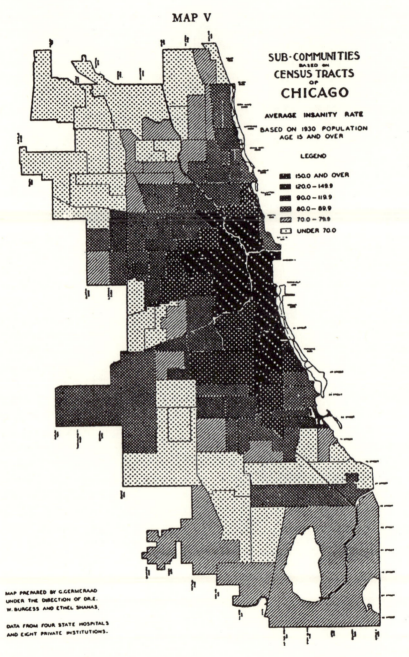

MAP V

SUB·COMMUNITIES
BASED ON
CENSUS TRACTS
OF
CHICAGO

AVERAGE INSANITY RATE

BASED ON 1930 POPULATION
AGE 15 AND OVER

LEGEND

150.0 AND OVER
120.0 — 149.9
90.0 — 119.9
80.0 — 89.9
70.0 — 79.9
UNDER 70.0

MAP PREPARED BY G.GERMERAAD
UNDER THE DIRECTION OF DR.E.
W. BURGESS AND ETHEL SHANAS.

DATA FROM FOUR STATE HOSPITALS
AND EIGHT PRIVATE INSTITUTIONS.

Figure 1.2: *'Average insanity rates' in Chicago.*
Source: Faris and Dunham, 1939.

suggest that if an individual develops a serious psychiatric disorder they become less able to maintain stable social relationships or hold well-paid employment, and tend to drift to the cheaper and more anonymous parts of the city. Strong evidence for a theory of social drift can be seen in the finding that maps of first psychiatric admission rates are considerably more random than maps of re-admissions. The slight patterns of concentration seen in first admission rates can also be explained by social drift on the basis that early pre-morbid aspects of disorder are similarly likely to lead to drift. Faris and Dunham originally argued against a theory of social drift on the basis that if social drift were the cause of the distribution for schizophrenia then it should also have led to a similar distribution for mania. However, most later researchers have argued that this difference would have been more plausibly interpreted as a reflection of the difference in the courses and prognoses of the disorders: schizophrenia is typically characterized by chronic decline while mania is often associated with a more positive prognosis and long periods of normal functioning.

So what has been learnt from more than fifty years of psychiatric geography? It has been clearly demonstrated that higher rates of psychiatric admissions are associated with areas that are poor, high in density, mixed in land use, and associated with other types of social disorder such as social delinquency, suicide and crime. Although there have been some methodological improvements, psychiatric geographies still rely on ecological correlations – though these are now often called *associative analyses* – and the central problem of inferring causal direction remains (Scobie, 1989). The widespread disappointment in the ability of psychiatric geographies to identify the cause of the patterns they reveal was summed up in a review by Kasl and Harburg (1975) who concluded, 'so far, ecological analyses have not yet illuminated anything about the aetiology of mental illness.' This has led many recent psychiatric geographers to shift their focus away from the study of aetiology towards the study of patterns of service use (Smith, 1984; Scobie, 1989). However, the conclusions of Kasl and Harburg are perhaps too severe in that psychiatric geographies provide researchers in other fields with a useful starting point in their studies, and sometimes with useful pointers for further research. Finally, there is evidence that if the ecological approach is combined with individual level data then extremely useful insights can follow (Bell, 1958). Daiches (1981) combined data from individually administered questionnaires with aggregate (ecological) level data and found that even after individual level characteristics had been accounted for, ecological level factors were still able to explain significant amounts of variance in individual level well-being. Unfortunately, Daiches' study is unusual, and overall, psychiatric geography has raised more questions than provided answers.

The New Town Studies

In 1938, a paper was published in the *Lancet* by Taylor documenting a phenomenon he called *suburban neurosis*. Taylor reported that the stresses experienced by the residents of new out-of-town housing estates, such as distance from employment, loss of familiar surroundings, and social isolation led to a higher incidence of neuroses, particularly in women. This paper marked the beginning of a protracted debate which has remained controversial for over 50 years (Freeman, 1984b).

Support for the occurrence of the phenomenon of suburban neurosis was provided by an extensive study of a new housing estate by Martin, Brotherston and Chave (1957). Martin, *et al.*, examined four different measures of the mental health of a London County Council housing estate with a population of around 17,000: mental hospital admissions, referrals to psychiatric out-patient clinics, general practitioner consultations, and self-reported symptoms. Age and sex specific mental hospital admissions were found to be 23 to 74 per cent in excess of national admission rates with especially elevated rates among women aged over 45. Referrals to psychiatric out-patient clinics were similar to national averages but the records were incomplete and were therefore an under-estimate. General practitioner consultations showed elevated rates of anxiety and depressive neuroses, sleep disturbances, palpitations, duodenal ulcers, anorexia, headaches and incontinence, again especially for women (with the exception of ulcers which were more common in men). Finally, a community survey of 750 families showed that 25 per cent of men and 40 per cent of women reported at least one of the symptoms 'nerves', depression, sleeplessness, or undue irritability. Martin, *et al.*, suggested that these rates were about 77 per cent higher than comparable national figures, though they noted the difficulty involved in finding a suitable control group. There was some evidence of a gradual amelioration with time in that complaints were most numerous among those who had come to the estate most recently. Martin *et al.* concluded that the population of the new estate were suffering from substantially elevated levels of neuroses, and that the characteristics of the population did not explain the excesses in disorder. They argued that the excesses appeared to stem from two factors: first, the effects of rehousing, and second, the conditions of life on the new estate which led to the attenuation of family ties and to loneliness and isolation. Martin *et al.*'s findings were broadly supported by Clout (1962) in a study of rates of psychiatric illness in a general practice in the New Town of Crawley. Clout found that patients from the New Town had higher rates of psychiatric illness than comparable patients from the old town, especially for anxiety reactions and in women of reproductive age.

However, an American study by Wilner *et al.* (1962) comparing the health of 300 families in a new project to 300 families who remained in a slum found evidence of slight improvements in mental health associated with the new project. Evidence was found for reduced accidents and improved physical health among the adults on the new estate, and there was evidence of a weak improvement in mental health and self-concept.

The debate became still more confused with the publication of a study by Taylor and Chave (1964) of the mental health of the residents of Newton (the new town of Harlow) with data from a community survey, general practitioner consultations, and psychiatric admissions. The authors conducted their research from the starting hypothesis that the residents of a socially planned community were likely to show a reduction in the incidence of neurosis. However, the results of the community survey showed that around 30 to 35 per cent of the sample reported at least one of the symptoms of nerves, depression, sleeplessness or undue irritability – very similar proportions to those reported by Martin *et al.* (1957) and to those in an exporting London borough (the control group). The rates of general practitioner consultations for neurotic complaints were substantially higher in the New Town than in the control group, leading Taylor and Chave (1964) to suggest that good social planning encourages these 'mixed neuroses to declare themselves'. The rates of psychiatric admissions, and especially for schizophrenia, were found to be much lower than in the control group. This last finding led the authors to suggest that the understanding of psychoses should be revised as they seemed to be more the reaction to the environmental conditions than had previously been thought, while neuroses were more the result of constitutional factors. Secondary reports of the results of this study are often confused and contradictory, but this is because the authors' conclusions do not sit easily on their results. A more plausible interpretation of the low rates of psychotic disorders would have been that people with serious psychiatric disorders were left behind in London; many people moved to the New Towns for jobs and to raise families – both factors negatively associated with psychotic disorders.

Finally, a study by Hare and Shaw (1965) attempted to replicate the work of Martin, *et al.*, (1957) on a new housing estate in Croydon, and a comparison group was provided by an old pre-1914 estate (Old Bute). Hare and Shaw found that once rates were age and sex standardized, few differences were found between the mental health of the populations of the new and old estates, although some elevation was found in the rates of neurosis and fatigue among women on the new estate, as in previous studies. A number of differences in physical health were found: residents of Old Bute had considerably more respiratory disorders (due to levels of pollution) and women in the new estate had more problems with high blood pressure and varicose veins. However, Hare and Shaw also noticed that considerably more households on the new estate had children – 78 per cent of households on the new estate had one or more children against only 34 per cent in Old Bute, and 37 per cent on the new estate had three or more children against only 21 per cent in Old Bute. Particularly in the light of more recent research on the elevated rates of mental illness in women with children (Brown and Harris, 1978) Hare and Shaw's results raise the possibility that the reason why women on the new estates suffered elevated rates of neuroses was because of the strain of raising children rather than because of experience of the estates *per se*.

Recently, a study of Thamesmead very reminiscent of the earlier New Town studies was published (Higgins, 1984) but it suffers from the same interpretive problems of the earlier studies. Higgins found that residents of Thamesmead, especially women of childbearing age, suffered from elevated rates of *emotional and mental illness* compared to a control population. The main conclusion of the new town and estate studies is that wherever one looks, a sizeable minority of the community will be found to have poor mental health. As Wing (1974, 1976) concluded, some individuals tend to be dissatisfied wherever they live, though the stated reason varies according to the setting. However, in terms of understanding the causal relationship between the environment and mental health, two sets of problems make interpretation very difficult. First, it is unclear to what extent and in which direction *selection processes* differentially sort the populations of new and old estates or projects. For example, the low levels of schizophrenia in the New Towns probably occurred as the result of psychiatrically impaired individuals being left behind in the old towns. We do not know whether similar selection processes operate on individuals suffering from minor psychopathology: if such selection was occurring then it could have concealed any negative effect that New Town living was having on residents. It is possible that sometimes a reverse pattern of selection was operating, with neurotic individuals choosing to move *to* the New Towns. Either way, the possibility of selection makes it difficult to judge who an appropriate control group should be. The second set of problems concern the imprecise identification of the *independent variables* and the extent to which they are compounded. How exactly is the New Town or estate different from the control area? Is it that the houses are better, that the transportation is superior, or that the air is cleaner? Is it that people are living in housing of a different design (eg, flats), that they have better employment, or that the schools are better provided? Some authors had the a priori expectation that the New Towns represented an improvement on the comparison areas, while others have assumed the reverse. The problem is that there is an enormous number of differences between the situation and setting of people living in a New Town or estate and those in the supposed control areas. The physical setting differs in a multitude of ways, some of which may be positive differences (larger houses, better schools) and some of which may be negative (distance from amenities, higher costs). Furthermore, the residents of New Towns have experienced the upheaval of a move to a new environment, new work, and the loss of familiar places, friends and relations.

Whatever the results of the New Town studies, it is difficult (in retrospect) to see what they can tell us about the relationship between mental health and the environment. So many potentially antagonistic variables co-vary across the comparison groups that any differences found are open to a multitude of possible interpretations. All that can realistically be concluded from the New Town studies is that the overall effect of New Town living is not as positive as many had hoped: there is evidence of slight improvements in physical health, of short to medium term adverse effects on mental health, and (possibly) of slight long-term adverse effects on the mental health of women, but the interpretation of these latter differences in mental health is extremely hazardous. If substantive progress is to be made on the causal relationship between mental health and the environment, researchers must be much more specific in their predictions and their methodologies.

Urban-rural Differentials

Many writers have, over the years, sought to pinpoint the distinctive features of urban life. Size, density, and heterogeneity of population are the most commonly cited. Most have emphasized the negative consequences of what are perceived to be characteristic of urban life: competition, lack of consensus and the loss of the bonds of solidarity that were thought to hold people together (Wirth, 1938; Fry, 1987). Others have emphasized the more positive consequences of the characteristics of cities: opportunity, choice, and the mosaic of subcultures (Fischer, 1982; Krupat, 1985).

One influential model of urban life has suggested that social and cognitive overload is the key to understanding the behaviour of the city dweller (Milgram, 1970). The overload model is congruent with that of environmental stress (see Chapters 2 and 3). It suggests that people have to learn to actively avoid social engagement, to narrow their attention in order to prevent themselves being overwhelmed by the buzzing confusion of the city. The counter argument is that such an environment is a stimulating and exciting one, and that many would happily trade the alternative – rural underload – for the stimulation of the city (Geller, 1980). It would be a mistake to make the a priori assumption that rural life is necessarily less stressful or better for mental health (Freeman, 1986). Clearly, this argument can be made in either direction and on a *post hoc* basis.

There is some evidence that certain types of mental illness, such as depression, may be lower in rural communities than in cities (for example, Brown and Prudo, 1981). Some researchers have reported these differences to be very large: in a study of North Carolina, rates of current major depression were found to be around three times more common in urban than rural areas (Crowell *et al.*, 1986). Others have reported that in many areas of the world, the prevalence of most disorders varies little across the urban–rural continuum (Webb, 1984). However, the empirical evidence on urban–rural mental health differences suffers from the same interpretive problems as the evidence from psychiatric geography and the New Town studies. There is a large amount of selection which occurs between urban and rural areas, but not in any simple form. For example, people suffering from schizophrenia may drift to urban cores within cities (and may have been less likely to have moved from rural areas in the first place). Similarly, people suffering from neuroses may avoid the bustle of urban living, either actively or passively attempting to reside in areas of low perceived stress (cf. the surprise results of Watkins *et al.*, 1981, described in Chapter 2). Differing levels of service provision, the problematic distinction between the urban and the rural in a modern industrialized nation and the possibility that urban and rural dwellers might express psychological distress in different ways confuse matters further. All this makes comparison of rates uninformative and even misleading.

On the whole, it is far more informative to try and decompose what is thought to characterize the urban, such as density, crime, noise and so on, and then examine each of these components in turn. This is what will be attempted in the present work.

Causes and Associations

The work on psychiatric geographies, the New Town studies and urban–rural differentials have all led to considerable debate but little progress. The methodologies of the three approaches differ, but all are characterized by poorly specified models of the environment-illness relationship and by correspondingly undiscriminating and non-specific methodologies. The net result is the documentation of many intriguing but generally uninformative associations. These associations are uninformative because they are open to so many radically different interpretations none of which the methods are adequately able to distinguish between. The most that can be concluded from the combined results of psychiatric geographies, the New Town studies and urban–rural differentials is that *if* there is a causal relationship between mental illness and the built environment, then it seems unlikely to be a very strong one. Reasonably enough, this conclusion appears widely held in the psychological and psychiatric communities – the aetiological relevance of the planned environment to mental illness is thought to be weak at most, and possibly nil (Mercer, 1975; Cochrane, 1983), and its consideration is absent from most psychiatric texts.

In the chapters that follow, the relationship between mental illness and the planned environment will be explored with a more specific and differentiated approach than that utilized in psychiatric geography or the classic New Town studies. The planned environment has so many aspects to it, many of which may have opposing effects, that it is unrealistic to expect to be able to set up research into its relationship to mental health without having first identified which aspects of the environment are likely to be relevant. Many associations exist between mental health and the environment, but how many of them, if any, are causal?

Two Recurrent Methodological Issues

The biggest problem that faces a researcher attempting to study the association between mental health and the social or physical environment is the interpretation of causal direction. Before embarking on the detailed literature reviews of later chapters, there are recurring methodological issues of which it is important to be aware. As we shall see, there are a plethora of studies demonstrating associations between poor mental health and environmental variables, but their interpretation is greatly clouded by two issues. These are (a) the occurrence of social selection, and (b) the response bias of subjects according to their mental state.

The Problem of Selection

Social selection refers to a process whereby individuals are sorted according to some social or individual characteristic. The phenomenon of social selection has already been mentioned in connection with the interpretation of psychiatric geographies, the New Town studies and urban–rural differentials. The discovery of an association between less desirable housing and the occurrence of mental illness, for example, might simply be dismissed on the basis that those prone to psychiatric impairment are also likely to be at a disadvantage in terms of social and residential progress. Hence, those with poorer mental health will effectively be selected or will drift into the least desirable and most unpleasant environments.

The occurrence of selection is widely accepted, and hence selection is often taken, quite correctly, as the default explanation of many mental health environment associations. The occurrence of social selection makes it extremely difficult to interpret the major strands of early work already mentioned on the relationship between mental health and the environment. Both the dramatic maps of disorder of psychiatric geographers (Faris and Dunham, *et al.,*) and the inconsistent results of the New Town and urban–rural differential studies can be accounted for in terms of social selection and drift. Of course, it is possible that some of the associations discovered by these studies were due to the environment causing mental ill-health, but these types of studies were unable to meaningfully separate between the two competing hypotheses (causation versus selection).

The influence of selection is complicated still further by the realization that it can operate in any number of directions. For example, whether we expect those with predispositions to mental ill health to become concentrated in urban or rural areas will depend on a range of social and economic push and pull factors. When all the best economic opportunities are seen to be in the cities, we would expect to see the most able individuals being attracted into the urban areas, while those with psychiatric problems would be left behind in the rural areas. However, where urban areas are seen to be less desirable, then a reverse pattern of migration and selection might be expected.

In sum, the occurrence of social selection presents a major methodological problem in the investigation of the causes of mental ill health. This applies not only investigation of the causal effects of the environment, but also to a host of other social factors such as income (does poverty cause mental ill health?); social relationships (do supportive relationships protect against mental ill health?); and employment (does unemployment cause mental ill health?). In each case, one can argue that the associations that are found result from social selection rather than causation. There are some ways of attempting to separate the effects of social selection and causation (Dohrenwend and Dohrenwend, 1974; Halpern, 1993) but in general, it remains a very serious issue and one that must be addressed in any comprehensive examination of the relationship between mental health and the environment.

The Problem of Response Bias

The second interpretive problem is equally serious, though it is one that tends to affect a different kind of study. Response bias is often a problem in social and psychological research, but in the study of mental ill-health it becomes a central concern. The problem is simple, though difficult to overcome. If a given subject reports suffering from depression, and also that his or her environment is unsatisfactory, how are we to interpret this? What weight should be given to an association between poor mental health and the reporting of a negative or unpleasant environment by the same respondent?

> Away I wander'd – all the pleasant hues
> Of heaven and earth had faded: deepest shades
> Were deepest dungeons; heaths and sunny glades
> Were full of pestilent light; our taintless rills
> Seem'd sooty, and o'erspread with upturn'd gills
> Of dying fish; the vermial rose had blown
> In frightful scarlet, and its thorns outgrown
> Like spiked aloe . . .
>
> (Keats, J., 'Endymion')

This excerpt from Keats' 'Endymion' encapsulates the issue – the perception and reporting of environmental variables is strongly influenced by the subject's mental state. If, then, an association is found between some measure of individuals' mental health and the reporting of problems with neighbours, passing juggernauts or perceived crowding, two interpretations are possible. One, that problems in the environment caused the mental ill health. Two, that the mental ill-health caused the environment to be *perceived* as a problem. The latter interpretation implies that the reporting of environmental problems is itself a symptom of disorder – a *bad mood* phenomenon (everything seems worse when you are already in a bad mood). This issue of response bias seriously undermines the validity of conventional cross-sectional self-report methodology in the study of the relationship between mental health and environment.

Unfortunately however, if transmission variables, such as appraisal or meaning, are important (see Chapters 2, 3 and 5) then the hapless researcher is left in the unenviable position of suspecting that the subjective assessments of environments are critically important, yet knowing that the meaning of these subjective assessments cannot be taken at face value.

An Illustration of the Problem of Response Bias: Picking Apart Subjective Appraisals

Before continuing, it may be helpful to provide an empirical example of the effects of response bias. The example will show how even a relatively simple subjective appraisal of the environment is affected by a wide range of factors and including mental health. This example will also illustrate the kind of multivariate analysis that is used extensively in the analyses presented in this book.

One of the pieces of research that is reported in this book is an analysis of the effects of road traffic and the problems associated (see Chapters 2 and 3). It is possible to use part of this analysis to explore respondents' subjective appraisals of their environments. If subjects are asked, 'How noisy is this place, how satisfactory is your house, or how dangerous is your road?', what affects their answers? Can subjects be relied upon to accurately appraise their environments? If it cannot be shown that subjects can reliably make such judgments, or if subjects' judgments are driven primarily by their mood or internal state, then doubt would be cast over the importance of the objective environment in the determination of environmental perception!

Two simplified viewpoints can be contrasted: first, that environmental appraisals are a simple reflection of the objective environment, and second, that environmental appraisals are principally a reflection of the subjects' mental state and world-view, and are incomprehensible without an understanding of personal meaning. Hence, for example, there are people doing work outside your window and you think, 'that noise is very loud.' To what extent is your perception determined by the actual level of the noise and to what extent by other factors such as your mood or the task you are trying to get done? Let us consider the relatively simple example of people's estimates of the level of traffic flow outside their homes.

It seems reasonable to expect that people's judgments of the level of traffic going past their homes should be fairly accurate, at least relative to other people's judgments of traffic going past their own homes. In this particular data set, this hypothesis could be tested quite simply as both subjects' perceptions and an objective, independent

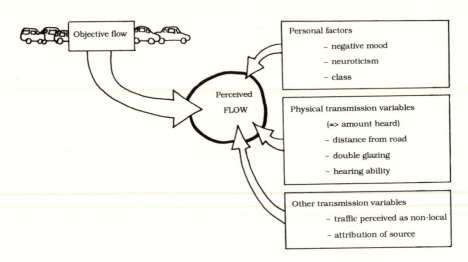

Figure 1.3: *Possible factors that might influence perceptions of traffic flow*

measure of the traffic count were available (n=6000). The Pearson correlation (a simple measure of association) between perceived traffic flow and the objective traffic count was .42 (a correlation can vary between 0, which would normally mean that the variables were completely unrelated, and 1 or −1 which would mean that the variables were perfectly associated). This correlation is highly statistically significant, but still only accounted for about 18 per cent of the variance or variability in the subjective assessments. This correlation was markedly improved by using the logarithm of the objective traffic flow measure. Sound is measured in a logarithmic scale (decibels) as indeed are most psycho-physical measures (Weber's Law), and this gives us our first clue to how respondents' judgments of traffic flow are formed. Once the logarithm of vehicular count is used, its correlation with perceived flow improves to a healthy .61 (or 37 per cent of variance).

This last correlation suggests that respondents' rating of traffic flow was, to a considerable extent, an accurate reflection of the actual traffic flow. However, one must still account for much variability. This suggests that there might be other factors that affected respondents' judgments apart from the actual traffic flow. This was tested by examining judgments of traffic flow once the actual or objective traffic flow had been controlled for. This was done through the use of the statistical technique called *multiple regression*. A regression equation was specified with perceived flow as the dependent variable and the logarithm of traffic flow entered as the first variable, thereby controlling for the variability in respondents' judgments that related to the actual traffic flow. The significance of the partial correlations of the variables not entered into the equation then indicated their independent effect on judgments of traffic flow – independent, that is, of actual or objective flow. This is shown for some selected variables in Table 1.1.

Table 1.1: *Dependent variable: perceived traffic flow*

	Correlation (r)	Partial (objective vehicular flow controlled for)
Lg (Objective vehicular flow)	**.61**[3]	–
Age	.05	.04
Sex	.07	.08
Income	.00 (ns)	−.01 (ns)
Class (white-collar)	.03 (ns)	−.10
School-age children	.01 (ns)	−.01 (ns)
Symptom level	.14	.12
Time in area	.03 (ns)	.04
Living room facing front	−.07	−.06
Double glazing	.01 (ns)	.02 (ns)
Barrier in front of house	.05	−.04 (ns)
Living in a cul-de-sac	−.31	−.01 (ns)
Land use (commercial)	.29	.05
Population density	.12	.07

n = 5371
3 [r^2 = .37; p<.0001]

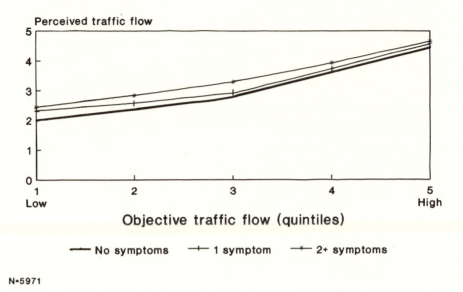

Figure 1.4: *Perceived traffic flow by objective flow and by symptom level*

Statistically controlling for the effect of objective traffic flow eliminated or strongly attenuated the effects of some variables, but left the effects of others unchanged. For example, there was quite a strong negative association between living in a cul-de-sac and ratings of traffic flow (−.31), but this association disappeared once the objective flow was controlled for. In other words, the perception of lower traffic flows in cul-de-sacs seemed to be an accurate reflection of actual flows. In contrast, the effects of mixed land use and population density were attenuated, but not eliminated by the controlling for differences in actual traffic flow. This may be because residents have a lower tolerance for traffic perceived to be due to non-residents (Appleyard and Lintell, 1972; see Chapter 2). Of particular interest here was the finding that the positive association with psychiatric symptom levels was little affected by the statistical control for the objective traffic flow. People with poorer mental health (who reported suffering from psychiatric symptoms), even when confronted with the same objective level of traffic, perceived the traffic flow to be worse (heavier).

It is possible to use the multiple regression to statistically control for other factors. Further variables were entered into the equation, and after each entry, the partial correlations of the remaining variables examined. The order of entry generally followed the pattern of individual descriptor variables first (age, sex and income); individual house variables second (for example, double glazing, house orientation); and objective street or area variables third (for example, road type). If, after controlling for other factors, an objective or area variable was still (or became) significant, possible mediators were then entered into the regression equation to see if these were able to account for the environmental variable's effect, in other words, were able to eliminate its partial correlation. In this way, a model of which factors influenced respondents' judgments was gradually built up.

The net result was a regression equation which indicated which variables, out of an extended list, had an independent affect on respondents' perceptions of the traffic flow outside their homes. A number of factors were indeed found to be influencing respondents' perceptions of the traffic flow over and above the actual or objective level of traffic. Higher levels of traffic were perceived by women; older respondents; those with living rooms at the back of their homes; those living in areas of mixed land use; those living in higher population density areas; and by those who also reported the road to be dangerous. However, even after all these variables were included, respondents' mental health (measured in terms of symptom levels) still significantly predicted their perception of the level of traffic outside their house. This residual has to be attributed to response bias. Even under objectively identical conditions, higher levels of traffic are reported by those reporting higher levels of symptoms than those reporting lower levels of symptoms.[2]

The Methodological Alternatives

The methodologies required to explore the causal relationship between the environment and mental health have to be able to disentangle the compounded threads of social, psychological and environmental factors. They also must be able to overcome the problems of social selection and response bias described above. Ideally, environmental psychologists would wish to study natural experiments in which random samples of the population were randomly assigned to a balanced range of environmental and social settings. In the absence of revolutions, these conditions do not occur. People are not passive agents in the selection of their environments, and unless blind to the determinants of their own well-being, it is a safe assumption that those individuals with the greatest resources (notably wealth) will end up living in the better environments. This means that, generally speaking, the quality of an individual's environment will be strongly determined by his or her financial resources, and differences in mental health could therefore be accounted for by the individual's general resources rather than environment *per se*. Fortunately, there are some strategies for overcoming this problem.

Identify a situation in which the link between income and housing quality is broken

The provision of state subsidized housing in many industrialized nations offers a partial example of a break in the link between income and housing quality: subsidized housing is provided for those below a certain income, thus weakening the low income–low quality housing link for those at the bottom of the market. A large number of the studies described in this book do indeed concentrate on residents in such public housing. However, at least in Britain, political and fiscal developments over the last decade have increasingly re-established the link between income and quality of the environment, as housing subsidies have been cut, the best state subsidized (council) housing stock sold, and public building programmes wound down. This may reduce the attractiveness of public housing as a setting for future research.

An alternative and clearer example of a weakened income–housing linkage is seen in Canadian public housing. Historically, there has been an attempt in Canadian housing policy to assess housing need independently from income. Public housing was therefore assigned separately from the determination of rent: if you are wealthier, you are simply required to pay a higher rental. Consequently, many of the methodologically stronger studies on the environment and mental health do indeed come from Canada (Booth, 1976; Gillis, 1977; Edwards, Booth and Edwards, 1982).

Study similar income groups in contrasting housing

If a comparison is restricted to within narrow income groups, then this effectively controls for differences due to income. This restriction is likely to reduce the range of housing types under study, but some variability will remain. This applies particularly in the public sector where housing design, for good or for bad, has been more varied and innovative than in the private sector. This can be seen clearly in the British New Towns, for example, where architects were explicitly encouraged to be innovative, and strikingly different designs can be seen virtually side-by-side. The New Towns have the added advantage of having relatively homogeneous populations, reducing sources of variability and increasing the ease with which comparisons can be made.

Some studies do exist on the mental health of New Town populations (see above), but the comparisons made have been between New Town residents and those dwelling in existing (source) urban areas rather than between residents living in contrasting areas *within* the New Towns such that all residents had experienced the same social upheaval. This latter approach would have been methodologically stronger. However, studies of this type have been conducted in military housing. For example, some of the studies presented in Chapter 5 compare the mental health of military families of the same rank but who had been assigned to different housing types (flats or houses). In such a study, the residents of the different housing types are very similar and have the same income and resources. This means that any differences in mental health are likely to be attributable to the differences in the environments rather than the populations.

Identify significant but 'invisible' variables

If variables could be identified that were causally relevant yet invisible in the sense that subjects were unaware of, or unable to assess, their influence, then a conventional cross-sectional study could be used with far more confidence. For example, in Chapter 4, one of the hypotheses examined is whether people who live on cul-de-sacs are friendlier than those who live on through roads. If this hypothesis was true, yet was something that, in general, people did not understand, then it would not be expected to have influenced their patterns of selection, though it might affect their mental health. Such a variable (living on a cul-de-sac or not) could be studied with more confidence than one about which people have strong opinions about the aetiological significance or (even if wrong) such as the difference between houses and flats.

The difficulty with this idea is that, even if aetiologically relevant but invisible variables do exist, they may be as invisible to the researcher as to anyone else. However, a careful reading of a literature does, at least occasionally, provide insights that are not entirely obvious. Either way, the issue of insight can be empirically tested, the critical factor being that the invisible variable should show no relationship with wealth. Clearly, people tend to use their affluence to escape negatively perceived aspects of the environment (aspects that are considered as stressful, anxiety provoking or depressing).

An example of a potential study of this type would be to examine the influence of the road network on mental health. Extending the idea that cul-de-sacs might have different socio-metric influences than through roads, one could explore the hypothesis that the characteristics of a road might influence factors such as crime level, safety of children, noise, pollutants, and patterns of neighbouring, but in ways that were not obvious to the residents.

Statistically control for the effects of income and other known correlates of mental health, and examine the residuals for the influence of environment

The problem with this approach is that it may suffer from the *partialling* fallacy. This means that a real effect of the environment on mental health could be concealed by the inappropriate controlling for other co-variates, notably income. It could be that the influence of income is itself, at least in part, mediated by the environment made possible by that income. This approach could therefore be described as conservative in that it is almost certain to underestimate the influence of the environment.

For some variables, researchers have concluded that income and its co-variates cannot be meaningfully disentangled (for example, the impacts of population density and socio-economic status; Galle, Gove and McPherson, 1972; see Chapter 3). However, for variables that incline towards invisibility (see above), the association may be low enough to allow for meaningful statistical control. The downside is that very large sample sizes may be required.

This more pragmatic approach can be strengthened further if the environmental variables used are objective, in other words, gathered independently of the mental health measures. This is essentially the design that was utilized in one of the studies re-analysed for this book (the Social and Community Planning Research study of road traffic and the environment by Morton-Williams *et al.*, 1978).

Employ a longitudinal design in which the subjects remain the same but within which the environment changes

A within-subjects design has the great strength of eliminating much of the variability introduced by compounded co-variates. In principal, such a study is ideal in that it can isolate the effects of a very specific environmental change or factor. The specificity of the design also increases its sensitivity, meaning that a smaller sample size is necessary than for an equivalent cross-sectional study.

A simple example might be a sudden increase in noise level associated with the commencement of building works. If a researcher could anticipate the increase, then residents could be questioned about their levels of annoyance, irritability and psychosomatic symptoms both before and after the onset of noise, and the two sets of results compared. Ideally, a second group of subjects living in an area unaffected by the noise would similarly be tested at the same times in order to provide a comparison group. If significant changes were found in the dependent variable (for example, mental health) in the first group but not in the second, then this would strongly implicate the aetiological relevance of the independent variable (noise, in this case). This classic experimental design was used as the basis for some of the methodologically strongest studies presented in this book (for example, the study of crowding by Wener and Keys (1988) or the case study of Southgate presented in Chapter 6).

The New Studies Presented in this Book

There are a number of new studies and analyses presented in this book, and these are presented alongside older work. The various studies differ in terms of their respective strengths, and each addressed a slightly different but complementary set of questions. In the end, if we are to understand the relationship between the environment and mental health, we must employ a range of methodologies and perspectives. If several different types of research methodologies lead us to the same conclusion, then our confidence in this conclusion will be greatly strengthened.

One of the new pieces of work presented in the book is a re-analysis of an existing but almost unused data set (Social and Community Planning Research, 1978). The original study was composed of over 7500 interviews from across Britain and was very unusual in that it contained independent, objective measures of environmental variables. A number of the objective environmental variables were re-analysed in relation to mental health variables; multivariate statistical techniques were used to explore the relationship between these and other potentially mediating variables. The example of response bias presented above utilized these data. Extracts from the re-analysis are reported in a number of places in the book, but especially concerning the effects of environmental stress.

The second study focused more on the planning process than the environment *per se*. The study consisted of a retrospective, longitudinal analysis of medical and official records in an attempt to reconstruct the social, medical and psychological impact of a controversial planning decision to demolish a housing estate that was proving difficult to maintain. This is reported in Chapter 6.

The third new piece of research was an in-depth study of an attempt to improve the quality of a problem housing estate, and its methodology involved both longitudinal and cross-sectional components. The study consisted of structured interviews of residents living in different phases of the estates redevelopment. The interviews were conducted in two waves, three years apart. The study provided a critical test and case study of the relationship between mental health and the planned environment. This study is reported in Chapter 7.

Summary

Mental ill-health is very common. At any one time, around one in three people are suffering from at least one psychiatric symptom, though typically such symptoms are relatively mild, such as headaches, tension or feelings of anxiousness or depressed mood. The purpose of this book is to examine whether the planned or built environment causes any of this mental ill-health.

Early studies, such as psychiatric geographies showing the spatial distributions of people suffering from psychiatric problems, demonstrated the existence of dramatic associations between the environment and mental illness. However, the inter-pretation of these associations was greatly compromised by the recognition of the occurrence of *social selection* or *drift*. People with poorer mental health were less likely to be economically successful and tended to end up living in less pleasant and desirable environments. The occurrence of social selection makes the causal interpretation of many associations between mental health and the environment difficult, and the interpretations of a number of major strands of early research – such as the New Town studies and the study of urban–rural differentials – are undermined by the uncertain influence of social selection.

An equally serious methodological problem confronting researchers working on the relationship between mental illness and the planned environment is the occurrence of response bias. How people see the world is affected by their mental state. Consequently, people with poorer mental health tend to see the world around them in more negative terms than those in better mental health. This was illustrated with a simple example of people's estimates of how much traffic went by the front of their homes. People with worse mental health perceived the traffic flow to be higher than those with better mental health even when the objective traffic flow outside their homes was identical. This type of response bias can make it very hazardous to infer causality from surveys of environmental perceptions that lack objective measures of the environment, as associations often arise between respon-dents' perceptions of the environment and mental health independently of any objective relationship.

Finally, some of the research strategies that can be used to control for the effects of social selection and response bias were described, and brief descriptions of some of the new studies presented in the book were outlined. As we shall see, by employing more sophisticated methodologies, it is possible to start to unravel the complex relationship between mental health and the environment.

Notes

1   Women are invariably reported in these community surveys as suffering from higher overall rates of psychiatric illness than men. However, it is noteworthy that drug abuse, personality disorders, and criminal offending, all of which are known to be more prevalent among men, are typically not included in the category of psychiatric illness as implied by these scales.
2   This result does not, however, exclude the possibility that there may also exist a causal relationship in the other direction, in other words, higher objective traffic flows causing higher symptom levels (see Chapter 2).

Classical Environmental Stressors

What is Environmental Stress?

The immediate environment can be a source of satisfaction but it can also be a source of irritation and annoyance. Frequently, of course, it is both. People living close by are in a unique position to provide certain kinds of satisfaction and support – a sense of community, help at short notice, looking over property – and yet their proximity also puts them in a position where they can impinge on our privacy, irritate us with their habits and generally spoil our living environment.

The potential spoiling of our environment by others and the ability of the environment to act as a stressor is the focus of the next two chapters. In this chapter, evidence will be reviewed on the potential influences on mental health of so-called classical environmental stressors – heat, chemical pollutants, and noise. In the next chapter, the influence of the more social environmental stressors on mental health – notably crowding and environmentally induced fear – will be examined. The discussion in Chapter 4 will culminate in the presentation of a general model of environmental stress and its effects. First, however, it is appropriate to consider in a little more detail what exactly is meant by *stress*.

The Stress Model

Simply put, *stress* is that which imposes demands for adjustment upon an individual. The term will be used here to refer to environmental demands, events or forces, as distinct from the *stress reaction* which will refer to the behavioural outcomes of the process. The stress model rests on the assumption that various adaptations to a range of changing environmental conditions share some common mechanism. The model is essentially a homeostatic one, where the person is seen as seeking to maintain a given state, though this state is taken to include psychological and social variables as well as more narrowly physiological ones.

The physiological component of the stress process has been emphasized in laboratory work by Selye (1978). When first exposed to a stressor, the body responds by mobilizing its coping abilities; bodily changes are triggered by the sympathetic adrenomedullary system, which inhibits digestive activity and speeds up metabolic activity, generally preparing the body for *fight or flight*. Longer adaptation in the face of threat is driven by the hypothalamo-pituitary adrenocortical system, maintaining a higher metabolic rate and blood glucose level, while also lowering levels of libido and eventually also depressing the activity of the body's immune system (Kennedy, Kiecolt-Glaser and Glaser, 1990). Consequentially, if this stress reaction is repeated often, or is overly extended, the organism may enter a state of exhaustion where adaptive reserves are depleted, physiological breakdown occurs, and the body becomes highly susceptible to disease (Baum, Singer and Baum, 1982). Selye called this the General Adaptation Syndrome (GAS).

Physiological models of the stress process recognize the occurrence of psychological activation of the GAS. The psychosocial and the physiological are linked in the stress process; we respond not only to immediate, present threats, but also to symbols of stressors, and to our expectations of them. Furthermore, psychosocial variables may sometimes evoke stress responses more damaging to the person than the aversive event itself, (for example, as in the case of certain phobias). The introduction of psychological or transmission variables enables the stress model to account for the otherwise imperfect match between the immediate environment and subsequent responses. Transmission variables are able to do this by emphasizing the process of appraisal and the relevance of coping strategies.

The detailed physiology of the stress process is of less concern here than its functional consequences. Of particular interest is the lack of specificity that the stress process implies – that widely differing stressors (such as pollutants, noise, fear of attack, and so on) can, through their mediation by a shared process, lead to essentially similar outcomes. As Freeman (1986) comments, 'the phenomenon is largely non-specific in both its determinants and its consequences . . . enhancing susceptibility to disease in general rather than having a specific aetiological role.' (p. 293)

The stress model, therefore, is an extremely economical theoretical device. It is able to account for the variance introduced by the imperfect environment–response relationship and it also accounts for why a large number of widely differing objective stressors lead to essentially similar general patterns of response – the stress reaction.

A few comments are in order on the kinds of outcome measures that researchers have used in the study of stress. Some authors just euphemistically refer to *stress-related outcomes* (mild, unspecified effects), while others have chosen to focus on dissatisfaction, mood, or symptoms, depending on their theoretical bias and the severity of the stressors under examination. Such outcomes can be loosely arranged into a hierarchy of severity ranging from specific dissatisfactions and concerns through affected mood, generalized dissatisfaction, anxiety, to the occurrence of psychopathological symptoms and clinically recognized psychiatric disorder (see Chapter 1). An implicit assumption of many researchers is that, generally speaking, the more severe a source of stress the more serious the outcome, though the relationship is heavily dependent on transmission variables such as personal vulnerability, the supportiveness of others and coping style.

Classes of Stressors

Divisions can be made between different general classes of stressors. They may be chronic or acute, and can vary in severity. Thus a simple classification can be made:

	Minor	*Major*
Acute	Daily hassles, e.g., problem at work, with car, etc.	Significant life events, eg., death of close friend or relative, etc.
Chronic	Many environmental stressors, eg., ongoing noise, pollutants, crowding, etc.	Major on-going difficulty, eg., long-term problem with health, poverty, etc.

Figure 2.1: *Classes of stressors*

Most environmental stressors tend to be minor but chronic, though in some cases their severity may become such that they may be described as major (for example, the very high crime levels in some areas). Also, it is worth noting that in certain cases daily hassles may have been provoked by environmental variables, such as crowding. Not all classes of stressors are as serious in their consequences, and in some cases the different classes of stressors are found to interact with one another. For example, there is some evidence to suggest that preceding life events can bring resilience in the face of daily hassles, although the reverse, daily hassles preceding life events, can lead to greater vulnerability, (Caspi, Bolger and Eckenrode, 1987).

Still, however elegant the theory, the task of systematically examining specific aspects of the environment to determine their salience as stressors can not be side-stepped. The next two chapters, therefore, will be concerned with reviewing the evidence of negative mental health outcomes from a series of potential environmental stressors: extreme temperatures, pollutants, noise, density and crowding, and environmentally induced crime and fear. However, two variables that will not be discussed much are urbanization (see Chapter 1) and urban relocation or slum clearance. Urbanization, as discussed in Chapter 1, is better understood as a cluster of many other variables which are best examined directly. Simple urban–rural differences are extremely problematic to interpret both because of selection and because urban and rural areas may differ on such a large number of variables that it is impossible to know which of any of these differences may have been aetiologically significant. Urban relocation or slum clearance, on the other hand, is discussed in the chapter on the planning process and mental health (Chapter 6).

All the stressors reviewed in this and the next chapter have been claimed, by one author or another, to have adverse effects on mental health.

The Seasons, Heat, Wind and Weather

There is a popular belief that seasonal fluctuations bring with them changes in mood and mental health. This belief has gained a boost in recent years from the recognition by psychiatrists that at least a proportion of the population regularly suffer from *seasonal affective disorder* (SAD), a constellation of depressive symptoms that occur during late autumn and winter, and that spontaneously remit in the spring. The disorder appears to be seen predominantly amongst women (who account for 80 per cent of cases), and at present the mean age of presentation is reported as 40, though this is expected to fall with better recognition of the disorder, (Kaplan and Sadock, 1988). Its symptoms include depression, fatigue, hypersomnia (excessive sleeping or sleepiness), hyperphagia (overeating), carbohydrate craving, and irritability.

Overlaid on top of this relatively specific disorder is the fact that physical complaints are far more common during the winter months. This is emphasized by the statistic that, for Britain alone, about 40000 more people die in the winter than in the summer (Lowry, 1991), and that for each degree Celsius by which the winter is colder than average, there are about 8000 excess deaths (Curwen and Devis, 1988). People also take more holidays in the summer. It is no surprise therefore, that virtually all medical or related utilization is higher in the winter. However, seasonal fluctuations could be attributed to several different factors.

Sunlight

As already noted, some people suffer from the condition known as SAD. This can be successfully treated with light therapy – exposure to bright light (approximately 2500 lux for a few hours every day) – so the shortage of sunlight is clearly implicated in the disorder, although the exact mechanism is not understood.

Sunny (but not too hot) days are associated with increases in altruistic behaviour and positive mood states; people are more willing to take part in questionnaires, leave larger tips and report higher satisfaction with life as a whole (Cunningham, 1979; Schwarz and Clore, 1983). Interestingly, however, there is consistent evidence that crime and suicides also increase over sunny periods. In the case of crime, this is almost certainly due to increased opportunities, and a similar positive association is found between moonlight and crime: for example, more murders occur during full-moons than at other times. The increase in the number of suicides is probably due to increases in the level of (stressful) social contacts, rather than anything to do with sunlight *per se*. Part of the effects may relate to changes in temperature.

Temperature

Rotton and Frey (1984) found that, even after partialling out (i.e. statistically controlling) the effects of the time of year and day of the week, temperature still had an effect on the daily number of psychiatric emergencies, there being more psychiatric emergencies on warm than cool days. Briere, Downes and Spensley (1983) found the same effect. Possible mediators of this effect have been suggested by experiments conducted in laboratory settings. Laboratory studies on the influence of temperature, specifically heat, on variables such as interpersonal attraction or aggression show an inverted *U-shape* relationship. Initially, generalized aggression and hostility increases linearly with temperature, but this relationship starts to reverse as temperature and the associated discomfort becomes higher still. This inverted U-shape relationship has been dramatically replicated in studies of real-world aggression: aggressive behaviours ranging from car honking in traffic jams to the occurrence of major riots are consistently associated with moderate to high ambient temperatures (Bell and Greene, 1982). A recent analysis of police records by Bell and Fusco (1989) showed this curvilinear relationship particularly clearly: the number of assaults per day increased sharply up to a peak rate at between 95 and 99 degrees Fahrenheit, and fell thereafter. It is thought that at very high temperatures, the trend towards overt aggression becomes supplemented with an avoidance response, hence the second half of the 'U'. This interpretation is supported by the increased variance that Bell and Fusco found at higher temperatures, and also in the finding by Harries and Stadler (1988) that the linear relationship between temperature and aggression was to be seen only in low to medium status areas: in high status areas, the existence of air-conditioning appeared to allow avoidance.

Evidently, although comfortably warm sunshine seems to bring improvements in mood and its absence leads to depression in some, the excessive heat and irritation of very hot days bring with them new stresses as evidenced by elevated levels of psychiatric emergencies and aggression. It is possible that it is the increased levels of aggression fostered by heat that leads to the need to handle extra cases as psychiatric emergencies. As we shall see, very similar evidence exists to that on heat for the effects of pollution on psychiatric emergencies and aggression, and the similarity of the effects are suggestive of similar underlying mechanisms.

Barometric Pressure

Barometric pressure also shows significant correlations with mental health and related outcomes. Low barometric pressure is associated with increased levels of depression, and with increased medical complaints in general (Briere, *et al.*, 1983). It is also associated with increased complaints to the police, poor classroom behaviour, and suicide (Fisher, Bell and Baum, 1984). However, barometric pressure is itself strongly correlated to other meteorological variables, and therefore the specific causal interpretation of these associations is difficult.

Wind

In certain regions, wind is believed to be the cause of many social and mental ills. Some planners have drawn attention to this in the context of modern cities, where increasingly tall structures are leading to severe winds at ground level, due to the downward deflection of higher gusts. However, though doubtless this extra gusting at street level can be inconvenient, it should not be confused with the type of winds that have been linked to more specifically mental and behavioural out-comes. Notable amongst these winds are the Chinook (in Colorado), and the Foehn (in

Europe). These warm, dry mountain winds are commonly linked by residents to depression, nervousness, pain, irritation, and traffic accidents (Sommers and Moos, 1976). Experimental evidence has lent some support to these beliefs; Muecher and Ungeheuer (1961) found that performance on various tasks was poorer on days of Foehnlike weather, while Moos (1964) found that accidents did indeed increase just before or during the approach of these winds.

The interpretation of these associations is again controversial. Rim (1975) found that during times of the hot, desert winds (Sharav) in Israel, subjects would score higher on neuroticism and extroversion scales, and lower on IQ and related scales. This has been interpreted by some as due to the high level of positive ions generated by the Sharav wind, as there is some experimental work that suggests that positive ions may disrupt performance and affect mental outlook (Fisher, *et al.*, 1984). This suggests that the adverse effects of these specific winds may be due to agents or pollutants that they carry, rather than the wind *per se*. Unfortunately, the statistical quality and detail of most of the studies are not of a sufficient standard to be able to dismiss with any certainty the aetiological relevance of other related variables, such as changing pressure, humidity, or temperature (Fisher, *et al.*, 1984; Campbell and Beets, 1981).

Putting it Together – Weather Patterns

As will have become clear by now, if we wish to progress in our understanding of the relationship of mental health to meterological variables, then more advanced statistical methods than simple measures of association must be used. Even the results of many types of multivariate analyses could be deceptive, as they might be attempting to statistically separate variables that cannot be meaningfully split; not only are the variables heavily compounded, but they also may be synergistic in their effects. Briere, *et al.*, (1983) recognized this problem in their study of psychiatric emergency room visits in Sacramento; rather than examine variables individually, they used factor analysis to identify recurring weather patterns. They found that there was a strong association between depression and one particular weather pattern – warm, low pressure, with cloud cover. This result is consistent with the other, more specific studies presented above, poorer mental health being associated with higher temperature, lower pressure and lower sunlight.[1]

In sum, the evidence suggests that fluctuations in the weather have fairly strong effects on mood in general and depressive states in particular. Increases in temperature are associated with increasing levels of aggression and (closely related?) psychiatric emergencies. In the absence of clear evidence showing mental health differences between nations with different climates, it must be assumed that individuals or cultures are able to adapt and that these are only medium to short-term effects, although even in very hot countries such as India, mood and ratings of others have still been shown to be worse on hotter days (Ruback and Pandey, 1992). Clearly, the weather *per se* is not planned (at least so far) but the temperature, humidity and colour temperature (degree of sunlight) of many environments are under our control, and this makes them relevant to the present work. Also, we must be aware of the influence of the weather if only to separate out its influence from that of other variables with which it is associated, for example, pollution or the timing of a survey.

Air Pollution

Pollution, in principal, is an unusually straight-forward stressor in that it is invariably appraised as negative. This does not always apply to other stressors, for example heat, noise or density, which may under certain circumstances be appraised as positive, (for example, the noise and density of a party, or the bustle of a busy market). For this reason, pollution is an interesting and informative stressor to examine.

Many pollutants have noxious smells and are mostly irritants in a very literal sense. The stress model suggests that such irritants, though unlikely to affect mental health by themselves, might affect mental health in conjunction with other stressors. A person already stressed by the irritation of a noxious pollutant might be more likely to show an adverse reaction to a further stressor or life event, or vice versa: it would be 'the straw that broke the camel's back'.

The major constituents of air pollution include nitrogen and sulphur oxides, photochemical oxidants (smog), carbon monoxide and particulates. Toxicological and epidemiological studies have revealed multiple health related effects of these agents. Prominent amongst these are associations with respiratory and cardiovascular diseases and especially the aggravation of pre-existing disorders (Evans and Jacobs, 1982). Despite the widespread legislation which has made smogs less frequent, air pollution continues as a serious problem, though today it is the less immediately visible agents that are of most concern. It has been suggested that many deaths in the USA are accounted for by air pollution (Mendelsohn and Orcutt, 1979) and a recent report in the UK suggested that around 10000 people per year were dying prematurely in England and Wales as a result of particulates (Bown, 1994). Air pollution is also estimated to cause billions of dollars of damage to property and agriculture every year. Lave and Seskin (1970) estimated that at least $200 million (in 1970 dollars) could be saved per year in US health costs, if air quality were improved by 50 per cent. A recent Royal Commission Inquiry in the UK concluded that air pollution from traffic alone was costing the country between 0.4 and 1 per cent of GDP, or around £40 billion per year (Royal Commission on Environmental Pollution, 1995).

High levels of pollution are known to affect behaviour, such as the level of outdoor activity, (though ironically, long-term residents appear to habituate, thereby exposing themselves to more pollution, rather than less, over the passage of time.) There is some laboratory evidence that people may be able to at least partially biologically adapt to the higher levels of pollution, but this evidence remains controversial (Hackney, *et al.*, 1977). Long-term exposure to pollution certainly leads to desensitization, and even denial; wherever people live, and to a large extent regardless of the level of pollution, they tend to rate the air quality in their own neighbourhood as significantly better than that of the surrounding areas (DeGroot, 1967).

In terms of methodology, there are two ways of examining the effects of pollutants. First, a comparison can be made between *areas* of high and low pollution. Second, a comparison can be made between *times* of high and low pollution. Comparisons across time tend to be easier to interpret.

Comparisons Across Areas

Suggestive evidence on the adverse effects of pollutants can be found in self-report studies in workplaces such as that of Klitzman and Stellman (1989). These researchers surveyed over 2000 office workers in four different sites. They found that, having controlled for age, sex, marital status and occupational group, self-reported aspects of the environment were strongly associated with satisfaction and mental health (the latter being measured by the Psychiatric Epidemiology Research Interview). Perceived air quality was one of the three aspects of the perceived environment most strongly associated with poorer mental health (the other two being ergonomic factors and noise). However, the problem with this type of study, as explained in Chapter 1, is that the causal direction remains unproven – perhaps those with poorer mental health just complained more.

It is clear that if we wish to establish the causality of the relationship between pollution and mental health, we must look to studies which included objective measures of air quality rather than just the perceptions of that quality. One such study was conducted by Bullinger (1989). He found that individuals living in a polluted area in Bavaria experienced consistently more negative moods than matched controls living in an unpolluted area (Bullinger, 1989). However, even in a study such as this, the causality of the relationship between mental health and the level of pollutants can be contested. Many characteristics of areas other than its level of pollution tend to co-vary, such as the quality of housing or the patterns of land use (see Chapter 1). The occurrence of social drift is likely to concentrate the less able and the psychiatrically impaired in less desirable areas such as those suffering from consistently high pollution. Furthermore, if chronic pollution affects the health of a population, then at least a certain amount of psychiatric fall-out is to be expected indirectly: major on-going difficulties, such as a long term medical problem and the financial hardship it brings, are a known risk factor for depression (Brown and Harris, 1978).

Some of these methodological factors were controlled for in a study by Evans, *et al.*, (1987) who looked specifically at the effects of ozone in Los Angeles. Subjects in different areas were interviewed twice and the average level of ozone in their area was measured during the period. Although no main effect was found for ozone on mental health, it was found that those people who lived in the more polluted areas showed more adverse reactions to negative life events. This finding is consistent with the stress model presented at the start of the chapter. Pollution, by itself, did not lead to poorer mental health, but when combined with other stresses, it did. The relationship was found to persist even when socioeconomic status, temperature and levels of symptoms at the first wave of interview were controlled.

Nonetheless, interpretive problems continue to compromise the usefulness of comparisons across areas. Methodologically, therefore, it is better to examine the influence of fluctuations in levels of pollutants across time and keep the area of study constant.

Comparisons Across Time

There is unrefutable evidence of the impact of fluctuations in pollutants on physical health – the last severe smog in London (1952, four years before the Clean Air act) is estimated to have led to an extra 3500 deaths over a period of a few weeks (Goldsmith, 1968) – but is there any evidence of a relationship between fluctuations in the level of pollutants and *mental* health? The answer seems to be *yes*. A series of studies by Strahilevitz, *et al.*, (1979), Briere, *et al.*, (1983), and Rotton and Frey (1984) all report the existence of small positive associations between the daily levels of pollutants and the number of psychiatric emergencies on those days. The correlations between pollutants and daily psychiatric emergencies are in the range of 0.1 to 0.25 and are strongest for the photo-chemical oxidants (CO and O_3) and nitrogen dioxide (NO_2), but are weaker and less consistent for sulphur dioxide (SO_2) and nitrogen monoxide (NO). Particulates and hydrocarbons have been found to have little or no association with psychiatric emergencies. The correlations are strongest in the study by Strahilevitz, Strahilevitz and Miller (1979), but this study can be criticized for failing to control for other related variables such as temperature or weather conditions. As we have seen, there is evidence to suggest that these variables are also related to psychiatric emergencies. The remaining studies, however, did attempt to control for these factors. Rotton and Frey (1984) statistically controlled for temperature and weather by partialling out their influences, while Briere, *et al.*, (1983) reduced them by sampling only the summer months. Despite these controls, positive relationships between psychiatric emergencies and pollutants persisted, particularly for photo-chemical oxidants.

More recently, Evans, Colome and Shearer, (1988) employed a structured interview to measure changes in symptom levels in the community with fluctuations in the level of ozone. It was found that, having controlled for age, socio-economic status and temperature, levels of anxiety were significantly higher on days of higher ozone levels. Levels of depression and hostility showed differences in the predicted direction but these differences did not attain statistical significance. Unfortunately, the authors only measured levels of ozone, and its concentration was not particularly high or varied.

These sets of results are particularly striking as the associations thus obtained are almost certain to be conservative estimates, due to the multicollinearity of, or degree of overlap between, the various factors. The weakness in some of the associations may also be due to the small amount of variability in the levels of many of the pollutants under study. Even if a pollutant is having a strong effect, the effect will not be detected if the level of the pollutant remains constant during the period studied. Furthermore, these studies have yet to address the complex relationships and interactions that exist between the pollutants themselves. The only negative association reported in the literature between a pollutant and admissions was found by Strahilevitz, *et al.*, for nitrogen monoxide and may have less to do with the pollutants' analgesic qualities (as suggested by the authors) than with its relationship to nitrogen dioxide, ($2NO + O_2 \Leftrightarrow 2NO_2$). Similar dynamic equilibriums exist between many of the other agents, for example, between nitrogen dioxide and ozone. These considerations make it difficult to pin a causal relationship on to any particular pollutant.

The weak associations between pollutants and psychiatric emergencies do not seem to be reducible to some other variable. The day-to-day correlations persist even after the related variables (such as temperature) have been statistically controlled for, though their magnitude is reduced. The implication of this finding – that air pollution can increase the occurrence of psychiatric problems – is a surprising one, yet the evidence appears strong. First, the correlations are consistent within and between studies. Second, we can discount the possibility that these studies are unrepresenta-tive because such studies are expensive and time-consuming to conduct, so any researchers, even with negative results, would have published their findings. Third, the most common problem that plagues much research into the effects of environ-mental stressors – selection and drift – does not apply to these particular studies. These studies are across time, not area or group, and therefore provide their own control. Fourth, the interpretation of causal direction, if not route, cannot be disputed; it cannot be argued that increases in admissions cause greater pollution. Thus we can say with some certainty that the association between psychiatric emergencies and the daily level of various pollutants is real, if weak.

Why might pollutants lead to increased anxiety and psychiatric emergencies? An obvious starting point is smell: many pollutants – especially the nitrogen and sulphur oxides – can be detected by their unpleasant smells. Bullinger (1989) showed that subjects reported higher levels of odour annoyance when the levels of sulphur dioxide in the community rose by even quite small amounts. Laboratory studies have shown that unpleasant aromas lead to lower levels of interpersonal attraction and higher levels of aggression (Rotton and Frey, 1984) and this raises the possibility that it is the social friction and aggression induced by pollutants that causes the increases in psychiatric emergencies.[2] However, some pollutants (notably carbon monoxide and ozone) are odourless but still cause irritation. Toxicological studies have shown that even quite low exposures to carbon monoxide can induce headaches, dizziness and nausea. Exposure to ozone causes eye and substernal irritation, and higher doses (0.5 parts per million) cause reactions including nausea, anorexia, pulmonary edema and respiratory disorder. Evidently, the effects of pollutants are unlikely to be reducible to their aromas. This last point is emphasized by the finding that subjects' self-reported mood (and performance on a concentration task) was a more sensitive indicator of objective levels of pollutants than subjects' reports of odour (Bullinger, 1989). A final possibility is that the association between pollutants and psychiatric emergencies is as much to do with the induced moods of clinicians and figures in authority as with the state of the patients themselves. The community based studies by Evans, *et al.*, (1988) and Bullinger (1989) suggest that this is unlikely to be the only factor operating, but it could be significant.

In summary, there is evidence that higher levels of pollution lead to more negative moods in the community and to higher levels of psychiatric emergencies. A similar pattern of evidence exists for the effects of heat suggesting that similar underlying mechanisms may be operating. The stress model would suggest that a high level of pollution (or heat), although unable to cause psychiatric disorders by itself, might be able to add to the adverse effect of other stressors over the threshold within which a given individual is able to cope, and where tested this has been supported (Evans, *et al.*, 1987).[3]

Noise

Noise, in lay psychology, is widely believed to have serious adverse effects on mental health. In most industrialized nations there are regular reports in the popular press of court cases concerning noise and, more dramatically, the occasional violent death of a noisy individual at the exasperated hands of a close neighbour. Indeed there are now active campaigning groups lobbying for reductions in noise pollution in most industrialized nations, and these are composed of both lay and professional members (Bronzaft, 1993). In Britain, The Right to Peace and Quiet Campaign (RPQC) has successfully persuaded the Department of the Environment to set up a Noise Forum which now meets every few months, and recent government regulations now strongly discourage the building of residential properties in noisy areas. The founder of the RPQC recently explained:

> 'You don't get used to noise. Unless someone does something about it, we're going to have more and more health problems. We're all going to be sent barmy one day.' (Valerie Gibson of the Right to Peace and Quiet Campaign, quoted in 1994, *The Big Issue*, **77**: 12, May.)

However, an examination of the influence of noise, unlike pollution, is inseparable from the detailed consideration of so-called transmission variables. The irritation caused by a pollutant is an essentially direct one; it depends very little on the interpretation of the stimulus – a bad smell simply is, more or less, a bad smell. Also, it cannot be argued that the symptom causes the stimulus in the case of a pollutant. The cause and effect is relatively uncontentious thereby easing the interpretation of associations. The same cannot generally be said of a given sound; an objectively similar sound may lead to dramatically different affective responses, even with the same person, if the context and appraisal differ. Noise is negatively appraised or unwanted sound, and this appraisal may depend on and influence the individual's internal state. Transmission variables mediate the transformation from sound to noise and account for the imperfect match between the two.

The influence of transmission variables is illustrated by the limited ability of noise indices to predict actual levels of annoyance, despite their internal reliability. The physical stimulus – the sound level itself – accounts for only a relatively small percentage of the variability in self-reported annoyance, usually 10 to 25 per cent (Cohen and Weinstein, 1982). Transmission variables such as sensitivity, attribution and appraisal of the meaning of the sound are very important in accounting for this discrepancy.

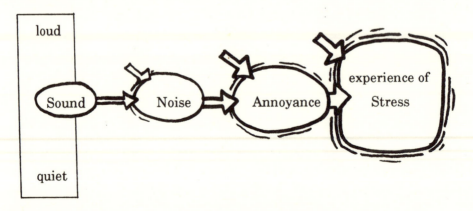

Figure 2.2: *A hypothesized relationship between sound and stress*

Auditory and Non-auditory Effects of Noise

There is no doubt that loud noise has effects on hearing. This fact was shockingly illustrated in a study by Rosen, *et al.*, (1962) which showed that 70-year old Sudanese tribesmen had hearing abilities comparable to those of 20-year-old Americans. This finding was reinforced by a 1972 Environmental Protection Agency survey that estimated that close to three million Americans suffered from noise-induced hearing loss.

The focus of this review will be on the non-auditory effects of noise, but it should be noted that even purely auditory consequences of noise may be able to have impacts on mental health, notably if they begin to affect the individual's communication with others. Surveys of mental hospital patients have revealed that age-specific hearing losses in patients are four times the age-expected rates found in the general population (Jeter, 1976). Deafness appears to be especially likely to increase the probability of developing a form of paranoia. Tarnopolosky and Clark (1984) report a similar association in a community survey, where they found that subjects with an impaired hearing capacity complained more frequently than normal of psychiatric symptomology. Ironically, it may be that a *reduced* sensitivity to *sound* brings with it an *increased* sensitivity to *noise*, as auditory discrimination (and communication) become progressively more difficult. To most people, however, it is annoyance that is the main and immediate consequence of noise.

Much of the irritation that noise brings has to do with the information it conveys rather than with the sound *per se*. Being able to hear neighbours' voices through a poorly insulated wall can be far more annoying and intrusive than an objectively louder, but impersonal, non-human sound. Studies on office noise, for example, have shown that hearing people talking is often reported as being a major source of disturbance and irritation while the noise of office machinery (except telephones) typically appears to cause little disturbance or irritation (Sundstrom, *et al.*, 1994). Laboratory work has also shown how it is particularly human voices, rather than noise in general, that interferes with subjects' performance on many cognitive tasks, (Salame and Baddeley, 1982). However, as irritation by human voices is effectively covered in the section on crowding, the present review will concentrate largely on non-spoken noise.

Noise and Helping Behaviour

Both experimental and field studies have suggested that loud noise reduces helping behaviour and induces a lack of sensitivity to others (Cohen and Weinstein, 1982). Subjects were found to be less likely to aid a person who had dropped a pile of books when a loud lawnmower was running than when it was quiet, and a cast on the victim's arm, though increasing helping under quiet conditions, made no difference when noisy (Mathews and Canon, 1975). Similarly, Page (1977) found that construction noise decreased the granting of small favours, especially reducing compliance to requests for verbal (as opposed to physical) aid. Moser (1988) has reported very similar effects from roadwork noise (drills). Moser found that higher levels of noise led to markedly reduced altruistic behaviour in passersby except for very low demand requests. The finding that people on busy streets are less helpful (Korte, Ypma and Toppen, 1975), engage in considerably less social interaction, and report such streets as lonely places to live (Appleyard and Lintell, 1972) may also in part be due to the influence of noise (see also Chapter 4).

There is some dispute as to what may mediate these effects. Alternative explanations include a narrowing of attention to avoid *overload*, the induction of a hostility to others through the negative effect generated by the noise (cf. experimental evidence on the influence of other unpleasant stimuli on interpersonal attraction), or finally, that the effects are simply attributable to the straightforward desire to escape, (cf. the relationship between heat and aggression). Of course, these explanations are not incompatible, and all are probably true to some extent. Still, is unhelpful behaviour enough to affect mental health?

Noise in the Work Place

To date, the best studied examples of the relationship between noise and mental health are those of industrial and office noise experienced in the workplace and aircraft noise experienced in residential areas close to airports.

Studies of industrial workers have shown that those exposed to higher levels of noise report an increased incidence of nervous and psychosomatic complaints, anxiety, and social conflicts both at home and at work, (Granati, Angelepi and Lenzi, 1959; Cohen, 1969; and Miller, 1974). More recently, McDonald (1989) in a survey of 900 blue collar workers found a large number of differences in psychological and mental health according to the noise level the workers were experiencing. He found that where the objective noise level exceeded 85 decibels (dBA) workers were twice as likely to report negative affect, 4 times more likely to report nervous reactions, 5 times more likely to report headaches, 10 times more likely to report after-work effects and 20 times more likely to report suffering from fatigue. Very much fewer symptoms were reported by those working in noise levels below 70 decibels (dBA). McDonald also found that those working in higher levels of noise reported more symptoms on the GHQ (General Health Questionnaire) (Goldberg, 1972), a short mental health check-list. However, McDonald found that many of the associations between symptoms and noise levels could be accounted for in terms of the quality of interpersonal relationships at work and the stress of the work, though it is extremely difficult to separate the effects of noise from this. It was certainly true that the effects were strongly mediated by levels of noise annoyance but, as we shall see later, the interpretation of noise annoyance can itself be surprisingly complex. It is noteworthy that the subjects' perceived *noise constraint* (their ability to control or avoid the noise) was more strongly related to noise annoyance than the noise level itself. This is consistent with laboratory work which suggests that subjects' perceptions of control over a stressor strongly moderates their reactions to it. Subjects in laboratory experiments who have been led to believe that they can turn off a source of stress show less adverse reactions to it.

Similar findings can be found with office workers, though the levels of noise and the associated stress reactions appear to be less serious. Klitzman and Stellman (1989), in a survey of over 2000 workers in four different sites found that complaints about noise were strongly associated with employee satisfaction and mental health (as measured by the Psychiatric Epidemiology Research Interview). These associations were found to persist, though attenuated, when statistical controls were introduced for sex, race, marital status, age and perceived psychosocial working conditions.

However, this study can be criticized for failing to demonstrate any objective differences in noise levels. Sundstrom, *et al.*, (1994) conducted a similar study of office workers but interviewed them before and after the refurbishment of their offices. Workers at 58 different sites were interviewed. Sundstrom, *et al.*, (1994) found that changes in the perceived noise level coinciding with the refurbishments were associated with corresponding changes in levels of environmental and job satisfaction, though not in changes in performance. Interestingly, where there were no changes in perceived levels of sound, satisfaction tended to have fallen. This may have been due to disappointed expectations.

However, as a number of reviewers have pointed out (Cohen and Weinstein, 1982; Smith, 1991), it is not possible to attribute with certainty the symptoms of workers in noisy environments to noise alone. Workplaces that are very noisy are also generally stressful in other ways – often hot, demanding, and dangerous. Furthermore, the lack of objective measures in many studies casts doubt on the strength of some of the reported associations as these may have resulted from response bias (for example, in Klitzman and Stellman, 1989). In sum, it is very likely that the symptoms derive from the stress of the workplace of which noise is only a part.

The Effects of Aircraft Noise

It is in studies on the effects of aircraft noise that researchers have been argued to have come closest to isolating the specific impact of noise *per se*. Studies have found associations between aircraft noise and a variety of health-related outcomes such as cardiovascular problems, hypertension, EEG disturbances, and drug taking (Knippschild, 1977; Cohen, *et al.*, 1980; Vallet and Francois, 1982). An early study by Abey-Wickrama, *et al.*, (1969) suggested that the noisier areas around London's Heathrow airport had higher psychiatric admission rates than the quieter areas. This study was soon challenged on the grounds that there were other differences between the populations of the areas that could have accounted for the differences (Chowns, 1970). A follow-up survey using improved techniques found a similar, though weaker, result (Herridge, 1974). Gattoni and Tarnopolsky (1973), repeating the original Abey-Wickrama, *et al.*, study but, using a larger catchment area, found small but not statistically significant increases in admissions from noisier areas. It was postulated that the effect of noise on admissions might have been an artefact of weaker methodology. The few surveys that had been done were also criticized because of the transparency of the hypothesis to respondents (McLean and Tarnopolsky, 1977): stronger associations were found when mention of aircraft noise is specifically made during questioning (Barker and Tarnopolsky, 1978).

A parallel literature developed in the United States, where an early study by Meecham and Smith (1977) seemed to show disproportionately high psychiatric admissions from the noisier areas around an airport at Los Angeles. It, too, was subsequently criticized on the basis that its pattern of results could have been explained on the basis of other confounding variables unaccounted for by the original authors (Frerichs, Beeman and Coulson, 1980).

In an attempt to clarify the issue Tarnopolsky and his colleagues (Jenkins, *et al.*, 1979) analysed data from 9000 admissions to three large psychiatric hospitals over a period of four years (the original studies had been based on only one hospital). Their findings initially seemed contradictory. Two of the hospitals showed the expected effect, while the third suggested that admissions were actually lower from high-noise areas. A closer analysis strongly suggested that the pattern of results was best understood in terms of the local population characteristics, and that any main effect of noise, if there was one, was being swamped by these other variables. However, there were some interesting interactions to be seen in the complex pattern of results, an association between noise and admissions being found only in certain population groups or districts. Those aged 45 and over, and to some extent the non-married, seemed more vulnerable to admission in noisy areas. Districts prone to show noise effects had high proportions of people living alone, immigrants, or professionals and managers (Tarnopolsky and Clark, 1984). [Note that these latter features refer to *areas* rather than subjects admitted.]

Evidently unsatisfied with these uncertain associations, Tarnopolsky, *et al.*, embarked on a string of still more ambitious and extensive work. An obvious criticism of the previous studies was that their outcome measure – psychiatric admissions – was too severe and insensitive a measure to pick up the subtle psychological effects of noise. With this in mind, a domiciliary survey of some 6000 people living in selected areas around Heathrow was conducted. The subjects were drawn from areas with varying (objective) levels of background aircraft noise, but matched in terms of socio-economic status, as measured by the head of household's occupation. Check-lists of 27 symptoms, of both chronic and acute form, were completed by each subject. Subjects were also directly asked how much they were bothered by aircraft noise, responses being coded from 0 – 'does not hear'; through 1–7, ranging from 'not bothered at all' to 'very much bothered'. Sure enough, being bothered by aircraft noise was strongly related to actual levels of aircraft noise, the proportion being 'very much bothered' rising from 8 per cent in the lowest noise area to 54 per cent in the highest. Yet the corresponding prevalence of symptoms seemed paradoxical. While it was true that 19 of the 27 acute symptoms were more common in the high-noise areas, this was true for only 4 of the 27 chronic symptoms. In terms of overall symptoms, only 4 of the 27 showed a higher prevalence in high aircraft noise conditions: burns/cuts/minor accidents (p<.01), tinnitus (p<.05), ear problems (n.s.) and skin troubles (n.s.). Twenty of the remaining 23 symptoms showed a higher prevalence in the *low* noise areas, and for 10 of these the differences were statistically significant at the 1 per cent level or less (Tarnopolsky, Watkins and Hand, 1980). In other words, people were generally *healthier* in the noisy areas! Standing side-by-side with this curious result, however, was the finding that regardless of area, it was those subjects who described themselves as annoyed by aircraft noise who were the ones suffering from high levels of symptoms. These confusing results can be summarized thus:

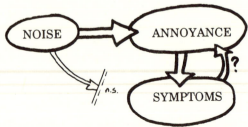

Figure 2.3: *The causal implication of Tarnopolsky et al.'s results concerning aircraft noise and symptoms*

Tarnopolsky *et al.*'s results were open to a number of interpretations. First, some people are far more sensitive to noise than others, in other words, are more annoyed by the same (objective) sound. The implication is that sensitivity leads to annoyance, and in some cases to symptoms, and that the importance of sensitivity is great enough to obscure the importance of the noise itself. Second, the fact that people in the noisy areas were not just equally healthy, but *more* healthy than the supposedly matched quiet areas suggests that selection had occurred. Despite the areas being matched by socio-economic status, it is noteworthy that there were considerably higher rates of home-ownership in the noisy areas (62 per cent vs 44 per cent in the low-noise sample), which is suggestive that the areas were considered more desirable, or at least had more committed residents. A more obvious interpretation of the result is that people who are easily irritated by noise are aware of it (note that self-report is how sensitivity is almost invariably assessed) and therefore avoid moving to an area where they know that there will be aircraft flying overhead. This (retrospectively) rather obvious interpretation is supported by the details of Tarnopolsky *et al.*'s results. Those with the lowest symptoms were those who reported little annoyance despite living in very high noise areas (imperturbables), while those with the highest symptoms were those that showed most annoyance despite living in relatively quiet areas (highly sensitives). Unfortunately, what this suggests is that until we identify what character-izes the noise-sensitive, we will gain little insight into the detailed effects of aircraft noise from community surveys, for there is little evidence of aircraft noise having a main effect, though much plausibility for it influencing residential selection. On the basis of these surveys, the only consequence most people appeared to suffer from aircraft noise was annoyance and it is only in a small minority (the noise-sensitive?) that noise might have been linked to actual psychopathology. Clearly then, it would be helpful to establish non-circular ways of identifying the noise-sensitive, and so it is to studies that bear on this issue that we now turn.

The Characteristics of the Noise-sensitive

In a minority of people, habituation to noise seems to fail (Glass and Singer, 1972). This raises the possibility that some people are considerably more sensitive to noise than others, and are consequently more adversely affected by it. This may help to explain the finding that certain categories of the neurotically ill show abnormal responses to noise. Hysterical patients in particular have been found not to habituate to repeated noise, while anxious patients have been found to show much greater responses of adrenal cortical and medullary activity, (McLean and Tarnopolsky, 1977; Tarnopolsky and Clark, 1984). These findings should alert us to the possibility that noise may have no main effect, in other words, that community surveys into the subjective impact of noise may give the impression that noise has no more than a very weak effect across the population, missing the possibility that this weak effect hides a distinction between a majority who are completely unaffected by noise, and a small minority who, for some reason, are hyper-sensitive and quite seriously affected.

Sensitivity is normally assessed by means of self-report scales which contain lists of statements that subjects mark according to how strongly they agree or disagree with the item. Items range from the direct, 'I am sensitive to noise', to the more subtle, 'In a library, I don't mind if people carry on a conversation if they do it quietly', or

'Motorcycles ought to be required to have bigger mufflers'.[4] The scales have acceptable reliability, and generally correlate well between one another, (see Stansfeld, *et al.*, 1985a, for a comparison). Subjects' scores on these scales can then be compared to their scores on other scales, for example, scales measuring aspects of their personality, their level of reported annoyance in noisy situations either in the laboratory or in a residential context, or their level of symptoms as measured by an interview or questionnaire. As ever, one has to be wary of (a) the potential overlap of such measures, especially between measures of general sensitivity and specific annoyance, but also between sensitivity and certain personality scales; and (b) of the danger of the hypothesis being obvious to subjects who will then attempt to answer in *desirable* ways.

Sensitivity to sound

It might be supposed that one of the reasons that certain people are more sensitive to noise than others is that they are objectively more sensitive to *sound*, in other words, they have unusually sensitive hearing. However, this does not appear to be the case. Stansfeld *et al.*, (1985b) found that a range of psychophysiological measures, including hearing threshold, uncomfortable loudness level and magnitude estimation, failed to distinguish women of high and low noise-sensitivity. They were selected as being high or low sensitivity on the basis of their answers on sensitivity scales administered some three years earlier; interviewers were blind to the category of subjects, and only a very small minority of subjects (16 per cent), when subsequently asked, remembered that the previous interview had been about noise. Another study, by Öhrström, *et al.*, (1988), found a similar absence of a relationship between various psychophysiological variables and sensitivity, though the researchers did find a small association between sensitivity and noise discomfort levels. However, this may have arisen as a consequence of the less rigourous methodology used: all tests and measures were done over two closely following sessions, leaving doubts as to the blindness of both experimenters and subjects. In sum, it would seem that sensitivity to sound *per se* (the sensitivity of people's hearing) does not predict sensitivity to noise as measured by self-report scales.

For an explanation of why some people are more bothered than others by the same objective noise, we will have to look beyond psychophysiological variables. This is consistent with the everyday observation that the elderly (despite objectively poorer hearing) are often vocal in their complaints about noise, and it points instead towards the importance of more social and psychological factors.

Attitude towards source

A number of studies have suggested that sensitivity to sound (and subsequent annoyance) is related to beliefs and attitudes towards the source of the noise. The classic example is a laboratory study by Cederlöf, *et al.*, (1961) which showed that subjects would rate a sound louder if it was attributed to a teenager's hot rod than if it was attributed to a taxi.

It is a common finding that those with a positive attitude to the source of the noise are less bothered by it than others who do not share this view. An example of this is that those employed by an industry or business are less bothered by the noise it produces than non-employees, even though they may be more exposed to it (Grandjean, 1974). [Almost identical results can be found in the literature on pollution – a strong negative association has been found between concerns about a pollutant and dependence on its source (Creer, Gray and Treshow, 1970).] It is difficult to attribute the noise toleration of employees to habituation. Long-term and community surveys have shown almost no evidence of adaptation to such noise. In fact, if anything, such studies suggest an increase in annoyance over time, at least in the sensitive (Jonsson and Sörensen, 1973; Weinstein, 1978). Finally, it has been found that those most annoyed by aircraft noise are also those most likely to be concerned about aircraft crashes (Tarnopolsky and Clark, 1984), and that propaganda aimed at altering people's attitudes in favour of the noise source reduced reported annoyance (Sörensen, 1970).

These findings have led some writers to label noise-sensitivity as a middle-class phenomenon. It is interesting that in a study by Tarnopolsky and Morton-Williams (1980), on the relationship between GHQ scores (Goldberg, 1972) and noise exposure, the only group within which a clear positive trend of increasing cases with increasing noise could be discerned was amongst those who finished full-time education at age 19+ and/or were in professional occupations. Stansfeld, *et al.*, (1985a) found a similar association with social class. Once again, the similarity between this and work on pollution is striking; lower socioeconomic groups consistently report lower awareness of and concern about air pollution (Swan, 1970; Evans and Jacobs, 1982). This is particularly striking given the fact that higher socioeconomic groups have, in general, both better health and lower contacts with such environmental stressors.

Personality

Various personality traits have been found to be associated with noise sensitivity, although there are some inconsistencies in the literature. Studies on student populations have found the noise-sensitive to be more likely to be introvert, with a greater desire for privacy, less secure in their social interactions, and tending to be of lower scholastic ability (Weinstein, 1978; Öhrström, *et al.*, 1988). Other studies have not always shown these relationships. In particular, the association with introversion has not been reliably found across studies (Davies and Hockney, 1966; Hockney, 1972), but this may in part be due to the differing ways in which experimenters have measured sensitivity. For example, Moreira and Bryan's (1972) failure to find an association could be attributed to their use of a psychophysiological measure of sensitivity – subjects' ratings of actual noises in the laboratory – a measure now known to correlate poorly with subjective measures of sensitivity (see above).

Recently, the concept of personality *hardiness* (Kobasa, 1979) has been shown to have a strong negative relationship to noise-sensitivity. A hardy personality is characterized by an internal locus of control (Rotter, Seeman and Liverant, 1962), a tendency to see difficulties as challenges rather than problems (Hahn, 1966), and the tendency to feel committed rather than alienated (Maddi, Kobasa and Hoover, 1979). Topf (1989) found a correlation of –0.51 (p<.001) between sensitivity to noise (using Weinstein's (1978) scale) and hardiness. Topf also attempted to predict the subsequent annoyance of her subjects (nurses) in the noisy hospital critical care unit in which they worked. She found, unsurprisingly, that annoyance was strongly

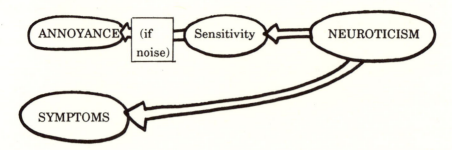

Figure 2.4: *An alternative model of the relationship between annoyance and symptoms.*

predicted by noise-sensitivity, but also that even when the influence of noise sensitivity was partialled out, hardiness (specifically commitment) retained some predictive power over noise-induced stress.

However, probably the most consistent relationship in literature on noise and personality is that of the positive association between sensitivity and neuroticism, (Broadbent, 1972; Francois, 1980; Stansfeld, *et al.*, 1985; Öhrström, *et al.*, 1988). Correlations between the two vary from around .25 to .45, and indeed some experimenters have suggested that the strength of the association would justify the inclusion of items on sensitivity to noise in future neuroticism scales (Nystrom and Lindegard, 1975).

If neuroticism is seen as a potential precursor or vulnerability factor for the development of more serious symptoms, then another interpretation for the strong links between annoyance and symptoms becomes possible (see Figure 2.4). In this view, the link between annoyance and symptoms becomes, if not spurious, at least indirect and non-causal. Annoyance effectively becomes just another symptom, though a symptom still dependent on the actual presence of noise. Sensitivity becomes synonymous with the general trait of neuroticism, perhaps now better called emotionality (cf., Cattell, 1965).

Is there a noise-sensitivity interaction?

The noise sensitivity interaction is important if sensitivity has only a main effect. This means that the sensitive report higher levels of symptoms regardless of the level of actual noise. This would imply that the symptoms of the noise-sensitive are not really the result of noise *per se*, but are just expressed as such. Stansfeld, *et al.*, (1985a) failed to find a noise-sensitivity interaction in the prevalence of symptoms; high noise-sensitive women in high noise areas did not have significantly more symptoms than those living in low noise areas.[5] However, these researchers only had a relatively small sample size (N=77).

In an extension of the study by Tarnopolsky, *et al.*, (1980), Watkins, *et al.*, (1981) examined a range of health related variables and their relationship to objective noise levels and annoyance. This study had a substantially larger sample size (approximately 6000) than in the Stansfeld, *et al.*, study. As in the earlier study by Tarnopolsky, *et al.*, Watkins, *et al.*, found that there was no interaction between noise and annoyance for most of their measures. Those who reported high annoyance were, in general, more likely to show illness behaviour regardless of whether they lived in a high or low noise area (a main effect only). This relationship held true for GHQ scores, out-patient attendances, general practitioner visits and the taking of prescribed medication. This pattern is suggestive of a vulnerability factor that operates regardless of actual noise. Higher rates of illness behaviour were found in the quieter areas, as mentioned earlier, this being suggestive of selection. However, a strong noise–annoyance interaction was found when examining self-medication. Identical patterns were found for both aircraft and traffic noise; the self-medication rate in the highest noise area rose from 8 per cent of those least annoyed to 33 per cent of those very annoyed, while annoyance produced no significant increase in self-medication in the low noise areas. The question arises, why was such an interaction not found for the other health measures? Surely, if noise sensitivity measures what we are told it does, then noise-sensitive people ought to be disproportionately more affected when living in noisy areas.

The simplest interpretation seems to be that both noise-sensitivity and psychopathology are symptomatic of a similar underlying trait. This may be neuroticism, emotionality, or simply the tendency or willingness to complain (cf., Weinstein, 1978), the term used perhaps depending more on our preference for labels than any

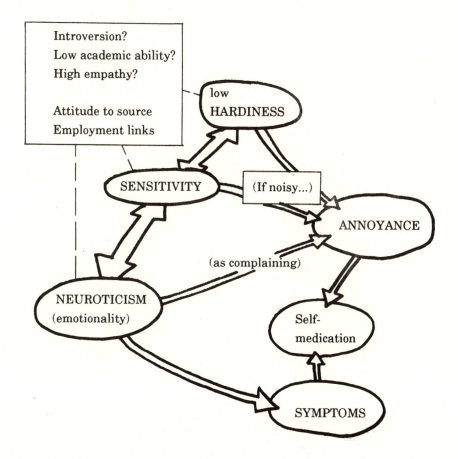

Figure 2.5: *The relationship between noise sensitivity and other variables*

substantive difference. This interpretation is very similar to one offered by Morton-Williams, *et al.*, (1978) in an investigation into the effects of traffic noise, and especially its impact on satisfaction. They noticed that an individual's level of 'nerves' was an excellent predictor of residential satisfaction, much better in fact than their own (objective) measures of the quality of the environment. Their reluctant conclusion was that there must be some kind of underlying 'personality variable such as aggressiveness or pessimism that tends to make some people generally more critical than others.'

On the other hand, noise-annoyance is dependent on the objective presence of noise and is mediated by sensitivity, as are certain other behaviours that are immediately under the individual's control, such as self-medication. It remains to be proven, however, as to whether this self-medication reflects subjects' treating of objectively worse symptoms, or instead just reflects subjects' differential attribution of the same symptoms according to the presence or absence of noise. In other words, perhaps those suffering from symptoms (which may actually have nothing to do with noise) but living in noisy areas attribute their symptoms to the noise and therefore judge self-medication, (as opposed to, say, going to the doctor), as the appropriate response.

Summary: Initial Conclusions about the Impact of Noise on Mental Health

In summary, on the basis of the evidence presented above, it can be firmly concluded that noise induces annoyance, especially in a noise-sensitive group of the population. However, the aetiological significance of noise in psychopathology has yet to be clearly proven. Sensitivity is related to other individual differences, personality variables, and beliefs held. Certain underlying traits appear to predispose an individual to develop psychopathology, and in this way both annoyance and symptoms may be seen as suggestive of a similar underlying factor.

Studies of workplaces have demonstrated that those working in noisier conditions tend to have higher levels of symptoms, but it is difficult to identify to what extent this is due to noise as opposed to the more general characteristics of the work associated with it. The evidence from studies of aircraft noise suggest that such noise can cause annoyance and dissatisfaction but not necessarily psychopathology or anything that would justify the term *mental ill-health*. Unfortunately, this latter body of research is seriously compromised by the problem of residential selection.

In total, the body of research, although extensive, raises as many questions as it answers. It can be argued that the large number of studies attempting to isolate the effects of noise by comparing the mental health of people who live in areas with high levels of aircraft noise with those who live in areas of low noise should be dismissed because of the uncertain effects of selection. Either way, we are still left with many puzzling questions about the relationship of noise to noise–annoyance and about the more basic question – does noise causally affect mental health?

In order to resolve some of these questions more satisfactorily, we need to turn to an alternative set of data and a new set of analyses. These are presented in the next section.

New Evidence on Noise: The Effects of Noise from Road Traffic

This section is based on the reanalysis of a dataset collected by 'Social and Community Planning Research; *Road Traffic and the Environment*. Colchester: ESRC Data Archive, 0000'

There have been a number of studies that have shown that adjacent transportation noise can have adverse effects on children. This work has tended to concentrate on the impact of noise on children's academic performance. Having controlled for factors such as social class and air pollution, the background presence of noisy transportation routes has been found to relate to poorer hearing discrimination and to poorer reading ability. These effects have been found both when the noise was experienced at home (Cohen, Glass, and Singer, 1973) and when it was experienced at school (Bronzaft and McCarthy, 1975). There is also some evidence that sustained noise can be causally relevant in hypertension: Cohen, *et al.*, (1980) found that children from schools in noisy areas had higher blood pressure than controls, and some evidence has been presented to suggest that noise may elevate the risk of cardiovascular problems in adults (Smith, 1991). However, unlike for aircraft noise, very few studies have attempted to examine the effects of road traffic noise on mental health. This is a surprising omission given the widespread and high levels of traffic in many urban areas.

It may be helpful to recap the methodological problems confronting environmental psychologists attempting to resolve the causality of the relationship between noise and mental health. We suspect that considerable slippage occurs between the environment as objectively measured and as subjectively experienced (see Chapter 1). The same situation – in this case, level of noise – can be appraised very differently by different people, and even very differently by the same person, depending on context or mood. The argument can be made that it is the individual's subjective appraisal of the noise that is critical for its behavioural and affective impact. This argument is very reasonable, but it brings with it serious interpretive problems in the understanding of causal direction.

The present study re-analyses an existing data-set to explore three related issues. (1) Are subjects' perceptions of noise distorted by factors other than the objective level of the noise itself? If perceptions are distorted, then by what? (2) Are there

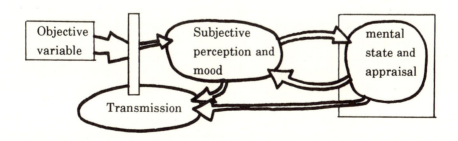

Figure 2.6: *The relationship between objective variables and subjective perceptions*

demonstrable relationships between the objective level of noise and self-reported symptoms? Can these be shown to persist once controls are made for individual background variables? (3) If such relationships can be demonstrated between the objective level of noise and symptoms, can evidence be found to identify what mediates this relationship?

Search and Selection: About the Data Set

A data set had been sought that would include some kind of mental health measure along with objective or independent measures of potentially salient environmental characteristics. Ideally, the data set would also contain information about possible (subjective and objective) mediators. A search of existing data sets was conducted to identify those with the necessary combination of variable types. Remarkably, very few met the criteria. However, a data set was identified that had been commissioned by the Department of Transport to study the noise, dirt, and inconvenience caused by different road types. The research was designed and conducted by SCPR (Social and Community Planning Research) between 1976 and 1978 (Morton-Williams, *et al.*, 1978).

The data set was fairly large: 5.4 Mega-bytes of information, 7540 cases, and 525 variables. The measures of mental health were crude but this was offset by the very large number of cases involved. The principal purpose of the survey had been to examine the inconvenience caused by road traffic and how this might relate to residential satisfaction. The mental health measures were included by the original authors not as dependent but as *independent* variables. The authors were concerned about personality variables acting as a source of response bias (Morton-Williams, *et al.*, see above). Little analysis was conducted using the mental health items, and no analysis was conducted using them as dependent variables. The relevant items were:

Have you personally suffered in the past month from:

Nerves or Nervousness	Y/N
Depression	Y/N
Undue irritability	Y/N
Sleeplessness	Y/N
Asthma	Y/N

Symptoms score = Total number of *Yes* responses

There are a number of reasons why we might expect road traffic levels outside of residential dwellings to have an effect on mental health. Higher traffic flows imply higher levels of noise and irritants, greater danger to young children and concern to their parents, and higher levels of crime due to the permeability of the neighbour-hood. In the remainder of this chapter, we will concentrate on the issue of noise. In later chapters references will be made to analyses of other environmental variables covered in the data set. Detailed questions had been asked about annoyance (bother) from noise, vibration, dust and dirt, difficulty crossing roads, problems with parking and so on. Information was gathered separately by the interviewers about the area, the type of road and the level of commercial activity, and objective traffic counts were taken. Background variables were gathered, such as age and sex of respondent;

household income; size and structure; and the presence or absence of school-age children. For a sub-set of the sample (1523 cases), extremely detailed traffic information was gathered including extended traffic counts and tape recordings of the noise level outside the house. (For the purposes of the present analyses approximately 50 variables were selected for detailed examination.)

The Original Analysis

In the original study, reliable relationships were found between the number of vehicles passing and respondents ratings of noise, dust and dirt, and vibration (Morton-Williams, *et al.*, 1978). The number of vehicles passing also showed a strong relationship with levels of annoyance. The authors divided areas into seven different types, each characterized by heavier vehicular flows and more serious traffic problems. The percentage reported as *highly disturbed* in these groups are shown below:

Table 2.1: *The percentage of residents who were 'highly disturbed' by traffic*

Area Type	1	2	3	4	5	6	7
Per cent highly disturbed	11	23	25	40	41	59	80

They found that in each group, 15 to 20 per cent more of those with high disturbance scores (than those with low scores) reported having one or more symptoms. In the lowest traffic groups, the percentage of the disturbed reporting symptoms was particularly high (54 and 60 per cent). This result showed that those reporting symptoms were considerably more likely to also report being annoyed. Those who described themselves as sensitive to noise were similarly more likely to report annoyance. The authors had found objective noise levels to be a poor predictor of residential satisfaction, and instead pointed to the importance of some kind of underlying 'personality variable such as aggressiveness or pessimism that tends to make some people generally more critical than others'.

The authors were attempting to identify the influences on residential satisfaction, and their results strongly suggested the relevance of personality. However, what was not investigated, perhaps surprisingly, was whether or not any relationship existed between symptom levels and the objective variables. The proportion of the disturbed in each area-type reporting symptoms bears no necessary relationship to the *total* number reporting symptoms in each area or at different objective levels of vehicular flow. The relationship between noise and symptoms is explored below.

The Relationship Between Symptoms and Background Variables

Before proceeding with the more detailed analyses, basic descriptive statistics of the symptoms measure were examined and the relationship of symptoms to key background variables explored (see Appendix). Just over 45 per cent of respondents reported suffering one or more symptoms. Of these respondents, 14 per cent reported nervousness, 17 per cent reported depression, 14 per cent reported irritability, and 20 per cent reported sleeplessness. These figures are within the range expected for a sample of the general population (Goldberg and Huxley, 1980). Correlations between items ranged from .24 to .47, and correlations between the individual symptoms and the overall symptoms score ranged from .57 (irritability) to .79 (depression).

Symptom levels have been widely reported to vary according to certain background variables, notably by gender, and to a lesser extent by income. These background variables provide a useful point of validation for the mental health measure. Women were found to report significantly more symptoms than men, and this was by far the most important of the individual background variables (r=.17, p.<.0001). This is consistent with previous work on gender differences in reported symptoms. Neither age nor presence of school-age children in the home had a significant impact on symptom levels. Both lower income, and blue- (as opposed to white-) collar occupational status were weakly associated with higher symptom levels scores, again consistent with previous work (Srole, *et al.*, 1962; Goldberg and Huxley, 1980; Cochrane, 1983). It was slightly surprising that there was no significant association between symptoms and having school-age children. This may be due to the crudeness of the symptom levels scale or to the measure *school-age children* having been a poor indicator of the classic risk factor of three or more children under 14 (Brown and Harris, 1978).

The Relationship Between the Objective Level of Traffic Noise and Symptom Levels

A number of different objective measures were available of both traffic flow and the objective noise level outside the home. These are shown in the table below. All of the objective traffic and noise level variables showed moderate, but highly significant, associations with symptom levels. The weakest association was with the untransformed, three minute traffic count taken by the interviewer, but as its distribution was highly skewed, it violated the assumption of normality, and the use of the logarithm

Table 2.2: *Objective traffic measures*

		Correlation with symptoms
Traffic flow	Extended traffic count (tape recording)	.064
log(Flow)	The logarithm of Tflow	.086
L10	Noise level in dBA exceeded for 10 per cent of the time	.153
LNP	*Noise pollution level* – an estimate of the average noise level plus 2.56s.d. [Takes account of the variability of the noise.]	.107
Count	3 minute traffic count (interviewer)	.037
Lg(Count)	The logarithm of count	.056

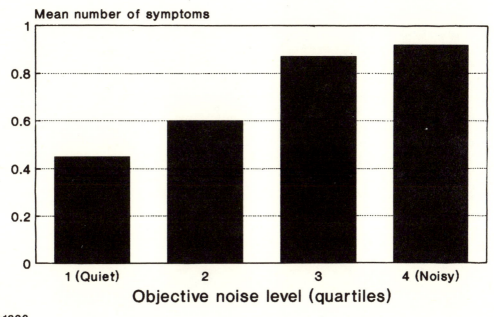

Mean number of symptoms

N=1206

Figure 2.7: *The relationship between the objective noise level outside the dwelling and residents' symptom levels*

was more appropriate. The strongest association (r=.153; p<.001) was with the noise level exceeded for 10 per cent of the time and taken from directly outside the dwelling (the measure called L10).

As can be seen from the graph (Figure 2.7), there was a clear relationship between the objective noise and traffic level and residents' levels of symptoms. People living in the noisiest 25 per cent of areas reported on average over twice the level of symptoms as those living in the quietest 25 per cent of areas. We can also confidently say that the independent variables (noise or traffic flow) were genuinely objective. It cannot be argued that the levels of traffic recorded resulted from the subjects' symptom levels or underlying neurosis as these were measured separately from the interview with the respondent. This is not to say, however, that the interpretation of the association is straight-forward.

First, the question arises as to why the different measures of traffic showed differing strengths of association to symptom levels. Weaker associations with symptoms of the untransformed measures of traffic count can be attributed to their skewed distributions, as shown by the improved strength of the correlation once the logarithms are used. The relative weakness of the associations with the three-minute count taken by the interviewer compared to the more extended taperecorded traffic count was presumably a consequence of the short-comings of the relative reliability of the two measures. However, both the measures of traffic *noise* showed stronger associations with symptom levels score than any of the traffic flow measures. This suggests that it was the traffic level as literally *heard* that was critical. Indeed, it was found that if the effect of the noise level outside the home (L10) was statistically controlled for, the positive associations of the other objective traffic variables with symptom levels were eliminated.

The fact that the peak noise level (the objective noise level exceeded for 10 per cent of the time) had a stronger association with symptom levels than did the *noise pollution level* (average noise level plus 2.5 times the standard deviation) is also interesting. This suggested that it was not fluctuations in traffic noise that were critical, but the absolute level of its (highest) intensity. Since the objective noise level exceeded for 10 per cent of the time (L10) seemed to be the most salient measure of noise, this was the measure that was used to represent objective noise level in the multivariate analyses that are described below.

Was the Association Between Traffic and Symptom Levels due to Compounded Background Variables?

The short answer to this question is 'no' – the positive association between objective traffic or noise levels and reported symptoms was not the result of compounded background variables. This was shown by statistically controlling for the influence of the relevant background variables and then examining the strength of the partial correlations of the objective traffic measures. For example, if wealthier people had lower symptom levels, and also actively selected to live in quieter areas, then controlling for the effect of income should have attenuated, or even eliminated, the effect of noise level. If this was found, it would have implied that traffic noise was simply acting as a proxy variable for something else (income, in this case). In fact, this did not occur. The partial correlations of the objective traffic variables to symptom levels, having controlled for sex, age, and income, remained largely unchanged. Controlling for length of residence also failed to attenuate the effect. Hence, the partial correlation of objective noise with symptoms after the background individual variables had been controlled for remained highly significant at r=.14 (p.<.0001).

Did the Reaction to Traffic Noise Depend Upon 'Sensitivity'?

The answer to this question seemed to be a guarded 'no'. The available measure of sensitivity was crude, but this was again partly off-set by the very large number of cases involved. Subjects were asked, 'Would you say you were more sensitive or less sensitive than other people to noise?' and could respond *more, less* or *same*. The majority of respondents rated themselves as *same* or *less* sensitive than others (44 and 38 per cent respectively) but around 13 per cent described themselves as more sensitive than others.

Two separate hypotheses can be distinguished. First, did people who described themselves as more sensitive show higher symptom levels in general, in other words, regardless of noise? The second hypothesis concerns whether sensitive individuals were systematically *more* adversely affected by noise than non-sensitives. The first hypothesis involves testing the significance of a main effect (symptom levels by sensitivity), having first controlled for the objective noise level. Overall, people reporting themselves as sensitive did report higher levels of symptoms (r=.174, p<.0001). Furthermore, once the objective noise level was controlled for, the partial

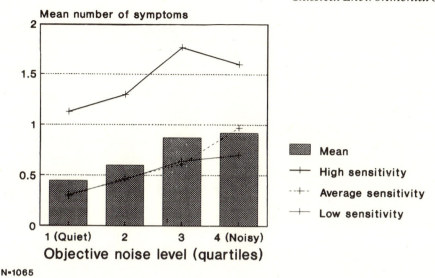

Mean number of symptoms

Objective noise level (quartiles)

- **Mean**
- **High sensitivity**
- **Average sensitivity**
- **Low sensitivity**

N=1065

Figure 2.8: *Graph showing symptom levels of noise by self-reported sensitivity*

correlation between symptoms and sensitivity rose to .26 (p<.0001). Those people who described themselves as noise-sensitive reported over double the level of symptoms as those who described themselves as being of low or average sensitivity. This result is consistent with the findings of Tarnopolsky, *et al.*, reported earlier – people who describe themselves as sensitive to noise consistently report higher levels of symptoms. Testing the second hypothesis involves examining the significance of the interaction between sensitivity and noise in relation to symptom levels. Classically, one might expect that in conditions of low noise, both the noise sensitive and the non-sensitive would report similar levels of symptoms, but that in conditions of high noise, the noise-sensitive would be disproportionately worse affected. This interaction was tested using an analysis of variance having first collapsed the objective noise level, a metric variable, into a smaller number of cells, (quartiles were used). The analysis of variance (ANOVA) showed that while both sensitivity and traffic noise each had strong independent effects on symptom levels, there was no significant interaction between the two.

Broadly speaking then, those describing themselves as sensitive reported higher levels of symptoms regardless of the actual noise level. It would seem that even when the noise level is extremely low, those reporting themselves as sensitive still report higher levels of symptoms. This finding suggests that, although sensitivity may be important in predicting symptom levels, it may have little to do with noise *per se*. Self-reported noise-sensitivity may be acting as a proxy variable for trait neuroticism, a conclusion consistent with the evidence presented earlier in the chapter.

It is worth noting that there existed a weak but significant negative association between objective noise level and sensitivity (–.074; N=1199, p.<.05). This is congruent with the conclusion that followed from the work of Tarnopolsky, *et al.*, (1980) that the noise-sensitive tend to avoid living in areas of high noise – a selection effect. This also accounts for the fact that once sensitivity is controlled for, the partial correlations of the objective traffic variables with symptom levels actually increase.

However, the strength of this selection effect seems to be far weaker for traffic noise than it was for aircraft noise.

What Mediates the Relationship between Traffic Noise and Symptom Levels? Is it Annoyance?

Having found an association between objective noise levels and symptoms, we need to establish what might mediate this effect. The obvious candidate for a mediating variable to explain the association is, of course, noise–annoyance. A simple model was provisionally postulated: noise, depending on the amount actually heard, could lead to annoyance and thereby to elevated symptom levels.

Two new variables were introduced into the analysis to test this hypothesis. They were both derived variables, summated from a number of more specific items and were: the number of traffic noises *heard* by the respondent, and the number of traffic noises that *bother* the respondent. The decision was taken to use the latter item instead of the more non-specific question – are you bothered by *general traffic noise* – because while many respondents answered *does not bother* to the general question, many more responded affirmatively to the more specific items. The Pearson correlations between the variables are shown below.

The simple associations were broadly consistent with the model. Furthermore, statistically controlling for the effects of annoyance *entirely eliminated the association between the objective noise level (L10) and symptom levels*. However, confidence in the interpretation that it was noise *per se* that lay behind this link was somewhat weakened by the finding that statistically controlling for the amount reported heard did *not* eliminate the association between objective noise level and symptoms or even association between noise levels and annoyance, though it did attenuate them. This could be interpreted in two ways, (1) that the variable measuring amount heard was of poor validity, or (2), that being bothered or annoyed by traffic noise depended on more than hearing the noise *per se*. Both interpretations were plausible, though the correlation of .48 between amount heard and noise–annoyance suggested that the *amount heard* variable must have at least some validity. The second interpretation,

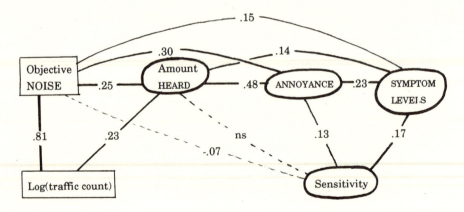

Figure 2.9: *A simple model of the relationship between noise and symptoms (Figures are Pearson correlations)*

that noise-annoyance was determined by factors other than noise alone, was explored through the use of further statistical modelling. This was done by temporarily considering noise-annoyance as the dependent variable and attempting to identify its determinants.

A regression equation was specified with annoyance as the dependent variable. The background variables of income, sex, age, sensitivity and amount heard were controlled for. It was found that while both sensitivity and amount heard had highly significant effects on the level of annoyance (multiple $R=.53$, $R^2=.28$, p.<.0001), even when they had been controlled for, the association between annoyance and the objective noise level was only slightly attenuated and the association between annoyance and symptom levels was virtually unaffected.

If instead of amount heard, the objective level of traffic noise was controlled for (in other words, entered into the regression), a very similar pattern of associations was found, with symptom levels continuing to retain a highly significant association with annoyance. In other words, noise–annoyance acted very much like symptom levels – it appeared very much like a symptom, and it had similarly broad determinants. Saying that noise–annoyance accounts for the association between objective noise levels and symptoms (which statistically it does) displaces the question rather than fully answering it. If noise–annoyance is itself only weakly determined by noise, then what else determines it? If we could answer this question then we would also have better understanding of the relationship between symptoms and noise.

So what are the Determinants of Noise-induced Annoyance, if not just Noise?

Once again, multiple regressions were used, but this time the range of variables examined was substantially broadened. The kind of technique used was similar to

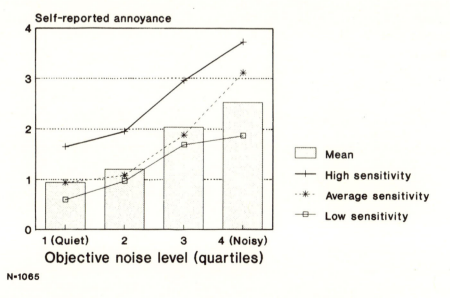

N-1065

Figure 2.10: *Graph showing annoyance by objective noise level by sensitivity*

that employed in the analysis of perceived traffic flow (see Chapter 1), but more extensive. First, the effect of objective noise level was entered into the equation. This was followed by sensitivity, the relevance of which had already been established.

At this point, the partial correlations (with annoyance) of other variables not yet entered into the equation were examined. The partial correlations showed that noise–annoyance was influenced by far more than the objective noise level alone. Other factors influencing annoyance included age (younger people were more annoyed), income (affluent people were more annoyed), ratings of the road as dangerous (associated with more annoyance), having problems with neighbours (associated with more annoyance) and symptom levels (those reporting symptoms were more annoyed). It was particularly striking that those with higher symptom levels were more annoyed than others, symptom levels accounting for a further 6 per cent of variance in annoyance after noise level and sensitivity had been controlled for. This could be interpreted as a response bias phenomenon (see Chapter 1) – people suffering from neurotic symptoms being more likely to be annoyed whatever the objective level of the noise.

Yet even with symptom levels controlled for, other factors remained significant. Higher levels of annoyance continued to be associated with: youth (younger people being more annoyed); the perceived dangerousness of the road; having problems with neighbours; residential dissatisfaction; cul-de-sac living (less annoyance in cul-de-sacs); and mixed land use (more annoyed if commercial land use present). The effect of age is interesting because it showed no association with symptom levels. Curiously, the association of age with annoyance actually became stronger once the objective noise level was controlled for. The reason appeared to be that for any given level of (objective) noise, older people were less annoyed simply because they heard less (the partial correlation between age and amount heard was –.17; p.<.001).

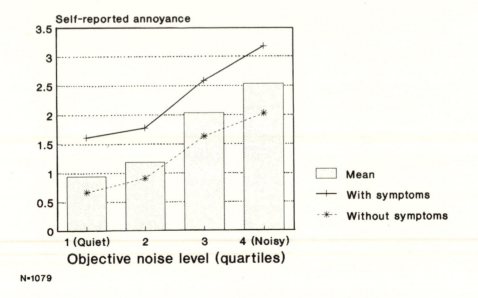

N•1079

Figure 2.11: *Graph showing annoyance by objective noise level by symptom levels*

The influence of the road's perceived dangerousness on levels of annoyance was perhaps unsurprising.[6] On those roads which were seen as being dangerous, residents were more annoyed by traffic noise. The relevance of factors like living on a cul-de-sac or land usage patterns could well have been due to attribution, as discussed earlier in the chapter and also in the discussion of the determinants of perceived flow (Chapter 1). People appear to be more annoyed by traffic that they perceive to be due to outsiders than by traffic that they perceive to be due to fellow residents. Suffice to say, an individual's level of annoyance from traffic noise is influenced by many factors beyond the noise's objective (or even heard) level. As we shall see, similar processes were found to mediate the impact of traffic levels on symptoms.

Controlling for the Amount Heard

An obvious method of testing the causal relationship between noise and symptoms was to control for the amount reported heard within the house. If it was the effect of noise *per se* which accounted for the noise–symptom level relationship, then statistically controlling for the amount reported heard should eliminate, or at least strongly attenuate, the association. If, however, controlling for the amount heard left the association unaffected then this would suggest that it was not noise *per se* that was important but was instead some correlate of the noise.

Another set of regressions was calculated with symptom levels as the dependent variable. Once again, salient background variables such as sex and age were entered first. This time, however, amount heard was entered next into the equation, and the partial correlation of objective noise level with symptoms was examined. Interestingly, the association was not eliminated. The partial correlation was attenuated, but only weakly, falling from .153 to .116 (N=1089; p<.0001).

This finding suggested one of two possibilities, as mentioned earlier. Either the measure of the amount heard had poor validity, or the positive association between objective noise level and symptoms was only the result of noise *per se* to small extent. The first interpretation was certainly possible. The measure in the SCPR survey of what was heard simply consisted of the question, 'When you are indoors, do you ever hear any of these noises …?' There then followed a list of possible noises, most of which concerned modes of transport, and the person's score simply consisted of the number of noises he or she heard. This measure may have been poor at discriminating between someone who was living in moderately noisy conditions and someone else who was living in very noisy conditions. Both might be able to hear a similar range of noises and would therefore score similarly on the scale, even though the objective noise level experienced differed widely. This means that the measure of how much people heard was probably rather insensitive. The second, but not incompatable interpretation would be that noise level could be acting as a proxy variable for something else. In other words, the elevated symptom levels could have resulted from something associated with the noise rather than the noise itself. If this was the case, then identifying and controlling for the other types of problems and aspects of the environment associated with noisy traffic should eliminate the association between noise and symptoms.

One alternative strategy of testing the causal relevance of noise to mental health

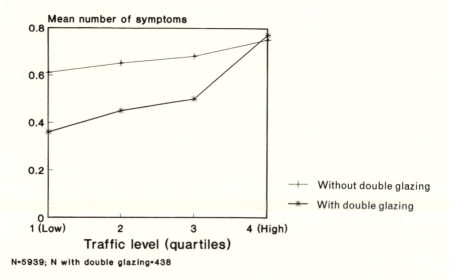

Mean number of symptoms

N=5939; N with double glazing=438

Figure 2.12: *Symptom levels of traffic flow with and without double glazing*

would be to demonstrate that the presence of a known noise reducer attenuated its impact. One such noise reducer is commonly believed to be double glazing. Subjects had been asked 'Do you have any double glazing?' Of the 6017 respondents, 7.4 per cent had double glazing. A weak but significant negative association was found between having double glazing and symptom levels (r–.036; p<.01).

This result, though weak, offers some further support for the hypothesis that noise *per se* affects mental health. However, other findings suggest that this finding concerning double glazing perhaps should be treated with caution. The presumption was that double glazing would reduce noise levels within the home, but unfortunately there was no evidence to support this claim. People with double glazing were no less likely to report hearing external noises than those without it. This could be another indication of the low validity of the hearing measure. However, people with double glazing were also no less likely to report noise – annoyance, in fact if anything, they tended to report higher levels of noise–annoyance (at any given noise level). It could be argued, therefore, that the negative association between symptom levels and double glazing had little or nothing to do with the quietening influence of the latter. The presence of double glazing might instead be seen as emblematic of a more adaptive and active subject responding to noise–annoyance, and it was by virtue of this active or internal personality that their symptom levels happened to be marginally lower, not because of the double glazing *per se*. The evidence concerning double glazing was therefore suggestive rather than conclusive.

Other Possible Mediators and Alternative Explanations of the Noise–symptoms Association

As already shown, a moderate but robust association was found between the objective traffic noise level and reported symptom levels. An attempt was made to trace the causal route of this association by systematically examining evidence for potential mediators and for other possible explanations of the association. For example, it could be argued that the association between noise and symptoms arises not because of the impact of noise, but because noise acts as a proxy for some other associated aspect of the environment, such as population density or danger from traffic. Some of these alternatives could not be explored within this data set as no suitable variables existed to empirically test them (for example, data on level of pollutants). Still, a number of alternative explanations did exist that could be tested.

A number of other objective measures of the environment were associated with noise levels, notably population density and land use (the presence of commercial land use on the same street). If the relationship between noise and symptoms was due to it acting as a proxy for these variables, then statistically controlling for them should have eliminated the association (partial correlation) between noise and symptoms. However, when these alternative variables were controlled for (plus age, income, sex and sensitivity), the partial correlation between objective noise level and symptoms remained significant, although it was attenuated (r=.07, p<.05). This was a conservative analysis given that one could make the reverse argument, in other words, that noise would have been a mediator of the influence of land use, population density and so on, rather than the other way around (this is discussed further in Chapter 3).

Another plausible alternative was that the association between noise and symptoms could be accounted for by other factors associated with traffic rather than

Table 2.3: *Correlation matrix*

	Rated danger	Time to cross	Spaces to play	Good for children
Danger	.			
Cross	**.384**	.		
Play	**−.126**	.035	.	
Good for children	**−.283**	**−.187**	**.158**	.
Noise (L10)	**.577**	**.606**	**−.172**	**−.388**
Flow (Lgct.)	**.565**	**.571**	−.036	**−.274**
Cul-de-sac	**−.245**	**−.174**	.002 ns	**.123**
Mixed land use	**.270**	**.321**	−.073	**−.212**
Population density	**.057**	**.069**	−.042	**−.090**
Age	**.053**	.023	**−.056**	−.016 ns
School-children	.016 ns	−.033	.024 ns	−.045
Sensitivity	−.000 ns	−.015 ns	.004 ns	−.004 ns
Symptom levels	**.111**	.039	**−.097**	**−.115**

[Figures in **bold** = p<.001]

noise. The most obvious such factor is the danger from traffic (the danger of being hit or run over). Two other possible factors were difficulty in crossing the road and the absence of areas for children to play in. Finally, a more general rating of the area in terms of how good it was for children was considered. Evidence from elsewhere suggested that this particular issue could be an extremely salient aspect of the environment (see Chapter 7). Difficulty in crossing the road was rated by the interviewer independently of the respondent by testing how long it took them to cross the road. The other three issues were rated by the respondents themselves and therefore concerned the respondents' perceptions.

As can be seen from the correlation matrix, all four variables were associated with symptom levels, though the association with difficulty in crossing was relatively weak. The correlational matrix revealed that all four variables behaved in broadly similar ways, especially rated danger and difficulty in crossing (r=.384). This was also confirmed by the use of factor analysis. Rated dangerousness, delay in crossing, and to a lesser extent, the rating of the road as a good place for children to live, were all closely related to the level of traffic noise (and to a lesser extent to the road being a cul-de-sac and to mixed land use). The perception of having plenty of spaces to play showed a similar but weaker pattern to the perception of the area as a good place for children.

The use of subjective appraisals, such as *this is a dangerous road*, re-introduced the problem of response bias that the use of objective residential variables had eliminated. However, at this point in the analysis, the existence of an association between noise and mental health was no longer in question; instead the search was on for clues about the causality of the linkage. This eases the pressure about the concern over causal direction as, in the light of earlier analyses, it can be taken as read that the mediating perception will be an emergent product of both external conditions and internal state.

Once again, regressions were used to test whether controlling for perceived level of dangerousness or the other variables eliminated the association between noise and symptoms. The analysis showed that the influences of the four potential mediators all had some independent effect on symptom levels, with the exception of difficulty crossing which was compounded and overshadowed by the effect of rated danger-ousness (see Appendix). This was confirmed by the use of a stepwise regression, the three variables danger, availability of play areas and the rating of the area as good for children all reaching the p<.05 criteria for entry into the equation [multiple R=.157; N=5348]. However, even when these variables were controlled for in a stepwise regression, the objective noise level still retained a small but significant association with symptom levels. This result, when combined with those presented above, suggested that noise did have a causal relationship with symptoms, albeit limited.

When noise-induced annoyance was added to the equation, it was found to account for further variance in symptom levels. Its entry (either early or late) eliminated any residial association between noise and symptoms.

Summary – Does Noise Affect Mental Health?

On the basis of the evidence presented above, noise does appear to affect mental health, but only to a very limited extent. Although there is a strong association between noise–annoyance and mental ill-health (r=.23), a significant part of this association appears to be due to response bias. People suffering from neurotic symptoms tend to report greater levels of noise–annoyance than people without symptoms even when the objective level of the noise is the same. There is a significant relationship between the objective noise level and mental health; the higher the noise level outside the home, the higher the number of symptoms reported by the resident (r=.15). This association persists even when individual background level variables such as age, sex, income and self-reported sensitivity have been controlled for, suggesting that the association is not the result of selection. This association was entirely eliminated once respondents' levels of noise–annoyance were controlled for.

However, the demonstration of an association between variables, even objective variables, does not demonstrate causality. A number of further analyses suggested that only a small part of the association between the objective noise level and symptoms was actually due to noise *per se*. A large part of the association seems to result from problems associated with the noise source (traffic). Prominent among these were concerns about safety from traffic, but it is possible that other unmeasured factors such as irritation from pollutants or fear of crime were also relevant. In later chapters we shall consider some of these covariates in further detail, such as crowding, fear of crime and the helpfulness of neighbours.

Finally, we must consider the possibility that part of the association may have arisen because of respondents double-guessing the hypothesis under examination and distorting their answers to conform to these. The simpler forms of response bias can be excluded as, given the secondary nature of the analysis, the original interviewers were clearly blind to the hypothesis in the present analysis. Similarly, we know that the objective noise level measures could not have been affected by the respondents' perceptions and symptom levels. However, in the final analysis we cannot exclude the possibility that some respondents who lived in noisy areas, having deduced that the study might be connected to traffic noise then disproportionately inflated their reporting of symptoms. In order to conclusively exclude this possibility a study would have to be designed that measured symptoms while giving respondents no reason to think that the study was connected to noise or the environment. It is to be hoped that such a study will be conducted in the future.

The most reasonable conclusion, based on the current data and state of knowledge, is that noise does have some effect on mental health, but that this effect is relatively limited, at least in most people, and in the range that it occurs in residential environments. A large part of the association between noise and mental health is due to other factors associated with the sources of noise. Having said this, it is also very clear that noise does cause a great deal of annoyance. This raises the question of why, if noise can cause so much annoyance, it generally leads to very little mental ill-health. This puzzling question will be returned to at the end of the next chapter.

Summary

In this chapter we have examined the relationship between mental health and a number of classical environmental stressors: heat and the weather, air pollution and noise. These variables are called stressors because all have been shown to trigger the so-called *stress reaction*, a generalized and apparently non-specific physiological response to certain types of (normally aversive) stimuli. The term *classical* is used to distinguish the stimuli from more social forms of stress, such as crowding, the effects of which depend more heavily on their social context and interpretation (see Chapter 3). However, as we have seen, even the effects of seemingly hard environmental stimuli depend to some extent on their interpretation.

Evidence was found to suggest that excessive heat, the absence of daylight, certain weather patterns and higher levels of air pollution can all have some effects on mental health. Evidence for these effects can be found from laboratory studies, community surveys and fluctuations in psychiatric admission rates. However, it was also found that one of the most infamous classical environmental stressors – noise – appears to have only a very limited effect on mental health. This is despite the fact that noise was shown to lead to considerable levels of annoyance in the community. These results raise the puzzling question as to why only some types of environmental stress seem to cause psychological symptoms, although all types of environmental stress can cause annoyance? This question will be returned to at the end of the next chapter, after we have had the opportunity to examine the influence of a number of other, more social, environmental stressors.

Notes

1   Breire, *et al.*, (1983) also performed a factor analysis on pollutants, but did not combine the two. This is frustrating, as it leaves us uncertain as to the relationship between pollutants and the weather. However, as the reported influence of weather is on depression and that of pollutants is more general or on schizophrenia (see later), the implication seems to be that the influences are independent. Future research should check the interrelationship directly.

2   Interestingly, Baron (1990) has also documented the converse result – increased levels of cooperation and reduced conflict as a result of the environmentally induced positive affect resulting from the introduction of a pleasant artificial scent.

3   We are now in a better position than ever before to resolve the relationship between pollution and mental (and physical) health. In recent years, a series of monitoring units have been set up across the UK (and other countries) by concerned local authorities. These now provide very accurate information about the local level of a whole range of pollutants on an hourly basis. This information could be directly collated with medical, community survey and psychiatric data.

4   These particular items are drawn from the well-used 21-item scale developed by Weinstein (1978).

5   Though having said this, the authors also mention that 'the association between High Noise Sensitivity and PSE [Present State Examination] total symptom scores in a one-way

analysis of variance remained highly significant in the high noise area and lost significance in the low noise area' [p.251]. Does this mean that there *was* an interaction but that it did not quite reach significance with their sample size (77 women in total)?

6   The wording of the question was, 'Here are some statements about this particular road, would you describe this road as . . . [statements follow] . . . A dangerous road to cross . . .'

Appendix to Chapter 2

Table A1: *The Pearson correlations between the objective traffic measures*

	Tflow	LgTf	L10	LNP	Count	Lgct	Symptoms
Tflow	.					.0.64	
LgTf	.78	.					.086
L10	.72	.85	.				.153
LNP	.47	.59	.65	.			.107
(Count	.83	.72	.65	.43	.		.037)
Lgct	.71	.90	.81	.58	.	.	.056

[All correlations between the traffic measures were significant above the .0001 level. For significance levels with symptoms, see text.]

Table A2: *Summary statistics of the symptoms measure*

Number of symptoms (value)	Frequency	Percentage	Valid percentage	Cumulative percentage
0	3897	51.7	64.8	64.8
1	1075	14.3	17.9	82.6
2	474	6.3	7.9	90.5
3	351	4.7	5.8	96.3
4	220	2.9	3.7	100.0
5	1523	20.2	Missing	
Total	7540	100.0	100.0	

Table A3: *Pearson correlations between symptoms*

	Nervousness	Depression	Irritability	Sleeplessness
Nervousness	.			
Depression	.47	.		
Irritability	.27	.38	.	
Sleeplessness	.25	.28	.24	.
Symptom score	.66	.79	.57	.61

Table A4: *Pearson correlations between symptom levels and background variables*

	Symptom levels
Sex (M = 1, F = 2)	.165
Age	.013 (ns)
School-age children	.018 (ns)
Income	−.041
Class (White- vs. blue-collar)	−.033

[N = 6001]

Table A5: *The relationship between the objective traffic measures and symptoms*

	r	Partial (controlling for sex, age, and income)	
Tflow	.051	.058	ns
Lgtf	.076	.080	p < .01
LNP	.096	.095	p < .01
L10	.140	.141	p < .0001

[N = 1053]
(NB. Small differences occur in the exact magnitude of r depending on the sample of cases taken.)

Table A6: *Self-rated sensitivity*

			Cases
Sensitivity:	(3)	More	1028
	(2)	Same	2290
	(1)	Less	2648
		Missing	1573
		Total	7540

Table A7: *The relationship between annoyance and other variables*

	r	Partial (having controlled for objective noise level and sensitivity)
Sex	.013 ns	.021 ns
Age	−.090	−.147
Income	−.012 ns	.070
School-age children	−.045	−.072
Symptom levels	.231	.250
Road 'dangerous'	.291	.190
Neighbour problems	.117	.131
Cul-de-sac	.111	.063
Mixed land use	.163	.119

Table A8: *Summary statistics on the road characteristics: rated danger, difficulty crossing, play space and suitability for children*

Road danger ('Danger'): '. . . would you describe this road as . . . a dangerous road to cross?'

		N
1	Describes this road	1798
0	Does not describe this road	4208
	Missing	1534
	Total	7540

Difficulty crossing (in seconds; 'Cross'). This was measured independently by the interviewer. Immediately after the interview, the interviewer attempted to cross the road, timing any delay with a stopwatch.

		N
0	No delay at all	5838
1	1–4	455
2	5–9	380
3	10–19	324
4	20–29	146
5	30–59	105
6	1 min or longer	139
	Missing	153
	Total	7540

Table A8 *continued*

Play space ('Play'): 'There are plenty of places near here for children to play'

		N
1	Completely agree	1788
2	Inclined to agree	1074
3	Inclined to disagree	1289
4	Completely disagree	1629
	Missing	1760
	Total	7540

Good for children: '... would you describe this particular road as ... a good place for children to live?'

		N
1	Describes this road	3898
0	Does not describe this road	2087
	Missing	1555
	Total	7540

Table A9: *Partial correlations to symptom levels, having controlled for:*

	Danger	Cross	Play	Good for children
(r to symptoms	.115	.047	−.091	−.115)
Danger	–	.105	.105	.086
Cross	.002 ns	–	.044	.025 ns
Play space	−.077	−.089	–	−.072
Good for children	−.089	−.108	−.101	–
Noise (L10)	.106	.153	.101	.098
Flow (Lgct)	.002 ns	.045	.061	.033

Table A10: *The relationship between symptom levels and the objective environment*

	Partial r (controlling for age, sex, income, and sensitivity)	lgtf	lgct L10	L10
Lgtf (traffic flow)	.106	–	–	–.076*
L10 (noise)	.169	.153	–	–
Cul-de-sac	–.060	–.030 ns	–.038 ns	–.021 ns
Mixed land use	.166	.140	.108	.103
Population density	.156	.143	.125	.125

[N = 1116]

NB. The size of sample here is mainly constrained by the use of the detailed objective variables. L10 and Lgtf, which were only gathered for 1450 cases. Missing values were deleted listwise to avoid instability.

*It is interesting to note that controlling for noise level actually resulted in a reversal in the direction of the partial of traffic flow, in other words, for any given level of noise, lower symptom levels scores were associated with higher traffic flows ($p < .05$). This could be the result of houses differing distances from the road. If the same level of traffic noise is recorded outside two separate houses despite the fact that house A adjoins an objectively busier road, then the plausible interpretation is that house A must be better protected or further set back from the road.

Table A11: *Pearson correlations between related objective variables*

	Noise	lg(Flow)	Cul-de-sac	Mixed land use	Population density
Noise (L10)	.				
Lg(Flow)	.854	.			
Cul-de-sac	–.254	–.327	.		
Mixed land use	.486	.443	–.212	.	
Population density	.251	.212	–.125	.101	

[N = 1116]

Chapter 3

Social Environmental Stressors

What is a Social Environmental Stressor?

A social environmental stressor is a source of stress that is inherently social, in other words, to do with other people. A classical environmental stressor, such as heat or pollution, may have originally been caused by people, but the stressor itself is essentially a physical agent devoid of social meaning. A social environmental stressor, on the other hand, cannot be meaningfully separated from the actions and perceived intentions of others. Of course, the distinction is not clear cut. For example, noise is generally classed as a classical environmental stressor, yet certain kinds of sound can be far more disruptive than others, even if their loudness is similar. Hence office workers find ringing telephones far more intrusive and stressful than other types of office machinery, and their presence has a far more negative impact on environmental satisfaction (Sundstrom *et al.*, 1994). Similarly, the human voice is far more disruptive of performance on many tasks than are random noises of similar frequency and amplitude (Salame and Baddeley, 1982). In retrospect, it might be more accurate to describe environmental stressors as being on a continuum between the social and the classical. However, it is still useful to be aware of the distinction, if only to remind ourselves of the wide range of phenomena that the term environmental stress encompasses.

In this chapter, we will examine the evidence concerning the major forms of social environmental stress – crowding and the fear of crime. We will be reviewing the literatures on these topics from a wide range of disciplines including environmental psychology, criminology and architecture. Where appropriate, references will also be made to new analyses of the Social and Community Planning Research (SCPR) data set on residential environments and mental health already mentioned in Chapters 1 and 2.

Crowding

Research on *Crowding* is outstanding if only for the degree of terminology-induced confusion it contains. In an effort to avoid a repetition of this confusion, perhaps it is wise to clarify a few terms before beginning.

First, *crowding* should be distinguished from *density*. Density refers to an objective measure of the physical space per person, either within the dwelling (household density) or within a locale (neighbourhood or population density). It relates to crowding, but is certainly not synonymous with it; it is a necessary but not sufficient condition. Crowding is to density, as noise is to sound, the latter in each case intended as a neutral, relative, objective description. The intervening transformation from objective environment (density or sound) to subject's perception (crowding or noise) depends on the subject's appraisal of the environment.

Second, a distinction is sometimes made between social and spatial changes in density. A doubling in social density would refer to a situation where the number of occupants doubled while the available space remained constant. A doubling in spatial density, on the other hand, would refer to where the number of occupants remained constant but the available space was halved. High *social* density, then, tends to refer to too many people, and high *spatial* density to not enough space. Following on from this is the observation that a lack of space *per se* is not enough to induce the experience of crowding. A person living alone in a small room experiences a high spatial density, but we would describe this as cramped rather than crowded. This emphasizes the important point that, unlike some environmental stressors, crowding is necessarily a social phenomenon (Epstein, 1982).

The Impetus for Crowding Research

The impetus for research into how high density affects humans came from three main sources: animal studies; the environment movement; and ecological analyses (Fisher, Bell and Baum, 1984). Studies of animal populations, typically within the laboratory, suggested that the consequences of high density could be disastrous, even when other aspects of the environment (notably food and water) were maintained (see Baum and Paulus, 1987, for a concise review). A dramatic and widely-quoted example was reported by Calhoun (1962). He placed a small number of male and female rats in a *universe* consisting of a 10 × 14 foot platform divided into four equal cells connected as in Figure 3.1. Calhoun found that as the population rose it brought with it disease, behavioural disturbances, and soaring infant mortality. The adverse consequences of the over-population were particularly marked in the central pens 2 and 3, where packs of deviant males became hyperactive, hypersexual, homosexual, and cannibalistic.

Calhoun later reported an even more dramatic, though less well known, study into the catastrophic effects of crowding resulting from unchecked population growth (Calhoun, 1973). A colony of mice were left in a large enclosure, protected from predators and supplied with sufficient food, water, and nesting materials for a population of over 4000. In fact the population never exceeded 2200, a peak which it reached within 500 days. After this the population began to decrease as successful reproduction fell, infant mortality soared, and *social pathology* set in. The pattern proved irreversible and the population continued to fall until, on around day 1660, the entire colony had become extinct. The last successful birth had been recorded on about day 600. The extinction had not been caused by a shift in climate, predation, or any other external factor. It appeared to be entirely due to crowding.

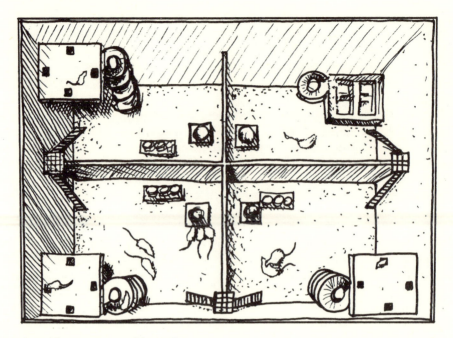

Figure 3.1: *The universe used by Calhoun*

Other researchers studying more naturalistic settings reported findings that seemed to be consistent with Calhoun's results, such as fluctuations with density in self-destructive behaviour (Christian, 1963; Dubos, 1965), decreased fertility (Christian, 1955; Snyder, 1966), and other physiological changes (Myers *et al.*, 1971). These studies, but especially that of Calhoun, were a major force behind the subsequent crowding literature, despite the fact that some of them were later criticized, not least by animal behaviourists themselves (Freedman, 1979).[1]

The second major impetus for density research was the growing awareness of human over-population stimulated by the environmental movement. The human population appeared to be continuing to grow at an exponential rate, doubling approximately every 50 years, with the greatest increases occurring in the areas least able to afford or support them (Fisher, *et al.*, 1984). This growth would be (and is) exacerbated by the simultaneous trend towards urbanization (Salk and Salk, 1981). Were Calhoun's results about to be replicated in the human population?

The third impetus, bluntly put, was the ease with which ecological studies could be conducted using density as a variable. Unlike many other environmental or social variables, population and household densities can readily be calculated from standard sources of information such as census data. This leads to easily derived correlations, but unfortunately such ecological studies can also be very misleading (see Chapter 1).

Yet whatever the reasons, a great deal of crowding research was stimulated. The methods used to study it fall into three broad types: laboratory work; ecological studies; and more ideographic approaches (typically community surveys). The latter two, both being naturalistic approaches, are best divided according to the setting under examination: family dwellings, dormitories and prisons.

Laboratory Studies of Crowding

Laboratory studies are very limited in the degree of realism they can introduce in the study of density effects, but against this they allow for the manipulation of variables and have therefore enabled the study of interactions that would otherwise have been very difficult.

These studies have confirmed the common assumption that high social densities (a lot of people in a small room) cause *negative affective states*; subjects find high social densities unpleasant and anxiety provoking (Evans, 1978). Indeed, the mere anticipation of crowding seems able to elicit this reaction (Baum and Greenberg, 1975). Laboratory induced crowding acts very much like other stressors already presented in its effects on attraction, helping behaviour and levels of aggression (see Chapter 2). Attraction for others is reduced, helping behaviour is inhibited, and both aggression and withdrawal increase, (though these changes are of small magnitude, as for other stressors).

One of the interesting findings of laboratory studies is the demonstration of the importance of subjective control (or its absence) in the experience of crowding. Subjects who feel they have more control over the situation, either because they have been told that they can press a button to escape it, or because they have a more internal locus of control in general (a personality trait), are less likely to experience high density as crowded (Sherrod, 1974; Epstein and Baum, 1978; Rodin, Solomon and Metcalf, 1978). Gender differences have also been revealed by laboratory work. In general, men appear to be more stressed by increases in spatial density, while women are more stressed by increases in social density (Ross, *et al.*, 1973; Fisher, *et al.*, 1984). Yet perhaps one of the most telling results of laboratory studies is the importance they suggest of group orientation. When the group is oriented towards cooperation for the task in hand, high density is far less likely to be felt as crowding (Marshall and Heslin, 1975). Indeed, it could be argued that it is differences in group orientation that lie behind some of the gender differences found in crowding. Men tend to cooperate in achievement-oriented group situations and women tend to cooperate in situations requiring socioemotional maintenance (Epstein and Karlin, 1975). Higher social density, for example, may make socioemotional maintenance more difficult due to the larger number of people involved. Density seems to intensify pre-existing, gender-based group orientations (Freedman, 1975).

However, the criticism remains that the artificial short-term conditions of the laboratory cannot really capture the essence of natural crowding. Laboratory studies may tell us something about the stress caused by a temporary invasion of personal space, but there is no a priori guarantee that this is the same thing as what is meant by crowding in a residential area or household.

Crowding in Family Dwellings

The group orientation of those sharing a family dwelling is clearly very different from that of subjects in a typical laboratory experiment. Household members are normally directly related or have specifically chosen to live together. Most households can be described as highly cooperative in the sense that the behaviour of their members shows a high degree of coordination and meshing. As we shall see, the contrast between the experience of density in family dwellings, student dormitories and prisons illustrates the critical importance of group orientation and individual sense of control as mediators of its effects.

Neighbourhood or population density

A number of early ecological studies (Schmitt, 1966) suggested that there were significant positive associations between population density and various measures of social pathology. Amongst the more sophisticated was a study by Levy and Herzog (1974) based on data from 125 geographic areas in the Netherlands. After having controlled for the economic strength of areas, religious diversity, income and household density, they found that population density was positively correlated (in order of increasing strength) with aggressive offences, total death rate, mental hospital admissions, general hospital admissions, divorces, fatal coronaries (male), delinquency, illicit births, and property offences. The strength of the relationship was particularly strong for the last three variables. This kind of study is very difficult to interpret, but it is typical in so far as it shows a cluster of social pathology variables correlating strongly with density at the neighbourhood level. It is reminiscent of classical geographical studies such as that of Faris and Dunham (1939) and equally difficult to interpret; is population density a cause or a symptom of the associated social pathology? Ecological associations can also be completely spurious. For example, one might find a strong ecological association between the number of office blocks in city districts and the numbers of drunks on the streets. However, this might be entirely spurious and could arise, for example, because of the locations of hostels and have nothing to do with the offices *per se*.

Researchers in other countries have not always been able to replicate Levy and Herzog's results. Galle, Gove and McPherson, (1972) using data from 75 community areas in Chicago found that any population density effects were eliminated when class and ethnicity were controlled for. Booth, in his extensive (1976) interview study, found no evidence for any effect of residential density. However, this study was based in Canada, so it might be argued that the base-line level of density was too low for an effect to show. Yet this cannot be argued for a study by Mitchell (1971) of mental health in Hong Kong, one of the most densely populated areas in the world. Despite a median density (43sq.ft per person) – four times that accepted as a minimum in European standards – Mitchell found few adverse affects.

Turning to Britain, it is possible to use the SCPR data set on residential environments to examine the effects of population density. The data set has already been described (Chapters 1 and 2), but suffice to say it contains data on 7500 respondents plus a range of independently gathered objective measures. Area population density was coded on a scale of one to five, ranging from under 0.25 persons per acre to conurbations.

It was found that the higher the level of population density that a person lived in, the higher the probability that he or she would report psychosomatic symptoms (r=.123, p<.0001). Controlling for the background individual variables of age, sex, income and self-reported noise-sensitivity left this association unaffected. Those who lived in conurbations and higher density areas reported higher levels of all types of symptom. Controlling for other aspects of the objective environment, such as the level of traffic and noise outside the home did attenuate the association between

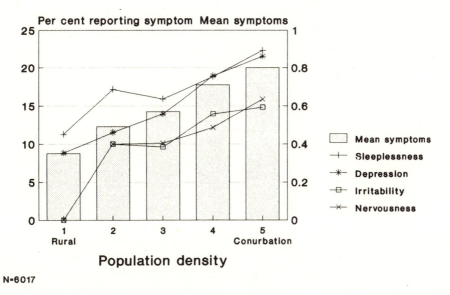

Per cent reporting symptom   Mean symptoms

Legend:
- Mean symptoms
- Sleeplessness
- Depression
- Irritability
- Nervousness

Rural — Conurbation

Population density

N=6017

Figure 3.2: *Average symptom levels by population density*

population density and symptoms, though it did not eliminate it (partial r=.066). [The Pearson correlation between population density and the objective noise level outside the home was .266, and between population density and the logarithm of the traffic flow was .111.] Further analyses suggested that part of the association between population density and symptoms was mediated by factors such as the behaviour of neighbours (neighbours were seen as less friendly in areas of higher population density, see Chapter 4), but none of the available mediators seemed able entirely to eliminate the association. This suggests that the residual association was due either to a methodological problem or to some other unmeasured factor which mediated the influence of population density. A possible methodological explanation could be that a subtle form of selection existed which was not eliminated by the statistical control of the background variables, but given the controls for income and sensitivity it is not clear what this would be. The second explanation would be that there are certain characteristics of more dense, urban environments that can affect mental health but which were not measured by the survey. We have already seen some possible candidates for this role (such as the irritation from pollution), but further possibilities include unwanted interactions with large numbers of other people (Milgram, 1970) and the fear of crime (see below). However, without the specific inclusion of these variables in data set it was not possible to test these hypotheses directly.

In sum, the evidence suggests that population, residential or population density does have an association with mental ill-health. However, this association does not appear to be invariant and does not seem to hold across all cultures or settings. Where an association has been found, as in the British data presented above, it remains unclear as to what may mediate its effects. This issue will be returned to in later sections. The complex cross-national pattern of results on the effects of population density has led many researchers to the conclusion that if density does have an effect, it is density within the house rather than outside that counts, and that even this must depend on cultural expectations.

Household density

The findings on the effects of household density (persons per room or dwelling) initially seem confused and even contradictory. Galle, *et al.* (1972) found household density to correlate highly with standard mortality, fertility, public assistance rate (children in care), and juvenile delinquency, but they found that the effect of density was inseparable from that of social class and ethnicity, making interpretation contentious. Booth (1976) found that household density had weak, positive associations with child ill-health and poor intellectual development, but found no significant relationships in adults. Levy and Herzog, on the other hand, actually found negative associations between their measures of pathology and household density: they attributed this to the *sanctuary* of traditional family life in Holland.

The contradictory pattern of these findings starts to make sense, however, if the assumption of linearity (i.e., of a linear relationship between density and its consequences) – is abandoned. Very low household density may indicate living alone, a situation which there is no reason to believe is optimal for mental health. People who are living alone, far from being protected from mental ill-health, may be at very high risk. Living alone may isolate people from potentially positive sources of social support (see Chapter 4) and may also have resulted from a recent traumatic event such as the death of a partner. A closer examination of Galle *et al.*'s study reveals that despite the strong correlations of delinquency, mortality, and public assistance rates with household density, it is the proportion of persons living alone that correlates most strongly with mental hospital admissions, and this persists after controlling for class and ethnicity. This is suggestive of a curvilinear relationship, with both very high and very low densities being associated with poorer mental health, (though the causal direction remaining unspecified).

This is exactly what was found in a study by Gabe and Williams (1987), who re-analysed some of the data from Tarnopolsky and Morton-Williams' (1980) study on aircraft noise mentioned earlier. A close examination of the relationship between household density (persons per room) and psychological distress (measured by the GHQ; Goldberg, 1972) of 452 British women revealed a highly significant J-shaped function. This persisted even after controlling for employment status, presence of children, social class, satisfaction with housing, number of persons and number of rooms.

This relationship was also found in an analysis of the SCPR data set of residential environments. Household density could not be calculated in exactly the same way as in the Gabe and Williams study (persons per room) as the number of rooms was not asked. Instead, the slightly cruder measure of persons per household had to be used as a proxy measure. Unlike that for population density, household size was, if anything, negatively correlated with symptom levels (r=−.035, p<.05, N=6017). However, the negative correlation between household size and symptom levels is misleading, as can be seen when the relation is plotted graphically (see below). The negative correlation was specifically due to the fact that those persons who live alone have, on average, significantly higher symptom levels than any other household type (Figure 3.3). This reproduces the J-shaped relation as reported by Gabe and Williams (1987). The effect was further explored by recoding into only two categories: living alone (1) and not living alone (0). Living alone showed a correlation of .073 with symptom levels (p<.0001). Those who lived alone were significantly older (r=.312;

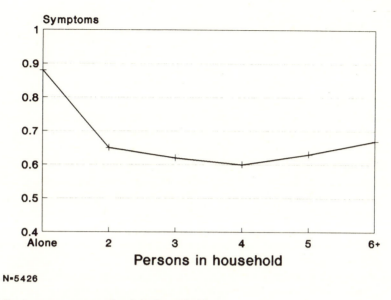

Figure 3.3: *Average symptom levels by household size*

mean =61.7yrs vs. 44.4yrs), had lived in the area for a longer time (r=.085), were more likely to be female (r=.105) and tended to have a lower income (–.110). However, controlling for all these factors did not eliminate the association (partial r=.054; p<.0001; the slight attenuation was specifically due to the influence of sex differences).

The elevated distress of those living alone may be the result of the recent loss of a child or partner, either by death or ambivalent departure, both of which might lead to depressive symptoms. This explanation would also provide an account of the negative correlation found by Levy and Herzog in Holland. However, it is difficult to account for the jump in GHQ score for those living with the highest household densities (greater than 1.5 persons per room) in the Gabe and Williams study in the terms other than the stress caused by these living arrangements, given the controls applied. This is reinforced by the finding that those with pre-school children, of low socioeconomic status, or unemployed are particularly likely to be adversely affected.

Still, against these data stands Mitchell's widely quoted study of Hong Kong (1971) mentioned earlier, in which household densities far higher than the worst found in Gabe and Williams' study appeared to lead to little emotional distress. Mitchell's study suggests a potentially nullifying influence of culture on the effects of crowding. However, this conclusion must be qualified by Mitchell's further finding that adverse effects *were* found when dwellings were shared by non-kin. Mitchell found that although density in general had no adverse effects, those living at high density on the higher floors of multi-storey buildings who were sharing their accommodation with non-kin did show poorer emotional health and increased hostility. This is consistent with the hypothesis put forward by Epstein (1982) that the high degree of cooperation found within families normally blunts the impact of crowding within the family dwelling.

In recent years, Mitchell's study on high household density has been supplemented by the publication of a number of studies on crowding conducted in India.
Evans and Palsane, *et al.*, (1989) conducted a survey of 175 male heads of households
using Dohrenwend's Psychiatric Epidemiology Research Interview (PERI; Dohrenwend, *et al.*, 1980). Persons per room varied from 2 to 11 with a mean of 2.8. They
found that higher levels of household density were significantly associated with
higher levels of psychiatric symptoms and lower social support, even having
controlled for income. They argued that the poorer quality of social relationships that
were found at higher household densities mediated the poorer mental health of the
residents. A slightly more recent study by Ruback and Pandey (1991) also reported a
significant association between household density and psychological health (r=−.11).
In their study of 481 people in six villages in the very dense region of Uttar Pradesh,
household densities ranged from 0.2 to 9 persons per room with a mean of 2.3. Again,
this level of density is around three times that found in the West. Ruback and Pandey
raise doubts about the use of conventional measures of income employed in studies
in India and therefore measured wealth by a detailed interviewer assessment of the
households' possessions. They found that there was a very strong association
between household density and their measure of wealth (r=−.54) and that when this
was controlled for the association between household density and psychological
health was no longer significant except for a persisting association between density
and physical symptoms in women. However, it could be argued that this more
rigorous statistical control for the influence of wealth may have resulted in a
partialling fallacy – part of the effect of wealth on mental health may have been
through the mediating influence of household density. Ruback and Pandey also
found that higher density was strongly associated with lower ratings of the house,
more frequent quarrels both inside the household and with neighbours and with
lower perceived control. The effects appeared to be worse on women than men,
perhaps because of the greater amount of time that women had to spend in the house.
The womens' mental health was also especially sensitive to the number of children
in the household – an effect that is also seen in the West (Brown and Harris, 1978).

Mitchell's finding that it was only on the higher floors that the adverse
consequences of density seemed to emerge, and Ruback and Pandey's finding that
the effects of density appeared to be worse for women than men due to the amount
of time that they spent in the household, provides another useful clue in the
understanding of the apparent inconsistency of household crowding effects. It may
be that even quite high levels of household density can be offset by the opportunity
and availability of escape. It will be recalled that in laboratory settings, simply
knowing that it was possible to escape (for example, by pressing a button) markedly
attenuated the impact of density. A study published by Magaziner (1988) offers further
support for this idea. Examining the pattern of first admissions to the 44 mental
institutions serving the 815 census tracts covering the Chicago area (and having
controlled for race and class), Magaziner found that living alone and density exerted
their own influences but that they also strongly interacted. The results are summarized
in Table 3.1.

As can be seen, the highest rates of admission came from areas where there was
a combination of both high internal (household) and high external density. This was
followed by the rates from areas of low internal and external density. The pattern of
results provides ecological evidence for the hypothesis that the effects of high

Table 3.1: *Mental hospital first admission rates per 1000 of population*

| | OUTSIDE (Units per structure) | |
	Low	High
INSIDE		
Low (10–46 per cent living alone)	1.24	0.79
High (0–10 per cent living alone)	0.99	1.41

Source: Data from Magaziner, 1988

household density can be offset by the opportunity to escape to a relatively low external density, and that similarly, the adverse effects of living alone can be offset by the activity of a higher density neighbourhood. Another interpretation of the latter, however, could be that those living alone in high density areas are doing so for different reasons than those in low density areas, for example, those living in low density areas being older and more likely to be living alone through bereavement. Confidence in the former interpretation is increased by the controls for race and class, by the use of first (rather than total) admissions, and by the exclusion of known skid row areas from the final analysis. Nonetheless, the results of this study should be treated with caution, given the ecological nature of the inferences. An analysis of the SCPR data did not show a significant interaction between household size and population density on symptoms casting further doubt on Magaziner's particular results.

So to summarize the findings on the effects of crowding in family dwellings, the following may be said: (i) There is some evidence to suggest a main effect of residential or population density on mental health, although this association is difficult to interpret and has not been found in all settings. Population or residential density has been found to correlate with a cluster of social pathology variables such as delinquency and crime – and it seems likely that density here may just be acting as another symptom of an area's problems rather than its cause. (ii) Provided the dwelling is not shared by non-kin, the effects of variations in household density appear to be limited, and furthermore, may be offset by the opportunity to escape into less crowded surroundings. (iii) Living alone is associated with poorer mental health leading to a J-shaped relationship with household density. This suggests that the use of simple measures of association to examine the relationship between density and mental health (or any other variable) can be very misleading in the study of crowding in family dwellings.

Crowding between Relative Strangers: Dormitories and Student Accommodation

In the previous section we noted that the effects of high densities were relatively modest in family dwellings, even at the very high levels found in places like Hong

Kong and India. People who care for one another often enjoy close proximity to one another, but when strangers are forced into the same situation they tend to find it very unpleasant. One only has to take a journey on a crowded commuter train to be reminded of this. Similarly, Ruback and Pandey (1992) interviewed passengers in Indian auto-rickshaws (tempos) at different levels of crowding. Sure enough, the larger the number of people in the rickshaw, the more unpleasant the passengers experienced it as being, the worse their mood and the more negative their ratings of the other passengers. No significant effects were found on psychological symptoms, but then the journey was only 20 minutes long. Of course, in a residential setting, the space must be shared over an extended period.

Unlike within family dwellings, relative strangers in student or dormitory accommodation can be expected to bring more individualistic orientations with them to their residential environments. As we shall see, how the environment is experienced depends largely upon whether an atmosphere of competition or cooperation develops, and this in turn depends on a number of factors including, but not only, residential density.

Among the methodologically strongest studies of crowding has been those provided by Lepore and his colleagues (Lepore, *et al.*, 1991; Lepore, Evans and Schneider, 1992). Lepore, *et al.*, conducted a longitudinal study of 175 students who were living at various levels of density (persons per room) in off-campus dwellings. The range of density was from 0.4 to 2.0 persons per room. Students were interviewed by telephone at two weeks, two months and eight months after moving into their accommodation. Mental health was assessed using the Psychiatric Epidemiology Research Instrument (Dohrenwend, *et al.*, 1980). The levels of crowding experienced by the individual students were extremely stable from the first to the third interview ($r=.88$, $p<.001$). Lepore, *et al.*, found that after 8 months, those who had been living in the more crowded conditions reported significantly higher levels of psychological distress, less perceived control and more hassles and disagreements with roommates. These differences could not be accounted for in terms of the students' psychological adjustment at the start of the study; there was no significant association between crowding and psychological distress when the students had been interviewed at two weeks after moving in. There was a significant interaction between hassles and crowding; hassles had a significantly worse effect on students in crowded than in uncrowded conditions. The results suggest that when students live in more crowded conditions, they experience a lower sense of control and higher levels of problems and conflicts with their roommates. These two factors lead to higher levels of distress.

Concerning dormitory accommodation, in a series of studies conducted at Rutgers University, New Jersey, Karlin, Epstein and Aiello (1978) found that students living in threes in rooms designed for two were more stressed, disappointed, and showed lower grade point averages than students living in twos. Complementing this, Baron, *et al.*, (1976) reported tripled students had less perceived control over their environment. These effects disappeared when the students were no longer living in high density rooms (Karlin, Epstein and Aiello, 1978). The authors attributed the phenomenon to *goal blockage*: having an extra person in the room led to resource scarcity, such as the opportunity to study. In this situation it was notable that while men attempted to pursue their goals in alternative settings, women tried to create a home-like environment. The women were eventually unable to sustain the cooperative groups, coalitions emerging instead. At the end of the semester, all of the tripled women disbanded their threesomes, though many of the tripled men remained together. These results are reminiscent of the laboratory studies on the effects of high social densities (see above).

However, the proviso needs to be added that threesomes are thought to be more socially unstable in general (ie, disregarding density) than two- or foursomes. Coalitions often form between two of the residents, leaving the remaining resident isolated (Aiello, Baum and Gormley, 1981). It is the isolate who bears the brunt of any shortage in resources. Thus it could be that rooms with four residents would actually lead to less crowding-related problems than rooms with only three.[2]

A clearer study of dormitory crowding in North American university campus accommodation has been presented by Zuckerman, Schmitz and Yosha, (1977). A comparison was made between two dormitory blocks. Block A housed 340 residents, its double rooms were of 198 sq ft, and its grid design *sociofugal* (reducing interaction). Block B housed 660 residents, its double rooms slightly smaller at 173 sq ft, and its starlike design *sociopetal* (increasing interaction). For all these reasons, the authors expected block A to be experienced as less crowded than block B. Forty residents (29 male, 20 female) in each of the dormitories were asked to fill out an individually administered questionnaire. As predicted, the residents of block B reported being less involved with their roommates ($p<.005$), being in a worse mood ($p<.01$), and experiencing their dormitory as being more crowded ($p<.005$). Yet perhaps the most comprehensive and important studies on crowding in dormitories have been those by Baum and his colleagues. They compared the behaviour and experiences of students living in dormitories of different designs and, using a range of techniques, attempted to identify some of the mediating factors. The principle comparison was between two dormitory designs of similar density, but in one (the corridor design) all the residents shared a large common bathroom and lounge suite while in the other (the suite design) each 4–6 students had their own bathroom and lounge. Residents of the corridor design reported more feelings of crowding and stress, complained more about unwanted social interactions, and were more hostile and withdrawn. (This work is also discussed in Chapter 4).

These studies strongly suggest that it is the large number of unpredictable and unwanted encounters with acquaintances and strangers that mediate the negative side-effects of higher social densities in dormitories and lead to the experience of crowding (Baum and Paulus, 1987). Common areas that are shared and used by large numbers of residents make it difficult to regulate when, where, and with whom students will interact, and it is this, rather than density *per se*, that leads to the experience of crowding stress. Interestingly, the negative effects were maintained or even increased over the course of the year; there was no evidence of habituation (Baum and Davis, 1980).

It is noteworthy that Zuckerman, *et al.*, found that the high correlations between perceived crowding and negative mood, and between perceived crowding and poor relationships with roommates, were almost as strong *within* dormitories as between them. This shows how crowding is related to personal and interpersonal affective responses even when the type of accommodation is held constant, indicating the importance of individual and social factors as well as that of the objective environment itself. This observation is further emphasized by other studies which have shown that *under certain circumstances* very few (or even positive!) consequences can follow from high density dormitory living, depending on the orientation of the group. In contrast with studies of college settings, a study of dormitory living conducted with naval personnel (Dean, Pugh, and Gunderson, 1975) failed to find any significant effects of crowding. Another study, by Smith and Haythorn (1972), of a simulated undersea laboratory, similarly found few main effects, but did find some important interactions with other variables, especially personality. Groups consisting of incompatible personalities showed significantly greater withdrawal under crowded than less-crowded conditions, while for groups of men with compatible personalities, increased density actually led to increases in time spent together in recreational activities. These failures to find main effects underline the importance of group orientation. Students in a college dormitory have tasks and orientations which are essentially individual; the naval ratings' orientations and purposes are shared.

Finally, MacDonald and Oden (1973) studied a group of five married couples, all Peace Corps Volunteers, who had volunteered to share an unpartitioned 30 by 30-foot room for 12 weeks of training. The couples not only failed to show adverse effects but showed enhanced marital relationships, were chosen as socioemotional leaders by other volunteers, and regretted leaving their accommodation more than the comparison group of those living in hotel accommodation. It was clear that these objectively crowded volunteer couples saw the adversity of the situation as a challenge rather than a crisis and developed a high degree of cooperation.

In summary, it seems that the effects of high density as experienced between relatively unrelated people in dormitories or student accommodation may or may not be negative depending on the details of the situation and the individual orientations of the residents. When the orientation is highly individualistic, or if there is a clash of personalities, then a lack of control over social interaction induced by higher densities can lead to adverse effects and the experience of crowding, but if the orientation of the residents is cooperative (typically as a result of a shared purpose) then few negative effects are seen. The latter is reminiscent of the situation in family dwellings: if the group is sufficiently cooperative in its orientation, and its members sufficiently committed to the project in hand, then high density dormitory living can actually lead to positive effects. Competition and individualistic orientations, on the other hand, are more reminiscent of the situation found in prisons, except that in prisons, escape is no longer an option. In principal, this is the situation within which density effects should be expected to have their clearest impact.

Crowding in Prisons

The densities found in prison environments are typically high, sustained for very long periods, unchosen, and inescapable. Researchers have studied spatial densities from as little as 19 sq ft per inmate, with simultaneous social densities of 70 or more to a dormitory (Baum and Paulus, 1987). This is the equivalent of more than 50 people living together in an average 1000 sq ft apartment, and all reluctant guests.

Among the most prominent researchers in this area have been Cox, Paulus, McCain, and their colleagues. Spanning over a decade, their research has been based on the archive data of nearly 200000 American inmates, supplemented by some 2500 interviews (see Cox, *et al.*, 1984, for a summary). By studying a large range of prison types with widely varying accommodation they have attempted not only to look for

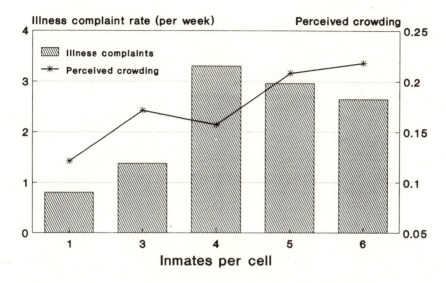

Figure 3.4: *Perceived crowding scores and illness complaint rates at Atlanta Penitentiary as a function. Data from Cox et al. 1984.*

direct associations between density and pathology, but also to identify the relative importance of its social and spatial components. They found that large institutions were associated with elevated rates of death, suicide, and psychiatric commitment. Without corresponding improvements in facilities, prison population increases were associated with sharp increases in suicide and other death rates, disciplinary infractions and psychiatric commitments. Population decreases were associated with corresponding falls in pathology. The style of accommodation was also found to be related to levels of pathology. Inmates in double cells, compared with those in single cells, had higher rates of disciplinary infractions, illness complaints and more negative ratings of their accommodation. Inmates in dormitories had worse rates than those in either single or double rooms, and especially for negative psychological reactions and illness-complaints. These effects were attributed to a combination of factors: the presence of (and threat from) other inmates, the lack of physical space, double-bunking, and the lack of privacy (Figure 3.4).

The importance of privacy has been underlined by the finding that the placing of cubicles in open dormitories significantly ameliorated the negative impact of dormitory living.[3] This finding points to the relative unimportance of spatial density, a suggestion further supported by comparisons between varying sizes of double and single rooms, which show little evidence to suggest that the size of rooms *per se* was important. It was also observed that density interacted with the presence of violent inmates, their presence exaggerating the negative effects of density still further. This raises the possibility that it is threat that leads to the severe experience of crowding in prisons, the negativity of its impact depending upon the potential seriousness of the concern.

The extensive results presented by Cox, *et al.*, are impressive, but certain criticisms and balancing remarks need to be made. Archival data, like so many sources, brings with it its own interpretive problems. For some of their case studies, Cox, *et al.*, were able to demonstrate that the density effects could not be accounted for by the influence of age, race, ethnic group, or inmate–security personnel ratio. However, it has been suggested that there remain other important factors that were not adequately controlled for, notably the level of pre-incarceration violence of prisoners. Cox, *et al.*, presented comparisons between prisons of equal official security ratings that show density effects, but some have questioned how well matched these prisons actually were. Selection may occur informally, certain prisons and types of accommodation being used for especially violent offenders. For example, it is plausible that potentially troublesome inmates are more likely to be placed in dormitories where they can be watched, than in the relative privacy and privilege of a single or double cell (though it is also possible to argue the reverse). Consequently, it has been argued by Innes (1986) that if the level of security was held constant, much of the variance accounted for by density might disappear (at least for violent behaviour). Innes has suggested that if this was done, the picture would become more complicated with certain low density prisons having quite high rates of assaults, (perhaps due to lower staff vigilance).

The observation should be added that the absolute levels of many of the forms of pathology in prisons are actually quite low relative to equivalent non-prison populations. For example, the absolute death rates due to illness and homicide are in fact significantly lower than would be expected for an equivalent non-prison population (Ruback and Innes, 1988). The average death rate for the parole population is two-and-a-half times higher than that of the incarcerated. This is not true of suicide rates, which are much higher than expected, but then it should also be said that these are actually most frequent in *single* cells, and the vast majority occur immediately following incarceration. However, these observations do not exclude the existence of density effects inside prisons, though they do suggest that Cox, *et al.*, may have overstated the absolute importance of their findings.

A well designed study has been presented by Wener and Keys (1988) which, although small in scale, is not open to Innes' criticisms of the larger scale, archive-based studies. The study compared two prison units, A and B, identical in design and management, differing only in population density levels. Data were collected both before and after a court order that led to a reduction in the density of the over-populated unit A but an increase in the density of unit B, such that after the change the density of both units was the same. Levels of perceived crowding, sick calls, and behavioural measures of the use of space were compared among the (randomly assigned) inmates of the two units. The results revealed both absolute and contrast effects of density on inmates. The level of isolated passive behaviour, perceived crowding and sick call rates all varied directly with density, and these were also affected by the direction of the shift. The perceived crowding and associated problems became higher in the unit that had experienced the increase in density (B) than for the unit that had experienced the decrease (A). This contrast effect was most marked for the perceived crowding measure but the absolute effect was more marked for the behavioural measures. The study provides strong backing for the earlier, but methodologically weaker, prison crowding research of Cox, *et al.* It also provides an insight into the process of the perception of crowding.

A study based on individual interviews by Ruback, Carr and Hopper, (1986) provides further insights into the mediating links between prison crowding and

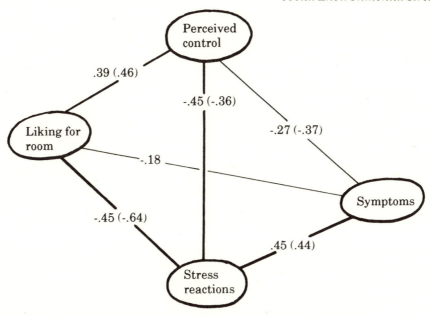

Figure 3.5: *The associates of crowding stress*
Source: Ruback, *et al.*, 1986. Bracketed figures are from the study of the smaller prison (181 inmates), unbracketed from the larger (623 inmates).

suggests the importance of perceived control in accounting for its negative impact. Ruback, *et al.*, found that inmates who perceived they had more control liked their room more, experienced less stress, and reported fewer symptoms than those who had less perceived control. A similar pattern of results was found in two separate prisons, one housing 181 male inmates, and the other housing 623. Single cells were strongly associated with liking for room, the experience of perceived control and with lower reported stress reactions. However, even when cell type was controlled for, some of the associations between the measures shown above retained significance. This result is very similar to that reported for students living in dormitories (Zuckerman, *et al.*, 1977).

Consistent with Ruback, *et al.*'s results is a finding by MacKenzie and Goodstein (1986) that inmates with a high external locus of control report significantly more anxiety, depression, and more conflicts with both guards and inmates. More specifically, it was found that it was the attribution that external forces were malevolent and punitive that was associated with the stress reactions. Of course, given the setting, such an attribution may be quite accurate. Innes' (1986) results on the association between the proportion of high security prisoners in a unit and its level of inmate assaults, deaths, and disturbances stand as a reminder of this.

The question arises, is the absence of perceived control and the experience of crowding a necessary condition for the stress reaction to occur, or are these perceptions simply other symptoms of the same stress reaction? This question is a particularly important one given that many people might feel that perceived control is not a sensible or desirable goal in the case of prisoners (Ruback and Innes, 1988). Correlational work showing that stress reactions are related to prisoners' *objective* housing conditions strongly implies that there are main and direct effects at work. Yet it has also been shown that when the objective conditions are controlled for, associations between the measures persist Zuckerman, *et al.*, 1977; (Ruback, *et al.*, 1986, for college dorms) and that relatively stable personality traits (loci of control) also contribute to the experience of crowding. Taken together these results indicate that the experience of crowding is influenced *both* by the objective conditions and by other, more individual, factors. The experience of crowding must be part cause and part symptom of the stress and symptomology with which it is associated. This, of course, closely corresponds to the conclusions already drawn in earlier sections (for example, for noise).

Towards a Model of Crowding Stress

Summarizing the findings in the literature, the immediate, objective consequences of density can be split into four components. Higher levels of density tend to be associated with the lack of physical space, the dilution of resources, the close proximity of others, and the occurance of more frequent and unregulated interactions with others. Each of these can be examined in turn, noting that their effects may not be equivalent and that density *per se* may not be their only source.

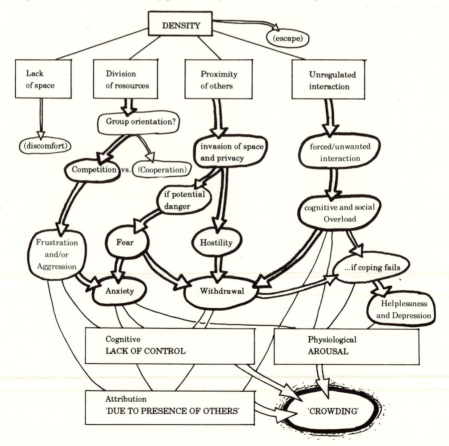

Figure 3.6: *The stressful consequences of density*

The lack of physical space

The conclusion of the research on this point seems relatively clear. Reduced physical space *per se*, has very few side-effects. It may cause discomfort, but it does little more; an individual moved to a smaller, but still single, room or cell, may well feel *cramped*, but not *crowded*. This underlines the social nature of crowding and density related outcomes.

The dilution of resources

This refers to the increased demand on an environment's finite resources, due to an increase in the number of users. So, for example, as the number of users increases, more conflicts may arise over which programme to watch on television, who sits in which chair, or who gets to use the desk space. A critical factor determining the negativity of the outcomes of these conflicts is the group orientation. Where a high degree of cooperation exists group members are able to mesh their behaviour thereby offsetting the impact of limited resources. The family dwelling is the obvious example of this. The prison environment, on the other hand, is an example of a more competitive environment where disputes may flare into open conflict. In such a setting, the outcomes of resource dilution are considerably more serious, resulting in frustration, withdrawal and outbreaks of aggression.

The close proximity of others

A third consequence of higher density is the close proximity of others. Its outcome depends largely on its appraisal. There are obvious examples of where close proximity would be considered positive; the physical closeness of a lover or good friend would not be labelled as crowding, but if it involves persons who are considered as unfamiliar or hostile then their presence will be appraised as negative or even threatening. The desire for *safe space* (Fry, 1987) has been compared by many to the territoriality seen in some animals. However, the introduction of this term brings with it more confusion than insight and its explanatory power is seriously compromised by the complexity and flexibility of human social behaviour. The prison environment exemplifies proximity as threat; the physical closeness of potentially dangerous fellow inmates can bring with it a very real sense of threat, and it is not surprising that this leads to anxiety. Yet even when the close proximity of others does not lead to a concern about personal safety, it is still often considered highly undesirable. This is normally expressed as limiting or invading privacy, but what does this mean? People selectively control access to their person and self, regulating both the input they receive and the information they divulge (Altman and Chemers, 1980). Clearly, the close proximity of others in the absence of physical barriers implies the loss of a principle method of such regulation. It also implies increased disruption from others, whether intentional or otherwise: interference with communication, concentration, and a source of irritation. In this situation the only alternative method of privacy regulation may be withdrawal, but this is not necessarily very effective and tends to be coupled with feelings of helplessness and lack of control, and it also undermines the opportunities for potentially positive social interation. As we shall see later (Chapter 4), some researchers have argued that this latter effect – the undermining of social support – may be as important a cause of the negative effect of high density as the stress itself.

The unavoidable and increased frequency of interaction

This can follow from the previous consequence of density, the close proximity of others, but can also arise independently. Dormitory designs identical in terms of the immediate proximity of others can still differ in the extent to which they oblige social interaction. Designs which lead to greater numbers of unwanted interactions and an inability to control who, when and where residents will meet each other lead to cognitive and social strain, and subsequently to a generalized hostility to others. Again, the withdrawal from, and hostility towards, other residents may also indirectly lead to the undermining of the positive experiences of being with others as well as being directly negative in itself (Chapter 4).

A few further general comments are appropriate. The impact of each of these four components can be greatly attenuated by the availability of escape and exaggerated by its absence. This again applies especially to the prison setting, but can also be seen elsewhere, as evidenced by Magaziner's data, or by Mitchell's finding that crowding only had an effect on people living above the sixth floor (where escape was more difficult). It should also be mentioned that there is very little evidence of individual adaptation to higher densities. In fact, in both prison and dormitory studies, the evidence suggests that people actually become *less* tolerant to crowding over time, and its adverse effects become stronger (MacKenzie and Goodstein, 1986; Baum and Paulus, 1987)[4]. Against this, however, is the observation that in general the effects of crowding are still quite mild, certainly in comparison to those seen in animals. It would seem that humans have social and cultural mechanisms for dealing with crowding, and this is supported further by the patchy evidence of racial differences in coping with density (Gillis, Richard and Hagan, 1986). Broadly speaking, Asians appear to have a greater tolerance of high density than those of Anglo-Saxon origin, with Southern Europeans lying somewhere in between. These differences echo cultural norms on personal space (Altman and Chemers, 1980).

A final point is simply to contest the common notion in the crowding literature that it is the perception of a situation as crowded that leads to its being experienced as stressful (for example, Fisher, *et al.*, 1984). A more plausible model is that the stress comes first, not second. Each of the components described above could be experienced as stressful, but it is only when negative arousal, lack of control and so on, is specifically attributed to the unwanted presence of others that it becomes experienced as crowding.

In summary, variations in density do have an impact on mental health. The concept of density can be pulled into its salient components and its impacts can be understood in terms of cognitive and social overload, control, spoiling and other general psychological processes. As we have seen, these impacts are mediated by many other variables, but their interactions are both comprehensible and traceable.

Crime, Fear, and the Environment

The literature on crime and the environment provides a parallel to that on mental health and the environment. Indeed sometimes the term *social pathology* is used to embrace them both, especially in the geographic literature (Wedmore and Freeman, 1984). This reflects the long-standing observation that psychiatric and criminological geographies often show very similar patterns. Areas with high concentrations of crime, especially violent crime, also tend to show high concentrations of other forms of social pathology such as delinquency, vagrancy, and large numbers of the psychiatrically impaired. Much of the co-variance between these various measures of pathology must be due to social drift or selection, but some of the co-variance *may* be causal (Levine, Miyake and Lee, 1989). It is also possible that the association reported above between population density and mental ill-health could be mediated the experience of crime and fear. Delinquency and property offences are especially highly correlated to residential density (Levy and Herzog, 1974).

This section will examine the relationship between environmental variables, crime, fear and mental health. As we shall see, the relationship between crime and fear is not straightforward: both crime and fear have environmental determinants, but not necessarily the same ones.

Environmental Criminology

Environmental criminology is the study of how the environmental context may foster or inhibit the occurrence of crime. Due to limitations of space, the following is an abstract of a more extensive literature review (Halpern, 1991) the salient point being that the level and distribution of many forms of crime are strongly influenced by environmental variables.

Robbery and personal attack

Violent and sexual assaults, and personal robbery and theft are crimes that are found particularly disturbing, though fortunately, they are also relatively rare. These crimes are strongly associated with city size, personal robbery, for example, being some 50 times more common in cities with populations greater than 250000 than in those with less than 250000. Within cities, attacks tend to be highly concentrated in the inner city areas (Walmsley, 1988). This concentration appears to be due to the convergence of three factors: the concentration of likely offenders (the less affluent); the concentration of suitable targets; and the absence of capable guardians. Violence at night is heavily associated with drinking, and it is found that most attacks occur on the principal routes that lead from drinking establishments to the late-night public transport facilities (Poyner, 1983).

Burglary

The average probability of a household being burgled in a year is estimated to be about 1 in 20 in the UK, and similar in North America. However, this rate varies enormously depending on neighbourhood and target specific factors. Poor neighbourhoods tend to have high rates of burglary as they attract younger and less ambitious offenders, the vast majority of whom have walked to their target, live locally, and often know their victims personally (Forrester, *et al.*, 1988). Wealthy but accessible areas also have elevated rates though they attract older, more professional offenders. Typical high-risk neighbourhoods also tend to be characterized by: the presence of more major thoroughfares, a larger percentage of commercial and mixed land use, more permeable boundaries, the close proximity of poorer areas, more multi-family units, higher levels of public parking and vacant land and lower levels of social cohesion (Reppetto, 1974; Bevis and Nutter, 1977; Greenberg and Rohe, 1984). In general, high risk areas show a high degree of accessibility and a low degree of homogeneity of land use. It is a controversial issue whether low levels of social cohesion encourage crime or whether low cohesion is just another consequence of the presence of strangers, the latter being the *true* risk factor for crime.

Specific target characteristics implicated in the occurrence of burglary include: the physical isolation of the property (for example, location in the country; less than five other houses in sight; set at a distance from the road in which the house stands), the property's accessibility (for example, located on the nearest major road; adjacent to private open space; access at both sides of the house from front to back), and the property's surveillability (for example, not overlooked at the front by other houses; majority of sides of house not visible from public areas; Forrester, *et al.*, 1988). When combined into a general scale of environmental risk, environmental aspects of the site account for more variance in burglary than any other variable (including occupancy patterns and rateable value, both of which are also important.) Winchester and Jackson (1982) found annual risk rates ranged from 1 in 1845 for the lowest scoring properties of the environmental risk scale to 1 in 5 for the highest scoring, (a multiplier of nearly 400).

Contrary to popular beliefs, apartments are at lower risk than houses (Winchester and Jackson, 1982; Reynolds, 1986). As for houses, accessibility is the most important risk factor (Waller and Okihiro, 1978; Newman and Frank, 1980).

Vandalism

In contrast to burglary, it is public areas that are most often the target of vandalism. Damage is concentrated in the communal and shared parts of housing developments (Wilson, 1978). Vandalism is a popular pastime of many children and teenagers (Gladstone, 1978) and therefore its occurrence is closely related to child densities (Coleman, 1985). The work of Newman (1973, 1980) and Coleman (1985) has shown that vandalism is far more frequent in some building types than others. Levels of vandalism vary with the number of dwellings per entrance, dwellings per block, number of storeys, the presence of multiple access routes and the spatial organization of the design. Newman and Coleman have argued that in general, criminal activity (and especially vandalism) is lowest in designs characterized by *defensible space*: space that is clearly subdivided into hierarchies of increasingly supervisable and private zones such that residents can recognize one another and feel willing and able to regulate the space outside their dwellings.

Newman's defensible space theory can be criticized on a number of points, especially concerning the role of resident intervention in the prevention of crime, and

Coleman's work can be criticized for its lack of statistical sophistication and its failure to control for background variables. However, it remains clear that vandalism is highly concentrated around the public and focal points of developments. This vandalism is of particular concern because it is perceived by many residents as an indicator of more serious crime and disorder. Managerial variables are also implicated in the occurrence of vandalism. It is believed that rapid repairs, resident involvement and the effective maintenance of facilities for children can help to reduce levels of vandalism (Mayhew, *et al.*, 1979; Newman, 1981; Poyner, 1983).

Fear and Other Psychological Consequences of Crime

... widespread anxiety over possible victimization takes a serious toll in the daily lives of many Americans. People are forced to change their usual behaviour. They stay off the streets at night, avoid strangers, curtail social activities, keep firearms, buy watchdogs and may even move to other neighbourhoods ... fear of crime is far out of proportion to the objective probability of being victimized. (Clemente and Kleiman, 1977: 519)

A simple phobic neurosis has three components: first, symptoms of anxiety identical to those of any other anxiety state; second, anxious thoughts usually in anticipation of situations the person may have to encounter; and third, the habit of avoiding situations that provoke fear. [Gelder, Gath and Mayou, 1983: 157]

The main psychological consequence of the occurrence of crime is fear, and many researchers feel that the fear of crime has become as serious a problem as crime itself (Clemente and Kleiman, 1977; Maguire, 1982). The impact of the fear of crime can be seen in several ways. First, as a chronic state of anxiety that compromises lifestyles and acts as a permanent source of concern. A comparison with phobic neurosis is tempting (see above). An examination of the Diagnostic and Statistical Manual (DSM-III-R) criteria for simple phobia reveals that all are met with the possible exception of 'the person recognizes that his or her fear is excessive or unreasonable'. Second, the fear of crime may act as a potent stressor and vulnerability factor for other more general types of disorder. It is chronic, intrusive, and emphasizes a sense of helplessness. White, *et al.*, (1987) in a study of 337 Black and Hispanic women, after controlling for demographic factors, found a broad negative association between perceived crime level and mental health using a variety of established scales (the Hopkins Symptom Check-list, the Zung Depression scale, and the Srole Anomia Scale). They also found a weak interaction with neighbourhood quality, the association being strongest in areas of highest housing quality. As usual with a correlational study of this type, the association between symptoms and perceived crime can only be suggestive, but the authors' finding that the association was strongest with somatization rather than depression lends some credence to the association being the result of more than just respondent bias. Finally, the social withdrawal that commonly occurs as a consequence of fear, as well as being negative in itself, deprives people of *positive* experiences and undermines local supportive networks.

The determinants of fear of crime can be divided into three broad types of factors: the experience of crime itself, both direct and indirect; individual vulnerability factors, such as age and sex; and indirect cues, such as degenerating neighbourhood conditions or *incivilities* (Baumer, 1985; Box, *et al.*, 1988). Crime itself is clearly a major source of the fear of crime. Curiously, however, the fit is far from perfect. A principal reason for this is that people learn about crime from several different routes: direct experience (victimization), informal contact with victims, and through the mass media.

The Psychological Consequences of Direct Victimization

As we have seen the occurrence of crime is not random and is strongly influenced by the environment. If the experience of crime leads to psychological distress, this could lead to elevated levels of distress in high crime areas. Yet surprisingly, many studies have failed to find a relationship between direct victimization and fear. Using data from national samples, Baumer (1985) found no more than a very weak relationship, while Box, *et al.*, (1988) actually found a slightly *negative* relationship between previous victimization and fear. The problem is that across the whole population there is a strong negative association between the probability of victimization and fear – the most common victims are young males, who are generally unafraid; and the most fearful are those least likely to be victims, such as older women. Furthermore, those who are most likely to become victims are also those least likely to show its effects. For example, women may be far more badly affected by an attack than men, but then on the other hand, women are also far less likely to experience an attack (perhaps due to rational avoidance). This means that the strength and direction of the association is very sensitive to the details of the controls applied.

Skogan and Maxfield (1981), and Tyler (1980) reported a more solid positive association between fear and victimization, but only after very careful controls had been applied. They point out that one must control not only for the characteristics of victims, but also for the characteristics of the offence, and for the form of the question. Some crimes, generally the rarest, are far more fear provoking than others. Unfortunately, most studies do not have data sufficiently detailed to be able to account for this, and this may explain the instability of the victimization–fear association in the literature.

Fear is not the only consequence of victimization. Maguire (1982) interviewed 322 burglary victims (in England), most of whom were seen between 4 and 10 weeks after the event. (Burglary is by far the most common of the 'serious crimes'.) Victims were asked to recall their initial feelings and the effect upon their lives in the intervening period. The most common initial reaction in men was anger (41 per cent), while women were more likely report shock or some form of emotional distress (49 per cent). To assess the longer-term effects of the burglary, a panel of 10 people from a variety of backgrounds were asked to rate the seriousness of the after-effects for each victim on the basis of their transcribed accounts. This showed that 35 per cent (114) of the sample suffered from *serious* or *fairly serious* lasting effects, and a further 31 per cent (100) suffered from *moderate* effects. The analysis also confirmed that it was women who were most likely to be worst affected – 34 of the 43 people described as having serious lasting effects were women. Interestingly, a disproportionate number of these were separated, widowed, or divorced. The description of those most affected is highly reminiscent of those who have been found to be vulnerable in the life events literature and is suggestive of a similar mechanism.[5]

It is notable that when asked, 'What was the worst thing about the burglary?' only 25 per cent of the victims selected loss of property. Instead, 60 per cent selected either intrusion on their privacy or general emotional upset as the worst element. Even those who said that the loss had been the worst thing were generally more concerned about sentimental than monetary value. The financial impact of burglary was of far less importance to victims than the emotional impact.

> I shall never forget it because my privacy has been invaded. I have worked hard all my life and had my nose to the grindstone ever since and this happens. Now we can't live in peace. I have a feeling of 'mental rape'. I feel a dislocation and disruption of private concerns. I have destroyed everything they touched.
>
> (Interview from Maguire (1982)

Similar findings have been reported elsewhere, though in less detail. A short analysis by an early Victim Support Scheme of their first 315 cases (Bristol VSS, 1975) suggested that about a third of all victims 'were upset to a degree which called for some help in restoring normal coping ability', and that 7 per cent had suffered 'severe and long-lasting impact, affecting their lifestyle'.[6] Maguire observed that the strength of victims' reactions had more to do with their image of the crime than the actuality. This applies very generally. Fear of crime is far more widespread than the occurrence of crime and it remains a remarkable fact that little of the variance in fear can be accounted for by direct victimization.

The Psychological Consequences of the Indirect Experience of Crime

Informal vicarious experience

Unlike the evidence on the impact of direct victimization on fear, the evidence on the impact of vicarious experience on fear is extremely clear. The more people hear about crime from their friends and neighbours, the more fearful they become (Tyler, 1980; Skogan and Maxfield, 1981; Taylor and Hale, 1986). Beyond this, the critical factor seems to be the identification with the victim. It is hearing about crimes that occurred within the locality that leads to fear (Box, *et al.*, 1988), and the more similar the victim is perceived to be, the greater the impact (Skogan and Maxfield, 1981).

As it is the crimes that are the most violent (and unusual) that are most talked about and that reach the largest number of ears, gossip therefore acts as a strong amplifier of the events that are the most fear inspiring. The paradoxical consequence of this potency is that those communities with the greatest social cohesiveness, (a possible factor in the reduction of crime), are also those that are most efficient at the spreading of fear. This almost certainly accounts for the initially surprising finding that elderly residents living in age-segregated accommodation actually report more fear than those living in unsegregated accommodation (Bastlin Normoyle and Foley, 1988).

Mass media

Although it is a widespread belief that the media presentation of crime is a significant source of fear, this has yet to be verified. Skogan and Maxfield (1981) attempted to test this hypothesis but were unable to find any association between different areas' media coverage of crime and fear. However, as media coverage varied very little between one area and another, one cannot conclude that it had no impact. All one can say is that it had no *differential* impact on fear. As the universal tendency of the media was to report the most fear inspiring crimes, the original hypothesis remains very plausible.

Against this hypothesis, work by Tyler (1980) suggests that individuals may separate judgments of wider crime problems from judgments of their own vulnerability. He found that while the mass media strongly influenced general estimates of the baseline crime rate, it had no influence on the sense of personal vulnerability. He suggested that individuals maintained two fairly separate levels of judgment – the general, which is strongly influenced by indirect experiences, and the personal, which is more strongly influenced by immediate experience. This hypothesis would account for why public campaigns concerning crime and fear appear to have so little impact on personal attitudes and behaviour.

Individual Vulnerability Factors

Individual vulnerability in relation to fear of crime is comparable to sensitivity in relation to other environmental stressors. Criminologists studying fear tend to divide vulnerability into two components: physical, which refers to the potential victim's perceived powerlessness to resist, and social, which refers to the extent to which the potential victim is exposed to risk (Skogan and Maxfield, 1981; Baumer, 1985). It is interesting to compare the vulnerability factors to the risk factors for mental ill-health.

Individual physical vulnerability

Of all vulnerability factors, the importance of gender has been the most consistently demonstrated (Clemente and Kleiman, 1977; Box, *et al.*, 1988; Lagrange and Ferrard, 1989). All reported studies have indicated that women experience more fear than men. Clearly, the fear of rape looms large in this discrepancy, though some have suggested that part of the difference is due to the reluctance of males to admit to their fear. The latter interpretation is weakened by the finding that more detailed questions also fail to remove the difference, and by the simple behavioural observation that men are much less likely to restrict their activity because of perceived crime. This is reflected in cognitive maps of fear; women are afraid of areas they know to be dangerous, while men are afraid of areas they don't know.

Age is another consistently reported risk factor, though recent work suggests that its importance may have been overstated in early work. The elderly, especially the over-sixties, are more fearful than younger persons, even when all other factors are held constant. This effect shows a strong (negative) interaction with gender. As people get older, the gender gap closes; men's fear starts to approach that of women. It would seem that as men age they feel increasingly vulnerable even though their *objective* risk actually falls. However, the elevated fear of the elderly is context dependent. Although the elderly are more fearful than younger people of walking alone at night, they report no greater fear than the young if the question refers to, for example, being in your own home at night (Jeffords, 1983). Hence there is some evidence that the size of the age differentials in fear have been inflated by the use of vague, suggestive questions in crime surveys such as: 'How safe would you feel walking alone at night?' When more specific questions are used, age differences become much smaller, though gender differences are unaffected (Lagrange and Ferraro, 1989).

Both gender and age show interactions with social vulnerability factors or exposures to risk. In high risk areas, the influence of gender and age are greatly attenuated as all groups show high levels of fear (Maxfield, 1984; Baumer, 1985). The attenuation is less for gender than for age: this may again be due to the special fear of rape, the occurrence of which does sharply increase in high-risk areas.

Social vulnerability

The most important social vulnerability factor, or non-demographic risk factor, is city size. The residents of large towns and cities are considerably more fearful than those of smaller towns. This effect persists after other individual factors are controlled for (Clemente and Kleiman, 1977; Baumer, 1985; Box, *et al.*, 1988). Income has also been reported as having some independent effect on fear, poorer individuals being more fearful (Clemente and Kleiman, 1977; Baumer, 1985). Race is more controversial. Though its raw association with fear is quite strong, it has little independent effect once income and area of residence have been accounted for (Clemente and Kleiman, 1977; Box, *et al.*, 1988). Belonging to an ethnic minority is heavily compounded with low income and inner city living, and it is not particularly informative to ask which one is primary.

The social vulnerability factors broadly reflect the occurrence of crime, though this is not true of the individual physical vulnerability factors. It is noteworthy that overall, the vulnerability factors for the fear of crime identified by criminologists bear a closer resemblance to the risk factors for sensitivity in general than they do to the risk factors for crime. Whether it is the publicity that surrounds crime or the apparent intentionality of the act, there is something about crime, and especially violent crime, that makes many people very afraid.

Incivilities

Physical incivilities refer to the signs of physical deterioration of an area – vacant property, unmaintained housing stock, graffiti and so on. Social incivilities refer to the unwanted presence of teenage gangs, vagrants, and the visible signs of criminal activity. Surveys on both sides of the Atlantic have shown that perceived levels of both social and physical incivilities are strongly correlated with the fear of crime (Lewis and Maxfield, 1980; Skogan and Maxfield, 1981; Maxfield; 1984; Box, *et al.*, 1988). The association remains after other relevant factors have been controlled for. Parallel positive associations are found in the literature between satisfaction with the residential environment – the perception of *civility* – and resident perceptions of

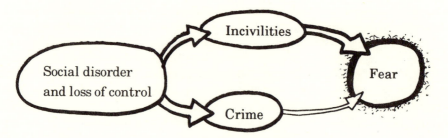

Figure 3.7: *The postulated relationship between incivilities and fear*

safety (Weidemann and Anderson, 1982; Baba and Austin, 1989).

The implication is that incivilities in an area are taken as indicative of higher crime levels (Taylor, 1987), though some researchers have argued that this is insufficient to account for the strength of the perceived incivility–fear linkage. These researchers argue that importance of incivilities lie in the fact that they come to symbolize not only crime, but the breakdown of the social fabric itself (Hunter, 1978; Figure 3.7).

An interaction reported by Box, *et al.*, (1988) is of interest here. It will be recalled that the experience of direct victimization, even after controlling for other factors, did not appear to have a particularly strong or reliable impact on fear, and this surprising result has attracted much attention. Box, *et al.*, found that the impact of victimization depended on the level of incivilities in the area. Victims report *lower* fear than non-victims in areas of low incivilities, but report *greater* fear than non-victims in areas of high incivilities. It seems that in areas of perceived safety (low incivilities) some kind of neutralization process occurs, but that in areas of high incivilities, this neutralization process is unable to proceed. The incivilities appear to act as a reminder or symbol of potential danger.

The preceding results are based upon *perceived* incivility and could still plausibly be attributed to respondent bias (the reporting of incivilities could be seen as a symptom rather than cause of fear). Until recently, very few researchers had attempted to use objective, independent measures of incivility. Though it is true that ecological studies had linked the presence of poor housing, changing land use, and rapid turnover to crime (Taylor, 1987), the equivalent links had not really been tested for fear. An exception was a study by Taylor, Shumaker and Gottfredson (1985). Street blocks were coded by teams of raters and a reliable measure of social and civil incivility measure was derived. The authors reported that after controlling for socio-economic characteristics, incivilities had a significant impact on fear in moderate income neighbourhoods, but not in high or low income neighbourhoods. However, it can be argued that by controlling for socio-economic characteristics in this study, the researchers inappropriately attenuated the effects of the incivilities themselves – a 'partialling fallacy'.[7] Nonetheless, the result appears to relate to those of a study by Maxfield (1984). Maxfield compared the impact of various risk factors for fear in three contrasting neighbourhoods of San Francisco: Visitacion Valley, Mission, and Sunset. The first, Visitacion Valley, was a stable but high crime area. The second, Mission, was a poor area with high turnover, much disrupted by the recent building of a rapid transit system, but it suffered an objectively low crime rate. The last, Sunset, was a wealthy and stable area with low crime. The descriptive data about the neighbourhood was gathered separately from the questionnaires on fear. Maxfield found that while broadly speaking, the same factors were related to fear in the different areas, their relative importance varied. Hence, fear was most closely associated with the perception of incivilities in Mission, the high turnover (and high objective incivility) but low crime area. In contrast, for Visitacion Valley residents the direct perception of crime problems was more important and incivilities less so. The relative importance of incivilities in Sunset was also low.

Maxfield's results show that the fearful attitudes of individuals living in different areas can, to some extent, be rooted in different sources. His comment that 'incivility has its greatest impact on fear in the area where it is most often perceived to be a problem' (p. 247) may seem rather obvious in retrospect, but it does emphasize how the relationship between objective incivilities and fear may depend on the context. The impact of incivilities will be most marked in areas of potential transition and in moderate income areas that had previously been marked by relative stability. It is in such areas that incivilities will cause most concern as they indicate a decline in the areas, even though these areas may not be the ones with highest crime rates or even the highest incivilities.

Recently, Perkins, Meeks and Taylor, (1992) conducted a detailed study of the relationship between objective incivilities, perceived incivilities and perceived crime. Detailed objective measures of various incivilities were gathered for 50 Baltimore neighbourhoods, and 412 residents were interviewed about their perceptions of their environments. They found that the objective level of incivilities in an area were strongly related to residents' perceptions of crime. Of the objective incivilities, vandalism was the strongest predictor of perceived crime levels (20 per cent of variance in perceived crime was accounted for by this), and this association was found, even having controlled for respondents' education, race, homeownership and block-size. Similarly, perceived crime was associated with fewer plantings (maintained gardens) and more bars on windows. Interestingly, in many instances the objective measures of incivilities were better predictors of perceived crime than the residents' own perceptions of incivilities. This result suggests that incivilities may mediate residents' perceptions of crime in an unconscious manner. In sum, although the study is not perfect – ideally the objective level of crime would also have been controlled for – it offers very strong support for the Skogan, Maxfield, *et al.*, hypothesis that the level of incivilities in an area mediate residents' perceptions and fear of crime.

The causal linking of incivilities to fear is reinforced by the complementary linking of civilities to the perception of safety. It is noteworthy that in the Perkins, *et al.*, study, the level and quality of plantings (a measure of civility) also had an independent effect on residents' perceptions of crime. Other studies have shown that subjects' ratings of the perceived safety of urban scenes (as shown in photographs) are strongly predicted by their rated level of maintenance and design (Shaffer and Anderson, 1983). Furthermore, such ratings have been shown to correlate well with independently gathered reports of the residents' own perceived safety (Craik and Appleyard, 1980).

Finally, there is evidence demonstrating that an area's level of incivilities is directly associated with the level of depression among its residents. Birtchnell, Masters and Deahl, (1988) found a strong association between an estate's Design Disadvantage Score, a measure developed from the work of Coleman (1985) on vandalism, and depression. This result is consistent with the hypothesis that incivilities can lead to psychopathology as well as fear, though by itself, of course, this association does not demonstrate causality. For this we will need more detailed studies which include careful controls for the effects of selection and detailed measures of the postulated mediating variables.

In summary then, incivilities are not so much a source of concern in themselves, but are emblematic of residents' worst fears. The potency of incivilities to affect residents' perceptions of an area depend not only on their perceived relationship to crime (higher incivilities indicating higher crime) but also because they play upon residents' fears of more general degeneration. It seems likely that the precise impact of (objective) incivilities depend also on the history of the area and the recency of the incivilities' occurrence. However, we shall have to wait for more extensive longitudinal studies before this can be known with greater certainty.

Other Neighbourhood Characteristics Associated with Fear

As already mentioned, levels of both fear and crime are significantly higher in larger than smaller cities (see above). Within cities, wide variation is found in levels of fear. A number of theories have been advanced to account for what makes the residents of one neighbourhood feel safe while those of another feel afraid.

Jacobs (1961) advanced the hypothesis that safety was gained from the *eyes on the street* and therefore suggested that the trend towards increasingly homogeneous land use, especially the segregation of the residential from the commercial, was going to lead to more rather than less fear. However, it may be recalled that one of the risk factors for crime identified by Greenberg and Rohe (1984) is the accessibility and permeability of an area. The principal reason for this is that it brings larger numbers of potential offenders to an area. This finding appears to contradict Jacobs' influential hypothesis. The competing hypotheses concerning fear were tested in an elegant study by Hunter and Baumer (1982). Based on a final sample of over 14000 respondents, they found that, in general, the perception of increased pedestrian traffic in residential neighbourhoods led to increased fear. However, they found a strong interaction with social integration: for those who were socially integrated, the volume of pedestrian traffic had no effect on fear, but for those who were not integrated, a very strong relationship was found. (Social integration was measured by agreement with the statement, 'feel part of the neighbourhood' and the ability to recognize other neighbours.) A similar pattern was found for stability, as measured by length of residence and home ownership. Increased traffic flow was strongly associated with increased fear in areas of low stability, but the association collapsed where stability was high.

This conditional relationship suggests that the fear of crime in residential areas is, to a large extent, the fear of strangers. Under no conditions was it found that increasing pedestrian traffic reduced fear. The authors suggest that the combined effect of increased traffic and low integration leads to fear through three links: (1) the presence of more *strangers*, (2) the undermining of the *assistance role* due to the low level of familiarity, and (3) the increasing *strangeness* of the street. Integration mitigates the first link by enabling residents to recognize more people, thereby reducing the effective number of strangers. Evidence for the second link can be derived from work within social psychology, including that on diffusion of responsibility (Darley and Latané, 1968). Contrary to Jacobs' supposition, experimental work (and real-life cases, for example, the murder of Kitty Genovese in which none of the many witnesses intervened) show how helping behaviour tends to *fall* as the number of observers rises (Myers, 1990). The third link refers to the increased unpredictability that the presence of so many others brings. It could be argued that this prevents the establishment of a *behavioural setting* (Wicker, 1979), a shared consensus of how one should behave.

Further evidence for the *fear of strangers* hypothesis can be derived from data presented by Fowler (1987). This study examined a large number of variables, some of which were objectively derived measures of neighbourhood characteristics. The variable of particular interest here is the area's concentration of use, a measure of the number of people using an area for residence, work, shopping or recreation.

The association between concentration of use and fear was found to be very strong (r=.47). Concentration of use was also associated with crime (r=.26), but the association with fear was substantially stronger. Its negative association with friendship and acquaintance suggests that these may at least partly mediate its impact on fear; greater concentration of use reduces the possibility of getting to know fellow residents, and this results in the perception of more strangers. Hopefully, Fowler will publish further analyses of this data. It could prove extremely illuminating to examine the interactions within it.

A final variable that has been reported as influencing fear of crime in residential settings is building size. Newman and Frank (1982) interviewed residents of 63

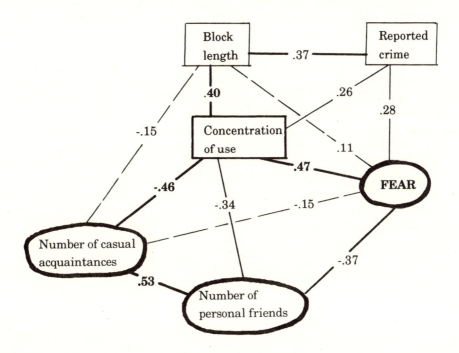

Figure 3.8: *The relationship between concentration of use and fear of crime*
Source: Data from Fowler, 1987

housing projects in order to test defensible space theory and examine the effect of building size. Although they found no final effect of building size on crime *per se*, they did find that it had a strong effect on fear. The larger the building, the greater the level of fear. Building size was also associated with a lower use of external space, a lower level of social interaction, less reported control over space outside the dwelling, and greater problems with building management. These results give the strong impression that defensible space theory may tell us more about the occurrence of fear than it does about crime.[8]

The effect of building size on fear is closely related to that of concentration of use or increased pedestrian flow. The sharing of communal areas and entrances with large numbers of others increases the proportion of strangers, lowers the sense of control, and undermines the development of a positive social atmosphere.

The preceding results give a fairly clear picture of what determines residents' levels of fear in their own neighbourhoods; they do not appear to support Jane Jacobs' famous *eyes on the street* hypothesis. However, before leaving this section, we should also consider the issue of fear as seen from the *stranger's* point of view. Although the presence of larger numbers of strangers (people from outside the neighbourhood) might make residents feel less at ease, the presence of other people might make these *strangers* themselves feel more safe. It may be helpful to think of this in terms of your own experience. If you think of your home environment and what it would be like with many more strangers present, you would probably think of this as being less safe. However, if you think of going to an unfamiliar part of town or to a public area such as a park, you would probably feel safer if there were more people around. This distinction or gestalt between *seeing* the stranger and *being* the stranger may explain the apparent tension between the view expressed by Jacobs, that eyes on the street should make people feel safer, and the findings of Hunter and Baumer that the presence of strangers makes residents more fearful. If instead of asking people about their level of fear in their own neighbourhood, as in the Hunter and Baumer study, we ask them about their level of fear when visiting other areas, then a somewhat different pattern of results emerge. Vrit and Winkel (1991) asked people to identify which areas of their city they considered unsafe (n=854). They found that the areas people perceived as unsafe tended to be quiet, deserted and poorly lit. Areas that afforded a poor overview were also considered unsafe. The perceived safety of areas bore only a very weak relationship with the objective crime levels of the areas. Hence from the point of view of non-residents or strangers, the absence of pedestrian traffic makes people feel less safe.

Fortunately, there are certain things that we can do that make both strangers and residents feel more safe. The best documented of these is to improve levels of lighting. Although improved lighting may not necessarily reduce the occurance of crime, there is little doubt that better lighting reduces levels of fear. In a second study, Vrit and Winkel (1991) demonstrated that by increasing the level of lighting in an area of high fear of crime, passersby felt significantly more safe (compared to passersby surveyed before the improvement), perceived the likelihood of being molested as being lower, and perceived the likely length of time before someone would come to help them if attacked to be lower. Other aspects of the environment that can make both visitors and residents feel safer include being able to see sources of light, feeling that help would be on hand in the event of trouble, and perceiving the environment as generally well kept and maintained. Nonetheless, it is important to realize that some factors that make residents feel safe may have the opposite effect on passersby, and this potential tension must be negotiated. Putting heads on the gates might make you feel safer if you are the resident but is unlikely to do so if you are the visitor.

Summary

Both crime and fear are determined to a very significant extent by environmental variables, though not necessarily by the same ones. Fear of crime has shown itself to be more than simply the fear of crime *per se*, and the fear of crime and crime itself are often only modestly associated.

Taylor and Hale (1986) contrasted three different models of fear of crime. They concluded that none of the models could be rejected. An attempt to summarize the multiple links between environmental factors, crime, and fear is made below. Crime, when experienced directly, impacts mental health as an unpleasant experience and acts very much as any other negative life event. Fear, on the other hand, can be

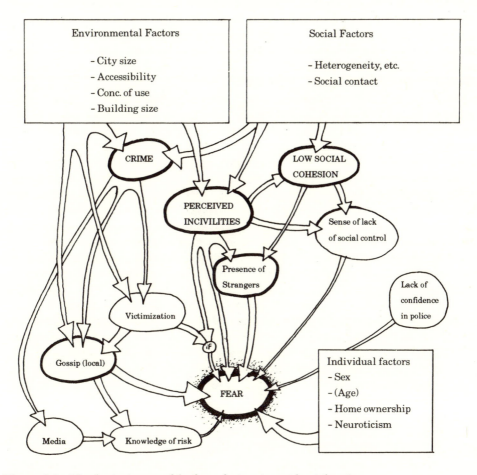

Figure 3.9: *The determinants of the fear of crime in residential settings*

thought of not only as a chronic stressor but also as bordering on psychopathology in itself. The principal determinants of fear are the personal and the vicarious experience of crime, social and physical cues from the residential context, and individual vulnerability factors like age, sex and personal exposure. For some low-risk, high-fear groups in the population, the extent of their fear may border on the phobic, and it is more social than clinical judgment that prevents us from labelling it as such. The social withdrawal that typically results from fear can also be expected to have a negative impact on mental health, especially if it cuts off the individual from potential sources of support.

Summary and Refinements to the Stress Model

Let us now attempt a brief summary of the literatures reviewed in this and the previous chapters. A general model of stress was presented. It was suggested that the impact of different aspects of the environment can be seen as unified by their sharing of a common psycho-physiological process – the stress reaction. Environmental presses requires the person or organism to adapt, and this adaptation or coping is mediated and motivated by a psychological and physiological state of arousal. If this state becomes chronic or severe due to chronic exposure and/or failure to successfully adapt, both mental and physical health tend to suffer.

The evidence for the impact of a series of environmental stressors on mental health has been examined. For pollution, the literature was limited but consistent with a weak causal relationship with poorer mental health. Toxicological studies showed pollutants to be powerful irritants, and studies of psychiatric admission rates revealed small but consistent positive associations with daily pollutant levels. Similar, but more fragmentary evidence was found for the influence of climatic variables on mental health. The evidence on noise was surprising in that although it showed noise to be a very strong source of annoyance, it showed that noise *per se* had only a very limited effect on mental health. When associations were found between noise and mental ill-health, these could largely be explained by problems associated with the noise source rather than by the noise *per se*. The evidence on density and crowding showed some adverse effects on mental health, but only under certain, quite narrow, conditions. This literature emphasized the social nature of crowding; the amount of physical space was of less importance than the number of persons, and social variables such as group orientation were found to be extremely important. Finally, the phenomena of fear of crime was examined. It was argued that criminal victimization acted on mental health much like any other negative life event, but that victimization was not enough to account for the enormous prevalence of fear, a fear that borders on the phobic. Both crime and fear were found to have strong environmental determinants, though not necessarily the same ones.

It would seem that, despite the implications of the stress model, stressors are not all equivalent in their impacts. Noise is a particularly interesting example. The evidence confirms it to be a classic environmental stressor. It leads to both heightened physiological arousal and a negative internal state (irritability, annoyance, and the desire to avoid it), but the evidence suggested that noise-induced annoyance rarely

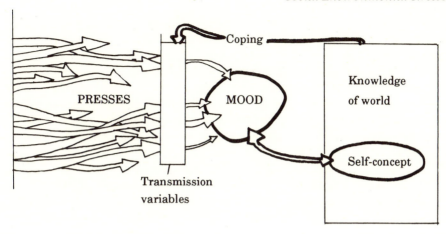

Figure 3.10: *A stylized model of the stressed individual*

led to actual psychopathology. Yet remarkably, there is evidence suggesting negative mental health impacts from obscure stressors such as low level pollutants and climatic change. Are these contrasting findings the artefacts of weak methodology or is there a plausible explanation? To help answer this, let us again consider the relationship between mood and mental health. A bad mood or negative internal state is not enough to merit the label of mental illness or psychopathology (see Chapter 1). A better suggestion would be that we only describe an individual as showing mental illness at the point at which his or her internal state or action acts to fruitlessly maintain (or even exaggerate) a negative internal state. A typical example of this would be where the failure of an expected method of coping leads to a generalized sense of helplessness or to a negative attribution of the self. The psychopathological lies in maladaptive *processes* rather than in the specifics of a given state.

With this distinction made, the failure of an environmental stressor such as noise to lead to any obvious psychopathology becomes more comprehensible. As it stands, the stress model fails to consider the relevance of the individual's own insights into aetiology or causes. All the environmental stressors studied can lead to annoyance, irritation and a negative internal state or mood. However, a key difference between the stressors is the ease with which they can be identified, and the ease with which the internal state can be causally linked to their occurrence. In the case of noise, the aetiology of the irritation can be described as transparent. It is obvious to the subject that the source of his or her annoyance is the loud noise outside or the frequent passing of aeroplanes above. This understanding of causality shapes the subjective experience of the internal state and guides the individual's subsequent attempts at coping.

A comparison can be made to the importance of cognitive interpretation in the experience of emotion. As demonstrated in the classic experiment by Schachter and Singer (1962), the subjective experience of a state of arousal depends on the individual's interpretation of its cause. Subjects were injected with adrenalin under the cover story that it was a vitamin compound. Some were accurately told of its effects (sympathetic nervous system arousal), while others were either not told or were misinformed (told to expect parasympathetic symptoms). They were then left in a waiting room with another 'subject' who was actually a confederate of the experimenter. The confederate would engage in euphoric or angry behaviour, depending on the condition. It was found that uninformed subjects showed and reported a high degree of corresponding euphoria or anger (depending on the behaviour of the confederate), while informed subjects did not.

Schachter's work built upon the earlier insights of Lange and others (Lange and James, 1922; Marañon, 1924) emphasizing the convergent importance of both physiological arousal and cognitive evaluation. Subjects label an internal state according to their understanding of its cause and this understanding is derived from the context and available knowledge. Thus emotional experience is conditional on arousal but is also critically structured by the process of cognitive appraisal.[9]

There is every reason to believe that similar processes operate to structure the experience of stress. The individual's attribution of cause may shape both the subjective experience of stress and the response to it. This is speculatively summarized below.

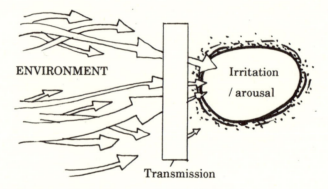

Figure 3.11: *Environmentally induced arousal*

Certain aspects of the environment, via the immediate interpretation of perception, lead to a state of arousal or irritation. The stress model is good at highlighting the importance of transmission variables at this level, but fails to recognize the equal importance of similar psychological slippage in the processes that follow it.

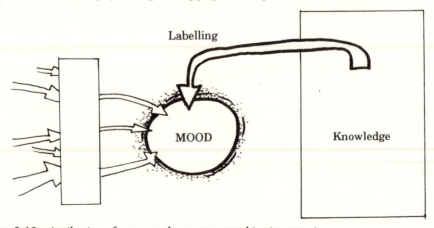

Figure 3.12: *Attribution of cause and consequent subjective experience*

The internal state or disequilibrium is then labelled and attributed a cause. This attribution will be based upon the individual's knowledge of the context and his or her understanding of the likely cause. The structuring of this subjective experience can be thought of as closely analogous to that of emotion in general. Hence, in the case of noise, the subject's internal state will easily be linked to its cause, and will be subjectively experienced as a highly specific, noise-induced annoyance. For other stressors, this causal link may be less obvious and the internal state incorrectly attributed to some spurious internal or external cause. This could lead both to the experience of an overly generalized and strongly negative mood (for example, anxiety or *nerves*), and to the attempted application of inappropriate coping responses. It is notable that studies conducted since the Schachter and Singer experiment have demonstrated that subjects show a negative bias in the process of identifying unexplained internal states; in other words, subjects are much more likely to experience unexplained arousal as a negative rather than a positive emotion (Maslach, 1979). If the individual has misunderstood the source of his or her negative mood, then the coping mechanisms applied are very likely to fail. This locks the individual into a potentially vicious circle of intensified action, failure and frustration in the short-term, and a negative reflection on self, demoralization and despair in the longer term.

To take the example of noise again, we can see that the transparence of the aetiology means that the subject is very unlikely to apply inappropriate methods of coping, and thereby is unlikely to experience the psychological fallout of subsequent failure. (This may not be true, of course, if the source of the noise is unpredictable and unresponsive, such as a difficult neighbour.) The effects of pollution, on the other hand, might be expected to be potentially quite serious. If a pollutant leads to an

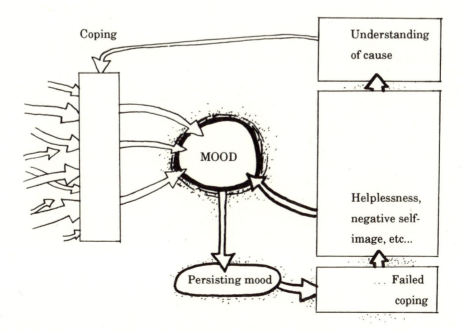

Figure 3.13: *Copng responses based on understanding of aetiology*

irritability the cause of which is not obvious (for example, ozone), not only is there room for error in the labelling of the internal state, but it is likely that the coping mechanisms employed will be inappropriate. The source of pollutant-induced irritation may be incorrectly projected onto other people, work or self. This will fail to deal with the actual source of the irritation and could also generate secondary sources of stress.

This adapted model of the stress reaction is able to account for the broad sweep of findings that have been presented in the previous two chapters. In fact, it would be difficult to account for these findings without such an adaptation to the theory. This model brings with it quite radical implications. It suggests that subjects' understanding of aetiology is of central importance in the subjective experience of stress and the likelihood of subsequent pathology. It would imply that the experience of a factor like crowding, for example, would have its greatest impact where individuals fail to identify its source as being density. The fear of crime is another example – the source of the fear is identified with the occurrence of crime, yet empirical work has shown fear to be only weakly determined by actual patterns of crime. The net result is disproportionate concern, and methods of coping that are often misdirected and ineffective.

The relevance of the model must apply to more than just environmental sources of stress. Consider the controversial example of post-natal depression. Its cause is typically attributed to hormonal imbalance, but this may not always be accurate, if at all. If instead its roots lie in an unexpected failure of support or a difficult change in role, then an incorrect attribution of cause could lead to the fruitless application of inappropriate coping and the type of vicious cycle as described above. (This argument would apply equally if the aetiology and misunderstanding were reversed.) It is interesting to note that in a recent longitudinal study by Downey, Silver and Wortman, (1990) it was found that among parents trying to come to terms with the sudden death of their child from unknown causes (the Sudden Infant Death Syndrome defined as the unexpected death of a child where no adequate cause of death can be identified) those parents who became most concerned with trying to attribute a cause of death were the ones who showed poorest subsequent adjustment and the highest level of distress. When attributional and coping mechanisms are employed where causation is uncertain or opaque to the subject, these mechanisms are likely to be maladaptive and to fail.

The superficial implication of this theory is that even if certain aspects of the environment lead to mental ill-health, this adverse effect could be offset simply by informing those affected about the precise source of their irritation. This would help by assisting the individuals concerned to apply the most appropriate and adaptive methods of coping. However, if the source of the irritation still remained or if no effective coping strategy was available other than removing the source of the irritation, then the desire to remove the source would remain. An accurate understanding of a stressor's aetiological relevance should reduce the extent of its pathological impact, but it may also simultaneously focus, not eliminate, its subjective undesirability and the determination to eliminate it.

Notes

1   It has been suggested, for example, that part of the reason for the behavioural sink in Calhoun's study was the use of solid food pellets that forced animals to remain in the central chamber while eating. It has also been suggested that the effects were more to do with group size than density *per se*.

2   There is some evidence of this from prison research: rooms of four lead to less control-related problems and less isolates (Baum and Paulus, 1987)

3   A similar ameliorating effect of partitions has been reported in student accommodation (Baum and Davis, 1980; see Chapter 4).

4   Cf. similar findings with dormitory noise (Weinstein, 1978)

5   Brown and Harris (1978), in their classic study on depression, noted that in the event of a major life event, those most likely to develop depression were those without a supportive confiding relationship. They also noted that part of the reason for the excess rates of depression in the working class women in their sample was due to the increased number of negative life events they had experienced; the larger number of burglaries that occur in poorer areas are presumably an example of such negative events.

6   [97 per cent of cases dealt with were burglary or theft.]

7   Taylor has been criticized for this error elsewhere (for example, in Taylor and Hale, 1986).

8   A paper by Bastin Normoyle and Foley (1988) failed to replicate this result for elderly populations, finding that for elderly tenants, increased building size (height) was *negatively* associated with fear. However, this result can be accommodated within the detailed predictions made by Newman in his earlier work (1981), where he argued that the elderly were a special case and well suited to high-rise living. (They have no children, high occupancy rates, and can organize to monitor the entry of strangers.)

9   Similarly, Rickels and Downing (1967) found that anxious patients, when given placebos that they were told were tranquilizers, actually experienced their symptoms as being worse. Storms and Nisbett (1970) reported a similar negative placebo effect for insomnia, but this result has proved difficult to replicate (Bootzin *et al.*, 1976).

Appendix

Table B.1: *Area population density*

		N
1	Under 0.25 persons per acre	240
2	0.25–0.624 persons per acre	558
3	0.625–under 10 persons per acre	1995
4	10 or more persons per acre	1143
5	Conurbations	2081
	Missing	1523
	Total	7540

Table B.2: *Household size (number of persons per household)*

		N	
1	One	661	
2	Two	1860	
3	Three	1371	
4	Four	1219	
5	Five	536	
6	Six	225	
7	Seven	94	
8	Eight	28	[Six or more 370]
9	Nine	13	
10	Ten or more	10	
	Missing	1523	
	Total	7540	

Chapter 4

Social Support and the Planned Environment

Introduction

This chapter focuses on how the social and physical characteristics of an area, building or space can influence an individual's social networks, the support they receive from others, and thereby their mental health.

First of all, an overview is presented of the concept of social support and its relationship to social networks and mental health. An examination is then made of the relationship between the social and physical characteristics of an area and the local patterns of neighbouring and support. Examples are presented of environments that appear to foster supportive relations and of environments that appear to inhibit supportive relations. Finally, conclusions are drawn and an attempt is made to define the *ideal neighbourhood*.

Social Networks, Social Support and Mental Illness

The term *social network* refers to the various persons with whom an individual maintains significant relationships including relatives, friends, fellow workers and neighbours. The social network is a topological description of the individual's social relationships and does not refer to the quality or supportiveness of those relationships. *Social support*, on the other hand, refers specifically to the quality of the relationships – the advice, encouragement, and assistance of all kinds that the social network provides the individual.

An extensive literature has developed over the last 15–20 years about the relationship between social support and mental illness. Brownell and Shumaker (1984) noted that some 450 studies were published in psychology alone in the two years after Social Support Networks was entered as an index term in *Psychological Abstracts*. There is widespread agreement that supportive social relationships are strongly associated with persons of better mental health, though the interpretation of this association remains controversial (Cohen and Wills, 1985).

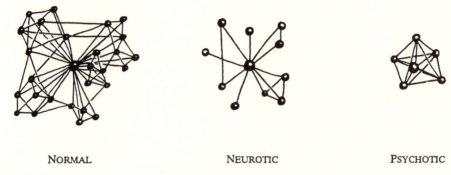

NORMAL   NEUROTIC   PSYCHOTIC

Figure 4.1: *The social networks of persons without disorder, and those suffering neurosis and psychosis*

It was noted some time ago that the mentally ill had social networks different to those of the general population. The social network of the average person was found to be of 25 to 40 people, 6 to 10 of whom were known particularly well, and the network was of moderate *density*. Density here refers to the level of interconnectedness of the network; in a normal network approximately 20 per cent of possible linkages exist (the persons know each other), typically forming the network into several clusters of six to seven people. It was found that persons suffering from neurosis, on the other hand, tended to have smaller social networks, normally of around 10 to 15 people, and networks of much lower density (interconnectedness). Persons suffering from psychosis were found to have very small and extremely dense social networks, normally of around four to five people, most of whom were kin (Mueller, 1980).

Clearly, a causal ambiguity existed concerning this data; was the form of the social network the cause or the result of the mental illness? Did persons suffering from neurosis have smaller, lower density networks than those not suffering because the impoverished social network had been the cause of their mental problems, or had the mental problems been the cause of the impoverished social network?

Later work demonstrating the effectiveness of experimental support interventions (for example, Levy, 1983) combined with careful longitudinal studies (for example, Holahan and Moos, 1981) strongly suggest that social support does protect individuals at risk, though undoubtedly, those suffering from mental illness may also undermine their existing social support leading to a vicious circle:

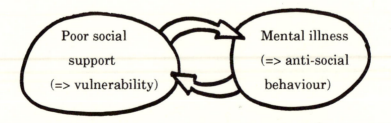

Poor social support (=> vulnerability)   Mental illness (=> anti-social behaviour)

Figure 4.2: *The relationship between social support and mental illness*

The concept of social support has attracted a great deal of attention because it seems to offer the possibility of prevention – if ways can be found to facilitate it (Greenblatt, Becerra and Serafetinides, 1982). It has been influential in the thinking that lies behind rehabilitation programs and half-way houses, of milieu therapy, and indeed behind *community medicine* (Greenblatt, *et al.*, 1982; Watts, 1983). What has not received detailed attention is the impact of the broader social and physical environment on social support. This is what will be considered here.

One of the most influential theoretical models of the relationship between stress and mental and physical illness has been the so-called Michigan model (Caplan, *et al.*, 1975). The Michigan model emphasizes two separate types of moderating variables between stress and illness: first, personality (Type A behaviour, hardiness) and second, the social environment, especially social support (Winnubst, Buunk and Marcelissen, 1988). Recent research has tended to see these two types of moderating variables as less distinct as researchers have become increasingly concerned with attempts to identify the causal antecedents of social support. In particular, interest has shifted to personality and other factors that lead to some individuals being more supported than others (for example, see Sarason, Sarason and Pierce, 1990). Individual and personality variables are clearly relevant; some individuals are more skilful at building and maintaining supportive relationships and also at illiciting support when needed. However, although these recent theoretical developments are extremely interesting, they give us few clues as to whether aspects of the planned environment can facilitate or inhibit social support. Clearly, any such influence should be seen as standing alongside the many other causal antecedents of support. It is certainly plausible that the planned environment exerts an influence over social support. Current research points to how certain types of interactions and emotional transactions appear to be more supportive than others, and if the planned environment can affect individuals' social environments and the form of their interactions with others, then presumably it can influence support.

Sources and Types of Social Support

Before directly considering environmental influences on support, it is important to recognize that within the term *social support*, different types and sources of support may be distinguished. A commonly made distinction is between *instrumental* and *emotional* support. Instrumental support refers to things such as material and financial assistance, practical advice, and help with looking after children. Emotional support refers to things such as encouragement, the opportunity to express feelings, and the affirmation of self-worth. *Informational* support (general information and referral sources) is sometimes also distinguished, though the way in which the term is used by most authors suggests that it can probably be included under the term instrumental support.

These different components of support tend to perform different functions and may come from different sources. It may be family or kin who offer long-term support and material aid, such as over financial problems, while friends may offer support over personal and social problems and protection from social isolation and boredom. Neighbours, on the other hand, may be the principle source of immediate and emergency help. Support from neighbours is often considered to be mainly instrumental, for example: the loan of equipment, help with children, retrieval of the cat, and so on. It is, of course, family members who offer the nucleus of both concrete and emotional support, at least for the majority of people. Nonetheless, the evidence indicates that it is the quality of support that is critical for the preservation of mental health during crisis, rather than from whom it comes, (i.e. kin or non-kin), (Lowenthal and Haven, 1968; Croog, Lipson and Levine,'1972; Gore, 1978; Brown and Harris, 1978).

Researchers' estimates of the relative importance of kin, friends and neighbours in the provision of social support vary widely. Some researchers suggest that the only really significant source of social support in terms of mental health outcomes is that received from a very close personal confidant, normally a partner (Brown and Harris, 1978; Harris, personal communication). Others have presented data to suggest that sources of support are considerably wider than this, but that they rarely include neighbours. McFarlane, *et al.*, (1981) for example, in a survey of 518 of the general population, found that subjects identified a median of nine people who regularly provided support with work, money, home and family, social and health problems, and a median of five to whom they would turn in time of crisis. Of these reported supports, only 2 per cent were neighbours (though this proportion was higher among women and the elderly). However, the insights gained from these studies are limited as the persons identified as sources of support depend largely on the type of problem about which the researchers happen to ask. What the studies do suggest though, is that for major personal crises, people seek the support of close personal confidants, while for less global and personal stresses, a wider supportive network is involved.

Perhaps in the past, notably before the time of mass transport and mobility, friends, family, and neighbours would have been local and highly interconnected, as is found in certain (vanishing?) working class areas and in traditional communities. Today it may be more realistic to speak of *communities without propinquity*, and the three groups with the differing forms of support they offer as relatively distinct. Relatives, friends and co-workers are often located outside the neighbourhood. This corresponds to a shift from place-based relationships to taste-based relationships, leading some social theorists to argue that 'in the sense of an embedded affinity to place, "community" has largely been destroyed' (Giddens, 1990: 117). Yet despite this shift, the close spatial location of neighbours still leaves them in a unique position to perform certain functions which other network members would find difficult. As Unger and Wandersman (1985) argue in their detailed review, 'neighbouring is more complex and more important than much recent literature implies' (p. 162). Furthermore, the reliance on distant sources of support may have costs both for the individuals and for the neighbourhoods in which they live.

Main Effect or Buffer?

Social support is widely thought of as acting as a buffer protecting against, or at least attenuating, the harmful effects of life events and on-going difficulties (for example, Brown and Harris, 1978). However, it is also possible to argue that the absence or disruption of a supportive social network has a direct effect on mental health. There is evidence to support both of these positions, and which one is preferred frequently depends on which aspect of support is being focused on (Geston and Jason, 1987).

When support is measured qualitatively from the recipient's point of view, the evidence tends to favour the buffering hypothesis. Yet when structural measures are used, the evidence tends to favour the direct, or main effect, model. Part of this difference could be explained by the methodological weaknesses of qualitative measures, and part by the insensitivity of structural measures. The applicability of the two models also appears to depend on the closeness of match between the form of support received and the specific nature of the stressor. Where the stressor is highly specific and the form of the support is closely matched, then the buffering model appears to apply. Where the stressor or the form of support is more general or less precisely matched then a main effect model appears to apply.

In this chapter, social support is being considered separately from the environment as stressor (see Chapters 3 and 4) but this is not intended to indicate that social support acts only as a buffer to other, clearly distinguished, stressors. The absence or disruption of different aspects of support can leave the individual more vulnerable to the effects of stress, but also may act as a stressor in itself. Of course, whether the disruption or inhibition of support affects the individual directly (as stress), or indirectly (as vulnerability to other stressors), its importance remains. The issue of whether the buffering model or main effect model is most appropriate in the context of neighbouring behaviour will be returned to later in the chapter.

Social Factors Affecting Neighbouring Behaviour

A number of surveys have shown that attachment to the neighbourhood and the quality of the relationship with neighbours explain a very large amount of the variance in residential satisfaction (Amerigo and Aragones, 1990). There is also evidence of an interaction with housing quality. If a person is in frequent social contact with his or her neighbours, then the objective quality of the dwelling makes only a small difference to the level of residential satisfaction. If, however, a person (in the same area) is not in frequent social contact with neighbours, then the objective quality of the dwelling makes a very large difference to residential satisfaction. Only when contact with neighbours is low do objectively poor dwellings tend to result in subjectively poor appraisals of the environment (Hartman, 1963). In other words, residents who are involved in their local community tend to be happy with where they live regardless of the physical quality of their homes.

There are a number of factors that are believed to influence the level and supportiveness of neighbouring interactions. It is widely believed that the level of *social homogeneity* within an area or housing development influences levels of neighbouring behaviour. Social homogeneity is thought to be a necessary pre-requisite for high levels of supportive neighbouring behaviour. Evidence for this hypothesis is discussed below. Evidence also exists to suggest that *age* is an important predictor of neighbouring behaviour. For both men and women, higher levels of neighbouring behaviour and a less dispersed social network are associated with increasing age (Keane, 1991). Part of this effect may be to do with reduced mobility, but much of the effect is thought to be the result of the length of residence in an area. This can be seen, for example, in an analysis of the SCPR residential environments data set. Neighbours were significantly more likely to be rated as friendly by older people, but this association was eliminated once length of residence was statistically controlled for. The phenomenon can also be seen in the New Towns. Although initially characterized as places with little neighbouring behaviour, the New Towns gradually changed as traditional patterns of neighbouring re-emerged, though as Peter Willmott has observed, 'it takes a very, very long time' (Willmott, personal communication). There are also thought to be *class* differences in patterns of neighbouring. Traditional working-class neighbourhoods are generally thought of as exhibiting higher levels of neighbouring behaviour than middle-class areas. The traditional pattern of highly supportive working-class neighbourboods may well have resulted out of the higher levels of hardship and thereby the enforced interdependence of poorer working-class families (Young and Willmott, 1957). In contrast, the higher levels of affluence and mobility of the middle classes seems to have reduced dependency on the local milieu. From this point of view, the emergence of the affluent worker and the modern welfare state seems likely to have de-emphasized neighbouring (Bilton, *et al.*, 1987; Giddens, 1990; Halpern, 1990). Finally, and perhaps most controversially, it has been argued that *physical design* can influence levels of neighbouring behaviour and support. Controversy has surrounded this issue partly because it has often been associated with *architectural determinism* (Mercer, 1975). However, there is no reason why links between the environment and behaviour should be seen as deterministic or exclusive of other influences. In the discussion below, the assumption will be that any such linkage is not exclusive. Indeed, as we shall see, effects of physical design on neighbouring are often only found when certain social preconditions are already met.

Social Homogeneity – A Planners' Dilemma

Planners are presented with a dilemma. There are a number of social and political reasons why *balanced communities* are considered desirable. Planners wish to avoid the situation where cities are divided into separate areas for the rich and poor, for Black and White, and for old and young. Once established, spatial divisions tend to prove extremely resilient and are often (literally) divisive. Against this, it is often more convenient to build environments for relatively homogeneous populations, and residents often prefer to live in such homogeneous areas. Many influential planners have argued that the level of social homogeneity in a community can be a far more important determinant of levels of friendship and positive neighbour relations than the physical design (Gans, 1961) and, as Wirth (1938) argued in his classic essay 'Urbanism as a way of life', heterogeneity of populations tends to undermine the bonds of kinship and neighbourliness. However good the physical design of an area or development, if neighbours feel they have nothing in common, then neighbouring relations are very unlikely to develop into patterns of support and are quite likely to develop into open hostility.

Yet social homogeneity also brings problems. If an area becomes reserved for the less affluent then the poverty of the residents means that the area will be less able to afford the maintenance of its amenities and a vicious circle becomes established. Spatial divisions according to affluence result in the areas with the greatest needs being the areas with the least resources to deal with those needs. Unfortunately, due to the fact that most urban areas are not undifferentiated masses, even when not explicitly intended, some areas tend to become *good* areas while others become *bad* (see Chapter 5 for a more detailed discussion of labelling). Divisions according to minority status can be similarly problematic, particularly given that they tend to be overlaid on patterns of socio-economic disadvantage. Ghettos develop, and these can concentrate problems as well as being flashpoints of conflict. Indeed, the higher the level of ethnic segregation, the greater the level of group conflict that seems to occur (Fisher, 1982). Divisions according to position in the life cycle also lead to problems. When areas become largely populated by residents at one particular stage in the life cycle, many long-term problems often follow. Many criticisms of the British New Towns have focused on this particular issue. When the age range of a population is relatively narrow, local population bulges develop. The young populations of the New Towns led to massive, temporary and uneven demand for primary schools, then for secondary schools, and finally for sixth form and technical colleges. Today the New Towns are faced with an enormous pressure for new housing as the second generation of the original settlers demand housing for themselves. This problem was forewarned by Young and Willmott back in 1957. Ironically, many of the young people now looking for housing in the New Towns will be obliged to move back to the areas vacated by their parents 20 to 30 years ago. This movement implies a repeat of the disruption of social networks that was one of the main criticisms of the original slum clearance programs that led to the New Towns.

For the preceding reasons, therefore, some planners have attempted to design communities and cities to be as balanced and socially undifferentiated as possible. For example, the planners of the American new town of Columbia, Maryland deliberately attempted to maintain a mix of housing types for different social groups within each neighbourhood unit so as to avoid socio-economic spatial divisions developing across the city (Hoppenfeld, 1971; Klein, 1978; Altman and Chemers, 1984). Another, somewhat older example of an attempt to avoid social divisions of space was the development of cites based on a grid design without a clear centre such as in Barcelona. It was an explicit intention in the use of the grid design in Barcelona that by so doing, patterns of spatial inequality could be minimized. If all areas were very much the same, there being no clear centre, no main street, and no obvious periphery, then, it was hypothesized, there would be no reason why one particular area should become gentrified while another became a slum. Attempts have also been made to avoid ethnic spatial divisions, though these have been less consistent and have wavered according to political opinion (Smith, 1988). Attempts at ensuring communities are balanced in terms of the life cycle have been relatively half-hearted, perhaps because of the long perspective needed. Housing has often been produced because of short-term pressures, and these have normally come from young couples with children – hence the problems of the British New Towns.

The Group Density Effect

The group density effect refers to a general phenomenon where the lower a group's population or neighbourhood density, the higher its prevalence of mental illness. As this phenomenon has already been discussed in some detail elsewhere (Halpern, 1993), I shall present it here in summary form only.

Wide-ranging evidence exists that for ethnic groups, the lower the group's *local* concentration, the higher its members' rates of first psychiatric admissions become. American evidence has shown within-group ethnic density effects for White, Black, Italian, Puerto Rican, Irish, German, Polish, Austrian or Hungarian, and Russian groups in various American cities (Faris and Dunham, 1939; Mintz and Schwartz, 1964; Levy and Rowitz, 1973; Rabkin, 1979; Muhlin, 1979). Similar but less detailed evidence has been published of within-group density effects for French and English speakers in Canada (Malzberg, 1964). Evidence on between-group differences is also consistent with the ethnic density effect, provided account is taken of the degree of group clustering, as it is the group's density at the local (not national) level that is critical to effect (Halpern, 1993).

The group density effect applies to group characteristics other than ethnicity. Similar evidence has been found for group density effects on the basis of occupation (Bell, 1958; Wechsler and Pugh, 1967) and on the basis of religious grouping (Rosenberg, 1962; Cairns, 1988). In sum, an enormous range of evidence suggests that when group concentration at the local level falls below a certain critical mass, the level of mental ill-health found in that group markedly increases. This applies whether the level of mental illness is measured through community surveys or through first psychiatric admission rates.[1]

The cause of the effect appears to be two-fold. Low local group density exposes group members to higher levels of stress in the form of prejudice, while at the same time providing relatively low levels of group support. The group density effect seems only to add to the dilemma facing planners – the tension between fostering homogeneous communities and the desire to create balanced communities. On the basis of long-term goals such as the reduction in prejudice, inequality and conflict between groups, one can argue that the spatial mixing of groups should be encouraged (Wilner, Walkley and Cook, 1955; Ford, 1973; Bethlehem, 1985). Yet the evidence suggests that, at least in the short term, low group density is deleterious to individual mental health. Fortunately, the conflict between these demands is not as severe as it at first seems. A close reading of the literature supporting group density effects suggests that the protective influence of the group does not require that the residents of a local area be entirely homogeneous for the benefits of group support to emerge. Once a critical mass is established – perhaps around 40 per cent of the local area – the benefits of group support seem to follow. If planners avoid extremes of both social homogeneity and heterogeneity then both sets of demands can be accommodated.

The Physical Environment and Social Support

> The category with which both the English and Americans were most in accord was that the layout of the estate or subdivision left something to be desired ... that 'someone' 'somewhere' could have done 'something' which would have achieved a better layout (Bracey, H. E., 1964: 67).

In the previous section it was discussed how the level of homogeneity can affect social relations and mental health. In this section, the focus will be on how the physical environment can influence social relations, if at all. Social support and the built environment can be considered in more than one context:

- Forms of housing – does the form or layout of housing have the ability to facilitate or inhibit group formation and thereby the probability of having friendly neighbours?
- Designs of work environments – can the design of the workplace influence group and friendship formation, and thereby support?
- The juxtapositions of housing/work/leisure – can the juxtapositions of environments, whether planned or accidental, have consequences for social support?

In this review, the focus will particularly be on how residential environments may influence support. First, I will attempt to show how the environment can influence the form of social networks and friendship formation. Then, I shall explore how the physical environment may affect the quality as well as the form of social relations. As we shall see, although there are very few studies which trace the link from housing type right through to social support, the literature strongly suggests that such a link does exist (Flemming, Baum and Singer, 1985). The possibility that the built form may affect behaviour beyond the specific context will also be considered. If an environment fosters the withdrawal of its users, can this coping behaviour then generalize to other contexts?

Physical Environments and Social Networks

Friendship and group formation is an obvious precursor to social support. A number of studies exist that relate the formation of social networks and patterns of friendship to the form of the physical environment. In general, the closer people live together, the more likely they are to become friends (Merton, 1949; Newcomb, 1961).

Byrne and Buehler (1955) found that amongst a college classroom of freshmen psychology students, new acquaintances showed a very strong tendency to be neighbours. They concluded, 'It is apparent that with the assignment of classroom seats, an instructor is arbitrarily determining future acquaintances to a significant extent.' (p. 148). As in the classroom, friendship among workers has been found to be closely related to proximity. People in both factories and offices converse with their closest neighbours and often choose to make friends with them. For example, Homans (1954) found that for clerks, the 'most important determinant of clique formation was the position of a poster's table during their first year on the job. [Those] who sat near each other then had many chances to interact and tended to become friends.' (p. 729). Similar results were found by Wells (1965).

Studies that have been conducted on the physical enclosure of work groups strongly indicate that these can facilitate friendship and group formation, (Richards and Dobyns, 1957; Wells, 1965). This facilitation is probably due not only to an increased level of interaction, but also to the privacy that the enclosure allows – enclosure fosters autonomy and allows the group to develop its own norms (Sundstrom, 1986). Similar results were reported by Blake, *et al.*, (1956) who found that barracks within which partitions (without doors) had been added, dividing the

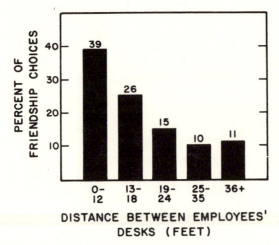

Figure 4.3: *Percentage of office employees chosen as friends as a function of distance between the employees' desks.*
Source: Adapted from Wells, B.W.P. (1965b).

otherwise identical barracks into six-man cubicles, served to increase the cohesiveness of the six making penetration by outsiders more difficult. Note, however, that the previous studies also indicate that if people are sufficiently incompatible, then no amount of proximity will induce their friendship, underlining the importance of homogeneity as discussed earlier. These studies shadow what one might intuitively expect: enclosure, either physical or symbolic, can catalyze group formation and cohesiveness. In principal, these friendships, if achieved, can offer a valuable source of support. Holahan and Moos (1981), using the work Work Relations Index (WRI) have shown that the quality of the work milieu with respect to its supportiveness, is predictive of psychological adjustment even after having controlled for initial levels of adjustment, life change and the availability of other sources of social support.

However, of all the studies conducted on the relationship between the physical environment and patterns of friendship formation, a 1950 study by Festinger, Schachter and Back of a residential environment is perhaps the most detailed and best known. The study consisted of an analysis of an isolated university housing project for war-veterans. The students were all married and lived either in two-floor reconverted navy barracks (Westgate West), or semi-detached, prefabricated bungalows that were arranged in U-shaped courts (Westgate).

Festinger, *et al.*, found that the closer the housewives lived to one another, the more likely they were to be selected as friends. The physical layout appeared to determine the number of people that residents met by chance (passive contacts), and it was these passive contacts of increasing length that formed the basis for the development of friendships. Festinger, *et al.*, went on to show that it was not simple proximity *per se* that was important, but *functional distance*. For example, in the case of Westgate West apartments, friendship was predicted better by the routing of the access stairs than by the closeness (distance) of the apartments *per se*.

Festinger, *et al.*, argued that the friendships were the building blocks of groups. It was found that similar attitudes towards the tenants organization were found within individual courts, but between courts marked differences emerged. In other words,

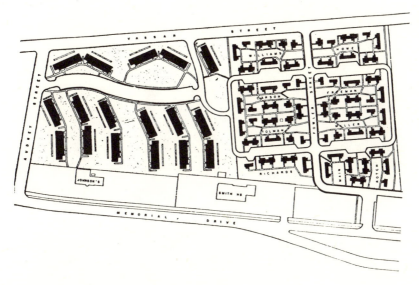

Figure 4.4: *The plan of Westgate and Westgate West*

there tended to be a consistency of attitudes within courts but not between them. This effect was not found for the Westgate West blocks, however, suggesting that group pressures were not operating within the blocks of apartments to the same extent as they were in the courts.

A similar study with similar findings was conducted by Caplow and Forman (1950) independently of Festinger, *et al.* Again the study was of a very homogeneous population of veteran students. Aged 21 to 39, the students were all married with children, white, transient, and with apparent status obstacles removed (occupation, income, family structure, and housing type). Caplow and Forman found that in the university village studied 'interaction rises to an extremely high level and organises itself with almost molecular simplicity in terms of the spatial pattern of the community.' (p. 366).

The two studies show, at least for relatively homogeneous populations, that the form of the built environment can strongly influence friendship and group formation. They show that once groups are established, they are able to exert influence over members through the friendship network. However, it should be noted that although friendship readily relates to social support, the relationship of group influence to support could be more complex. While group pressures and support may be helpful over a specific crisis and may serve to reduce social deviancy such as criminal behaviour, these pressures to conform may sometimes be experienced as unwanted attention and an extra source of stress (particularly on one who's behaviour is socially stigmatized).

A criticism of the studies presented above is that the situations studied are sufficiently extraordinary that their relevance to normal residential situations may be limited. Homogeneous populations with random assignment to dwellings are far from typical. It could be argued that the built environment will only show such effects in the complete absence of other influences, and hence is of little importance outside of

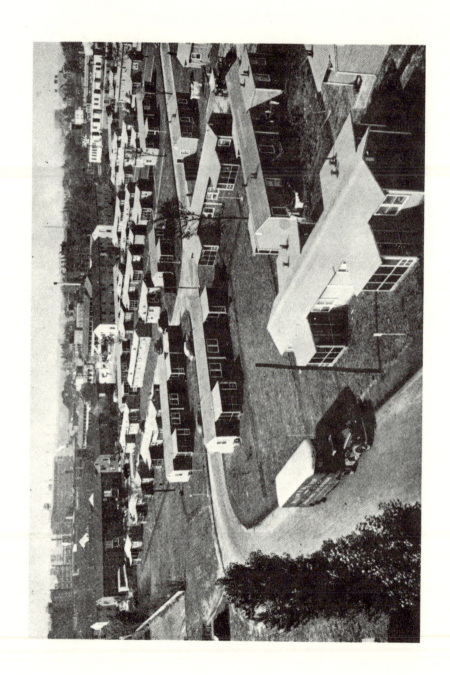

Figure 4.5: *View of Westgate and Westgate West*

the college campuses and army barracks of academic studies. A second point is that although the evidence shows that the environment may influence *who* your friends are and, therefore, where your support might be received from, it does not demonstrate in itself that the degree or quality of support is influenced by the environment. This requires evidence from other studies.

Example 1: Supportive Environments

It needs to be demonstrated that the environment influences not only the form of social networks, but also their size and supportive qualities. The studies by Festinger, *et al.* and Caplow and Forman suggest that levels of supportive neighbouring were higher in courts and along enclosed sidewalks, but these studies were of unusual and highly homogeneous populations as mentioned above. Among the few studies of environmental influences on neighbouring in more general populations, one finding has been that developments with larger numbers of dwellings tend to have a more negative impact on patterns of neighbouring. The larger the number of dwellings in a development, the lower the number of neighbours that are known and the lower the level of attachment to the community (Frank, 1983; Lefebvre, 1984). This result suggests that where developments are divided into smaller numbers of units, more positive neighbouring might be expected. The hypothesis is confirmed and illustrated in data from a fascinating study by Willmott (1963) of a large development outside London.

In *The Evolution of a Community*, Willmott presented a detailed study of Dagenham – a suburban housing project built by the London County Council in the 1920s, and housing some 90000 people. Willmott noticed that there were wide variations in the sociability and patterns of neighbouring in different parts of the development. In particular, he noticed that different kinds of streets seemed to have distinctive social atmospheres. The small cul-de-sacs or *banjos* and some short, narrow streets, had more of a sense of community and the residents of these streets were generally less reserved. In contrast, on the wider and longer roads, fewer people were found who knew many of their neighbours or who described their fellow residents as friendly. Willmott's findings were illustrated with detailed interview material.

> 'We know everyone in this part,' said Mrs Carson, who lives in a cul-de-sac. 'Everybody's friendly. They will always do a good turn. If you're queer or anything like that, they'll knock at you're door and say, "Don't go out today; I'll do your shopping for you."'

> 'They are all very nice in this turning,' said Mrs Farley, who also lives in a banjo. 'If anybody wants anything done we'll all sort of muck in and help. If people want the gas man let in, or if anybody's ill and wants some shopping done, or anything like that, we all sort of help one another.'

A similar situation was found in those narrower streets, which were either short in themselves, or which were effectively made short by intersecting roads. Neighbours offered not only instrumental support, but also a sense of belonging:

'They're very friendly in this street,' he said, 'we know nearly all of them. If they thought you were in trouble they'd go out of their way to help. There's nothing they wouldn't do. I'd hate to leave this little street.'

This stood in contrast to the longer, wider streets where significantly more people thought others in their street were 'unfriendly'. A Mrs Salmon compared the longer avenue she lived in with her previous street:

'Apart from people on either side of you, you're only on good-morning terms with the rest. But when we lived in Poplar it was a small turning. There were only about 40 houses in the turning and everybody knew each other.'

Willmott found that on longer streets or main thoroughfares, people interacted less, and knew less about each other, and took less interest in the road as a whole. In his reporting of the study, Willmott did not deny the influence of other factors on neighbouring patterns, such as differences in the length of time people had lived in an area, differences in people's ages, and differences in social status; but he concluded that, for this 'relatively homogeneous [working class] community', it was differences in street design that were 'the major determinant' on patterns of neighbouring (Willmott, 1963: 82).

Willmott's finding in Dagenham that cul-de-sacs seemed to be friendlier places to live was tested by using the SCPR residential environment data. In SCPR data set, 18 per cent (1332) of the respondents lived on cul-de-sacs as opposed to through roads. The difference between these two road types was not as neat and tidy as in the study of Dagenham alone, and many of the roads technically defined as cul-de-sacs might actually have been very large roads, while many of those technically defined as through roads may have been relatively quiet, short roads. Residents had been asked, 'Here are some statements about this particular road; would you describe this road as a road where the neighbours are helpful?' Residents could respond 'Describes this road' or 'Does not describe this road'. Despite the simplicity of the distinction between road types, residents on cul-de-sacs *were* significantly more likely to have described their road as being one on which the neighbours were helpful (83 per cent compared with 78 per cent on through roads). This difference, though modest, remained significant even after the effects of sex, age, length of residence and presence of children had been statistically controlled for.

Willmott did point out that it was not only cul-de-sacs but also other short and narrow roads that appeared to foster friendlier and more supportive neighbouring relations. This suggests that it may have been the absence of outside traffic rather than the living on a cul-de-sac *per se* that may have led to the difference. This can be tested fairly directly in the SCPR data set by statistically controlling for the level of traffic in the road. Sure enough, when this was done, the difference in the level of rated neighbour helpfulness between cul-de-sacs and through roads was entirely eliminated. In fact, it is clear that the level of helpfulness in any road is significantly predicted by the level of traffic through it – the correlation between the logarithm of the traffic count (an objective measure) and the rated friendliness was $-.12$ ($p<.0001$). The less traffic on a road, the more likely residents were to describe the neighbours as helpful.

Of course traffic is noisy, and noise is known to reduce helping behaviour (see

Chapter 3). There was a similar negative association between the level of the noise outside the dwelling and rated neighbour helpfulness of the road (r=–.15). This raises the possibility that some of association between traffic noise and mental ill-health reported in Chapter 3 may have been mediated by the effect of traffic noise on neighbour helpfulness. This issue will be returned to later in the chapter, but for now it will suffice to note that people living on quiet roads and cul-de-sacs had significantly fewer symptoms than those living on through roads. This association was not eliminated by statistical controls for age, length of residence, income and so on, but it was eliminated by the statistical controlling for the influence of traffic flow or traffic noise.

Before concluding that we should build only cul-de-sacs, we should note that there may also be costs involved in such a layout. There may be a tension between friendly neighbouring and privacy. Hence in the absence of a fairly homogeneous population, or amongst residents who are particularly seeking privacy (the contemporary middle-class?), small cul-de-sacs may actually be disliked (Kuper, 1953; Mayo, 1979). When social interaction is unwanted, then it is likely to be experienced as the absence of privacy rather than as a positive source of support. Social interaction is more likely to be experienced as unwanted when a community is more heterogeneous (see above).

Example 2: Unsupportive Environments

The evidence presented so far suggests that it is possible for the built environment to facilitate supportive patterns of neighbouring, at least for certain homogeneous populations. The question arises, however, can an environment do the reverse, can it inhibit friendship and encourage *atomization*?

The first example is simply the converse of the positive example of cul-de-sacs or other quiet roads presented above. If we can use the SCPR data set to divide road types according to how busy they are, we can see at a glance that busy roads are significantly less likely to be described as helpful. People who lived in the noisier roads (the noisier 50 per cent of roads) were twice as likely not to describe the neighbours on their road as helpful (30 per cent) as those living in the quieter roads (15 per cent). Still, we should note that this means that even in the noisier roads, 70 per cent of residents described their neighbours as helpful.

The SCPR data also supports the common perception that helpfulness varies according to population density. In areas of low density (fewer than 0.624 persons per acre), 87 per cent of residents described their neighbours as helpful. This figure fell to 74 per cent in urban conurbations. The association between population density (or urbanism) was attenuated, but not eliminated, by statistical controls for the level of traffic on the street. Multiple regression analyses suggested that, as for the relationship between traffic and mental health, part of the negative association between population density and mental health (see Chapter 3) was mediated by the helpfulness of neighbours. This is not, of course, to say that other factors were not also mediating the association.

Interestingly, a neat example of an environment selectively isolating certain individuals can be found in Festinger, *et al.*'s study of Westgate. When studying the attitudes of individual residents, Festinger, *et al.*, found that although most individuals

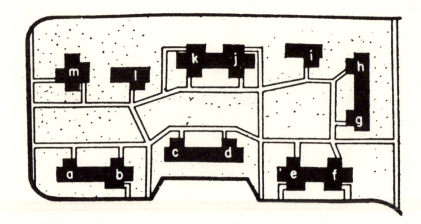

Figure 4.6: *Plan of Westgate Court*

held the same attitudes as other residents on their court, a minority of residents held views that deviated from the norm. It was found that a major factor contributing to *deviancy* (deviation from the group norm) was the physical isolation of some dwellings. Some of the houses on the courts did not face inwards towards the court but being, as it were, on the ends of the 'U', faced outwards towards the road (for example, house 'm' in figure 4.6). In these dwellings the number of passive contacts and friendships with other residents were significantly lower. The low level of friendship with the residents in the end dwellings resulted in an undue concentration of *deviates* in these dwellings – presumably it was more difficult for the group to exert influence on people in these houses.

The next question is, can the design of an environment act to isolate not just a minority of residents, but the vast majority? A study by Yancey (1971) of an ill-fated project called Pruitt-Igoe near downtown St. Louis, Missouri, suggests that it can. The Pruitt-Igoe project was opened in 1954, and consisted of 43 11-storey buildings; some 2762 apartments. It covered 57 acres, and housed more than 12000 people. Yancey found that although residents had similar numbers of friends to non-project populations, these 'bore little or no relation to the physical proximity of families to each other'. It will be recalled that Hartman (1963, see above) found that the perceived quality of residents' dwellings tended to take second place to the quality of their relations with other residents in determining residential satisfaction. Pruitt-Igoe offered a shocking example of this phenomenon. Although the vast majority of residents were satisfied with their apartments (78 per cent versus 55 per cent living in the nearby slum), less than half were satisfied with living on the project (49 per cent compared to 74 per cent in the nearby slum).[2] The project was characterized by an extreme atomization of the residents, who seemed largely hostile to one another, and heavily reliant on the police for the resolution of even the smallest conflicts. *Social support* was out of the question; as one typical resident explained when asked about her neighbours:

'They are selfish. I've got no friends here. There's none of this door-to-door

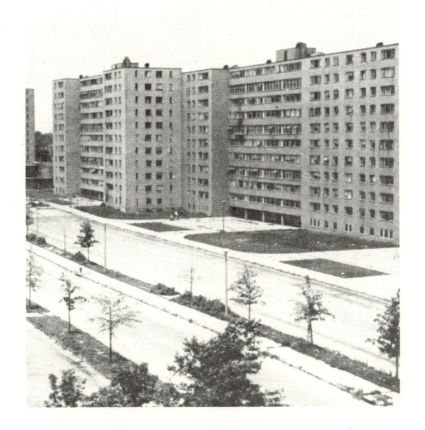

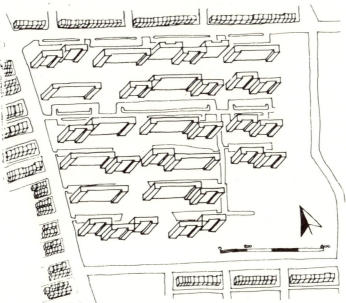

Figure 4.7: *Pruitt-Igoe*

coffee business of being friends here or anything like that. Down here, if you are sick you just go to the hospital. There are no friends to help you. I don't think my neighbours would help me and I wouldn't ask them to anyway. I don't have trouble with my neighbours because I never visit them. The rule of the game down here is *go for yourself* (Quoted in Yancey, 1971: 175).

Yancey attributed the atomization, and hence the physical danger and deterioration of the project, specifically to the design. In particular he noted that:

Pruitt-Igoe provides no semi-private space and facilities around which neighbouring relationships might develop. There is a minimum of what is often called *wasted space* – space within buildings that is outside of individual family dwelling units (Yancey, 1971: 172).

Ironically, this efficiency won praise in an early review of the design (Architectural Forum, 1951). By 1970, only 16 years after it had been opened, 27 of the 43 buildings were totally vacant. Two years later, accepting the non-habitability of Pruitt-Igoe, officials demolished the entire project (Krupat, 1985).

Some have suggested that an alternative explanation of the project's atomization could have been that as so many of the residents were on welfare (which they were afraid of losing), they feared becoming friendly with neighbours in case they might be turned in to the authorities over some minor violation. Hence withdrawal into the single-family dwelling unit and hostility between neighbours. But then why particularly at Pruitt-Igoe? For example, the project studied by Wilner, *et al.*, (1962) of new public housing in Baltimore stands in sharp contrast to Pruitt-Igoe, for despite being a project with a similar population, its design appeared not to inhibit interpersonal interaction. The Baltimore project was of six 11-storey blocks, with 10 flats per floor but, unlike Pruitt-Igoe, there was a deliberate inclusion of semi-private space, most notably, a common play area (16×30 feet) on each floor. Wilner, *et al.*, found an increased amount of neighbouring, visiting, and mutual aid amongst persons moving from a slum into the project.

Yancey's interpretation is also supported by a study of social behaviour in physically contrasting low income neighbourhoods in New York. Holahan (1976) found that the design of (external) public spaces in housing projects had significant influences on residents' socializing behaviour, and suggested that many of the faults of large projects could be attributed to the design of their public space, (particularly the inability to support functional activities). His field work led him to emphasize the importance of functionally, not just aesthetically, evaluating design. If public and semi-public spaces were not appropriately designed, these could undermine the success of the project no matter how good the quality of the apartments themselves.

Closely related to Yancey's discussion of the potential importance of semi-private space is Oscar Newman's notion of *defensible space*: Yancey in fact used the term before Newman's famous (1973) study was even published. Defensible space refers to areas shared by small groups of neighbours who use the space regularly and come to control it, or in other words, who come to regulate its use. Newman argued that such areas, where surveillance and control are possible, have lower crime rates than areas not under the informal control of residents. (See chapter 4 for a more detailed discussion of the defensible space thesis and crime.) The salient idea here is that these

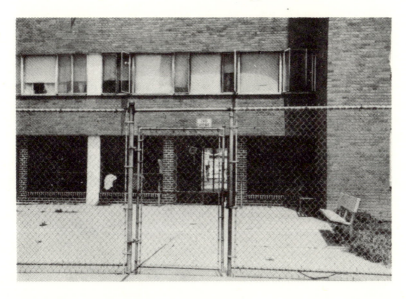

Figure 4.8: *View showing the retained construction fence at Pruitt-Igoe (Newman, 1973; reprinted with permission of the author)*

spaces can encourage group formation and supportive patterns of neighbouring. That the built form can facilitate or inhibit small group formation, neighbourly support, and thereby control (over space and its users) is an explicit theme throughout the many examples presented in Newman's work. Newman also refers to the Pruitt-Igoe project. He documents a chance alteration to a part of the project which is particularly interesting because it took the form of a quasi-experimental intervention. One of the buildings at Pruitt-Igoe was scheduled to have maintenance done, but in order to protect equipment and materials from theft and people from injury, a fence was installed around the entire building. Keys to the gates were given only to residents and some construction workers.

During the six months the construction lasted, residents found that crime rates and vandalism were dramatically reduced, and residents also began to sweep their hallways and pick up litter. When the construction ended, residents petitioned to have the fence remain. Two years following the construction, the fence remained. The crime rate for that building was 80 per cent below the Pruitt-Igoe norm, and the vacancy rate was 2–5 per cent against the Pruitt-Igoe norm of 70 per cent.

The example of Pruitt-Igoe stands as the classic example of how the physical environment can undermine the supportive social relations of residents, and its subsequent demolition testifies to the seriousness of the consequences.

Problems Arising from the Juxtaposition of Built Environments (Mixed Land Use)

Further tensions are introduced by juxtapositions of environments designed for different uses – work, shopping and residential. A number of factors such as the economic value of land, cultural preferences and planning guidelines lead to varying levels of mixing between land uses. As we shall see, the various juxtapositions of environments built for different uses can have unintended effects on the social interactions and mental health of those who live with them.

This issue has already been touched on in regard to the juxtaposition of residential areas housing people with very different social characteristics. Relatively socially homogeneous neighbourhoods, in terms of class, race or religion, may lead to some social and mental health benefits inside the neighbourhood. However, where such homogeneous but contrasting neighbourhoods meet, problems frequently arise. For example, where an affluent neighbourhood adjoins a relatively poor neighbourhood, high levels of crime (mainly theft) tend to occur. Similarly, where neighbourhoods become segregated by race or religion, the boundaries between the communities can become sources of major conflict.

The spatial concentrations and distributions of social and ethnic groups are often largely beyond the control of urban planners. This is not true, however, of the spatial relationship between residential and commercial areas. In most planning systems, planners make clear distinctions between land uses, and changes of use normally require formal permission from the planning authorities. The planning systems of different countries differ in the shades of distinction that they make between land uses, but at their heart there is always a distinction between residential and commercial uses.

The spatial relationship between residential and commercial areas can be an extremely sensitive local issue. This is especially so where large shopping or other commercial areas are close to, or are embedded in, residential areas. Is there any evidence that these spatial relationships make any difference to the quality or form of neighbouring behaviour?

There is surprisingly little research on this topic, but a useful starting point is provided by an American study which examined the influence on residents of having a shopping area at the end of their street. Baum, Aiello and Davies (1979) found that the presence of shopping at the ends of residential streets was associated with more frequent unwanted social contact, less group use of shared space, and inhibited group formation. Residents complained of a lack of control – the space that neighbours might normally use for interaction was instead subject to use by strangers. Consequentially, residents not only experienced more stress, but tended to withdraw from neighbourly interaction.

Baum, *et al.*'s study is interesting, but it can be criticized for its relatively small scale and consequently limited sample size. Fortunately, it was possible to examine this issue through the much larger sample contained in the (British) SCPR residential environments data. For each respondent's dwelling, the land use within 200 yards of the dwelling was assessed by the interviewer independently of the respondent. The information was coded into four categories of land use (Table 4.1). The findings confirmed those of Baum, *et al..* in America. The higher the level of commercial land use in the area, the less likely residents were to rate their road as one 'where the neighbours are helpful'. Although 82 per cent of people living in entirely residential areas described their neighbours as helpful, this fell to just 58 per cent in areas of extensive commercial land use. This effect was not eliminated by controls for background individual variables such as age, income or length of residence.

Table 4.1: *Neighbour helpfulness by land use within 200 yards of the respondent's dwelling*

		Per cent describing neighbours as helpful	N
1	Entirely residential	82.2	4111
2	Mainly residential, but some commercial/industrial	76.8	2740
3	Half residential, half commercial/industrial	69.3	379
4	Mainly commercial/industrial, some residential	57.6	208
	Missing		102
	Total	79.0	7540

Unsurprisingly, mixed land use was again highly associated with higher traffic levels (r=.40). However, unlike for the effect of living on a cul-de-sac, controlling for the level of traffic attenuated, but did not eliminate, the association between commercial land use and reduced neighbour helpfulness. Mental ill-health (mild psychiatric symptoms) was also found to be more common in areas of mixed land use, even having controlled for income, age, sex and self-reported sensitivity.

These findings, especially when added to the evidence presented in earlier chapters, suggest that mixed land use and the extra traffic that it brings can have a negative impact on residents' neighbouring behaviour and on their mental health. The potentially negative impact of mixed land use has already been raised in the environmental criminological literature, where higher levels of mixed land use were found to be associated with higher levels of fear among residents. This raised level of fear appeared to be due to the large number of strangers that non-residential land use can bring into an area. Its relevance was also mentioned in Chapters 1 and 2 in explaining some of the excess variance left in perceived traffic flow and levels of annoyance once the effects of objective traffic flow and noise had been controlled for.

However, as is often the case, there is a second side to the coin. While the presence of commercial land uses in residential areas tends to have an adverse effect on neighbouring behaviour, it should not be assumed that the separation of residential from commercial areas is itself unproblematic in terms of social relations. In fact, the contemporary tendancy to spatially separate commercial and work areas from residential neighbourhoods on a very large scale has been argued to have had many negative effects on the community and social lives of individuals. It is now common, if not the norm, for the workplace to be far removed from the home, necessitating extensive commuting. French studies (quoted in Baldwin and Bottoms, 1976) have shown that for matched groups of workers, time spent playing with children, the children's relationships with their parents, the conjugal relationship and the amount of leisure time are all directly and adversely affected by the length of the journey to work. The impact of commuting on family and community life has led to damning critiques of the building of large out-of-town developments and suburbs. The city of Paris is famous for its self-contained urban districts where workplaces, residential dwellings and places to eat all co-exist within small areas such that residents can live and work within relatively small neighbourhoods. So perhaps it is unsurprising that it has been French researchers who have been especially concerned about the effects of commuting on communities and have linked commuting to widespread reports of the negative impact of French out-of-town developments on mental health (Lefebvre, 1984).

In as far as commuting undermines family and local relationships, it clearly has a negative effect on the social support available to, and given by, the commuter. Unfortunately, commuting can also have a destructive effect on the business locale, which is not lived in, and on the areas in between which, used as passageways, can cease to be *places* (Wedmore and Freeman, 1984). Sadly, it may be that because of the scale on which people have sought to protect their residential environments from the presence of outsiders, and especially from commercial activity, they may have inadvertantly undermined much of the social benefits that they (or others) had hoped to gain from these arrangements.

The Relationship between Neighbour Helpfulness, Neighbour Problems and Mental Health

As we have seen from the examples and data presented above, neighbours can be a positive source of support. However, we have also seen from these examples and from the previous two chapters that neighbours can be a considerable source of stress and irritation.

The unique ability of neighbours to be either a serious source of stress or an invaluable source of support was elegantly captured in a study by Ebbesen, Klos and Konecni, (1976). Ebbesen, *et al.*, examined the relationship between physical distance, frequency of face-to-face contacts, and the probability that individuals would be chosen as friends or enemies in a middle- to upper-middle income condominium complex. Consistent with previous research, it was found that the probability of being a friend increased as the distance between people's dwellings decreased – in other words, the closer people lived together, the more likely they were to become friends. However, Ebbesen, *et al.*, also discovered that there was an even stronger relationship between distance and selecting people as *disliked*; the probability of being disliked increased sharply as distance between people's dwellings decreased. Ebbesen, *et al.*,'s results illustrate very clearly the issues raised in this chapter. People living close by can be a positive source of friendship and support but, given their proximity, there is a very real risk that the neighbours will end up as a permanent source of stress, especially if the option of avoiding them is not available.

Returning to the SCPR data, we have already shown that there was a negative association between the rating of the neighbours on a road as helpful and symptom levels. There are also a series of associations between the rating of the neighbours as helpful and the characteristics of the environment. Multivariate analyses suggested that these associations between the objective residential environment (traffic flow, land use and population density) and symptom levels were partly mediated by the rated helpfulness of neighbours. Yet the question arises as to whether these effects resulted from the positive benefits that follow from generally positive neighbouring

Table 4.2: *Cell count of neighbour problems by neighbour helpfulness*

		Neighbour problems?		
		No	Yes	
Neighbours helpful?	Yes	4312	363	78.1%
	No	994	257	21.1%
		91.7%	8.3%	100.0%

relations, or whether they resulted from the negative impact from the occasional troublesome neighbour.

It was possible to compare these two alternative possibilities by introducing a new variable from the SCPR residential environments data set into the analysis. As well as being asked whether they would describe their road as *a road where the neighbours are helpful,* subjects had also been asked, *Is there anything you particularly dislike about living in this area?* This gave residents the opportunity to express any problems they might be having, or have had, with their neighbours. Complaints about the neighbours or about the *type of person* living nearby were coded as a neigbour problem.

In total, less than 1 in 10 people reported having problems with their neighbours. Clearly, the vast majority of respondents rated their neighbours as helpful and unproblematic. Unsurprisingly, a smaller proportion of those who described the neighbours on their road as helpful complained about them, 7.8 per cent, compared with 20.5 per cent of those who reported their neighbours as unhelpful. Nonetheless, there was considerable independence between the two variables. Eight per cent of those describing the neighbours on their road as helpful also reported having neighbour problems, and similarly, of the 21 per cent of people who did not describe their neighbours as helpful, nearly 80 per cent still reported having no problems with their neighbours.[3] Both having helpful neighbours and neighbour problems were significantly related to symptom levels (Table 4.3).

The associations between the two neighbouring variables – helpfulness and problems – and the objective residential environmental variables were examined. These proved extremely interesting. All of the residential environmental variables were significantly associated with the level of reported helpfulness of the road. In every case, busier, higher traffic environments were associated with lower levels of reported helpfulness. Neighbour problems, however, showed no consistent relationship to the environmental variables. Higher population densities (i.e. conurbations) were moderately associated with more neighbour problems, but the only traffic

Table 4.3: *Associations of the neighbouring variables with symptom levels*

	r	Partial r (controlling for age, sex, income and sensitivity)	
Neighbour helpfulness	−.110	−.118	(p < .0001)
Neighbour problems	.132	.123	(p < .0001)

variable (lg[traffic count]) that showed a significant correlation with neighbour problems suggested that higher flows were associated with marginally *lower* levels of neighbour problems. Neighbour helpfulness seemed to be influenced by aspects of the residential environment, while neighbour problems seemed to be relatively independent of such factors, presumably depending more on the individuals than the environment involved. The contrast, at least in retrospect, is intuitively plausible. If higher traffic flows reduce contact between neighbours, then this might reduce sociability and helpfulness, but without necessarily influencing the level of actual neighbour problems (perhaps even reducing them).

The independence of the two neighbouring variables was confirmed through a series of multiple regressions. When attempting to predict levels of symptoms, neighbour helpfulness and neighbour problems were found to have independent effects. However, as suggested by the simple correlations, while neighbour helpfulness did attenuate the influence of the environmental variables (hence suggesting that it might mediate their effects) neighbour problems were independent of them (with the exception of population density, which it slightly attenuated). The bulk of the variance accounted for by the residential environment in symptom levels was still mediated by the other variables (annoyance, etc.), but neighbour helpfulness helped to account for some of the effect. The independence of the effect of neighbour

Table 4.4: *Pairwise correlations between helpfulness, problems and other variables*

	Helpfulness	Problems
Age	**.053** ***	.003
Sex (Male = 1, female = 2)	.006	.019
School-age children	.012	−.007
Income	−.001	−.012
Class (0 = blue, 1 = white)	.023	−.031 *
Length of residence (area)	**.041** **	−.003
Objective noise	**−.145** ***	−.003
Lg (traffic flow)	**−.117** ***	**−.030** **
Cul-de-sac	**.041** **	.016
Mixed land use	**−.103** ***	.006
Population density	**−.117** ***	**.095** ***

[Unmarked = ns, * = p < .05, ** = p < .01, *** = p < .001; correlations with p < .01 marked in **bold** for clarity.]

problems suggests that having a neighbour who causes you major problems depends on the luck of the draw. Your environment – at least in terms of the variables measured here – can help, or hinder, how well you get on with your neighbours in general, but if there is one of them you just cannot stand, then you would probably have disliked him or her wherever you had lived.

Finally, it was found that there was no significant interaction between the two neighbouring variables and symptom levels, in other words, there was no evidence to suggest that the helpfulness of neighbours in general was able to buffer the adverse effects of some neighbours in particular. Instead, the effects of the two variables were found to be additive. This supports a main effects model for neighbouring behaviour on symptoms.

Further Evidence

As we have seen, there is substantial evidence to suggest that the physical environment can have real and significant effects on group and friendship formation, and on patterns of neighbouring behaviour. However, there remain further questions to be answered. We need to understand the details of the psychological processes involved and, in particular, we need to be able to understand what makes an environment unsupportive and how specific resultant behaviours can potentially affect mental health. The final studies examined in this chapter are of particular interest because of their multi-method and multi-level approach and their considera-tion of psychological processes. The studies go beyond asking if an environment can influence residents' behaviours in that particular setting by examining if the respondents' behaviour can be affected more generally, in other words, across settings. This is very important – if a design can foster withdrawal and hostility, and if this behaviour was found to generalize, then residents would not only lack social support in their immediate environment, but would find themselves with generally impoverished social support. Some of the studies below have already been mentioned briefly in Chapter 3 in the section on crowding, but now they will be explored in more detail.

Baum and Valins (1977) reported a series of studies examining the behavioural consequences of different dormitory designs. Two principle designs were studied. The first was a double-loaded corridor design, which housed students in groups of about 34 per floor. The bedrooms (shared by two residents) were arranged on either side of a long hallway (see below). A large bathroom area and a lounge area were shared by all 34 residents. As access was provided by the hallway, it was used by all floor residents.

The second dormitory was a suite design, which housed equal numbers of residents per floor, but broke the shared spaces on the floor into smaller units. Several suites were arranged along a central hallway, again shared by all floor residents. However, lounge and bathroom areas were provided within each suite, which consisted of two or three double-occupancy bedrooms grouped around a central lounge area and a small bathroom. In the corridor designs 34 people shared all living space outside the bedroom, whereas in the suite design, much of the living space was shared by not more than six people. However, the overall density of the two designs was the same.

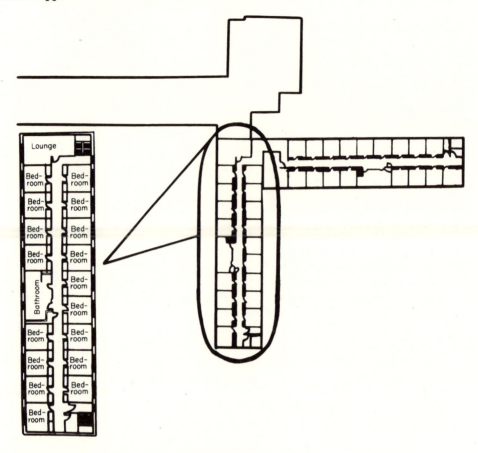

Figure 4.9: *The corridor design (Baum and Valins, 1977)*

Despite there being no significant initial differences between the student populations, sharp differences were found between the helpfulness and general atmosphere of the corridors. Corridor residents complained of unwanted social encounters, and reported less control over when, where, or with whom an interaction might occur. They reported more frequent passive contacts (usually in the hallways) and were more likely to feel that contact was excessive. The design of the corridor seemed 'responsible for promoting excessive, unwanted, and uncontrollable inter-action amongst neighbours'. Corridor residents exhibited more withdrawal and were more likely to attempt avoiding contact with neighbours. Group formation in the corridor dormitories was also inhibited.

The description of the withdrawal and hostility of the corridor residents is highly reminiscent of the withdrawal and hostility of Pruitt-Igoe residents described by Yancey, though somewhat milder. It is also easy to see similarities between the residents' experiences and the social overload and anonymity of the city dweller, as described by Stanley Milgram (Milgram, 1970; Wedmore and Freeman, 1984). The intensive contact of the corridor design, unlike the suite design, was not transformed into friendship. Contacts were divided between too many, and they were experienced as uncontrolled and stressful.

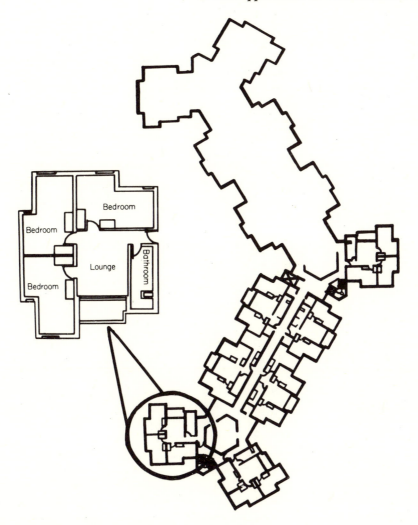

Figure 4.10: *The suite design (Baum and Valins, 1977)*

Baum and Valins also found that the withdrawal of corridor residents generalized to quite separate environments. In a seemingly unrelated situation, corridor and suite residents were required to wait a few minutes in the presence of a confederate (waiting for the start of an experiment). Corridor residents were found to sit further from the confederate, avoid eye contact, and initiate fewer conversations. Yet despite these coping behaviours, corridor residents remained significantly more uncomfortable than suite residents, even after several minutes (self-report data were later gathered). In another experiment, subjects were awaiting an aversive dental procedure. While waiting alone, corridor and suite residents experienced comparable discomfort, but when waiting with a confederate, suite residents experienced *less* stress while corridor residents experienced *more* stress. In a final two experiments, residents had to engage either in an exercise requiring competition or in one requiring cooperation. The results showed that having to compete (reducing interaction) as opposed to cooperating, or being ignored as opposed to being attended to, was more stressful for suite residents but less stressful for corridor residents. In other words, corridor residents actually preferred to be ignored. Evidently, corridor residents not only showed withdrawal in the context of the dormitory, but found interaction with strangers aversive in general. Again, the generalized coping strategy is highly reminiscent of the descriptions of the residents of the ill-fated Pruitt-Igoe project (Yancey, 1971) and indeed, of the residents of many other problem estates (Reynolds, 1986).

Similar, but less detailed, case studies of student dormitories that appear to undermine supportive behaviour have been reported by other researchers. Newman (1973) described some new, double-loaded dormitories at Sarah Lawrence College in Bronxville, New York, where:

> students in the new dorms feel isolated without any sense of community. It is claimed by college counsellors that the students easily fall into patterns of antisocial behaviour.

The atomization and alienation of the new dormitories, in contrast with the old dorms, was sufficiently serious for the college to be forced to seek their conversion to offices and classrooms. Another example mentioned with respect to crowding, has been reported by Zuckerman, Schmitz and Yosha (1977: 107). Zuckerman, *et al.*, compared two dormitory blocks. Block A housed 340 residents in a grid design described as *sociofugal* (reducing interaction). Block B housed 660 residents in a star-like design described as *sociopetal* (increasing interaction). Forty residents (29 male, 20 female) in each of the dormitories were asked to fill out an individually administered questionnaire. As predicted, the residents of block B reported being less involved with their roommates (p<.005), being in a worse mood (p<.01), and experiencing their dormitory as being more crowded (p<.005).

Baum and Valins' work has recently been replicated and extended by Evans and his colleagues. It may be recalled from the section on crowding that Lepore, *et al.*, demonstrated that students living in higher household densities for a period of eight months had higher levels of psychiatric symptoms than equivalent students living in less crowded conditions. This was despite the fact that when the students had moved into the accommodation there were no significant differences between the groups in their levels of psychiatric symptoms. In a follow-up to this study, Evans and Lepore (1993) examined the behaviour of the students in a separate laboratory experiment. Students were asked, in pairs, to perform a series of essay writing tasks. However, one of the pair was a confederate, and the situation was manipulated so that in some conditions the subjects were told that they had performed worse on the essay writing test than the confederate while in others they were told that they had performed better. The purpose of these manipulations was to examine (through a two-way mirror) the supportive and other behaviours of the subjects (the students from the crowded or uncrowded accommodation). Raters of the behaviours were blind to whether the subjects had come from a crowded or uncrowded household. Evans and Lepore discovered that those from crowded accommodation were (a) less likely than those from less crowded accommodation to seek, or respond to, support from the confederate after receiving a disappointing test score; (b) were less likely to offer support to the confederate when the confederate received a disappointing score; (c) were rated as more withdrawn than those from less crowded accommodation. In the analysis of the results, the researchers found that partialling out subjects' levels of withdrawal reduced the relationship between crowding and social support to insignificance. On this basis they argued that the crowded household conditions led the students to employ withdrawal as a coping strategy. Unfortunately, this coping strategy undermined the students' ability to give and receive social support from others. This lack of social support seemed to have been a major contributor to the negative effects (such as psychiatric symptoms) of the crowding.

The work of Baum and Valins, and Evans and Lepore shows how the physical environment can induce withdrawal and reduce social support in the home setting, and also how this behaviour (coping) can generalize to affect residents' social support in other contexts. This research is very significant because not only does it give us insights into the processes by which the environment can affect social support and mental health, but it also shows us how the individual's response to the environment can act to generalize and amplify its effects.

These studies of student populations illustrate many of the phenomena reported earlier in the chapter with non-student populations. The simple presence of others is not enough to ensure positive and supportive social relations. Indeed, the presence of many others can lead to poorer social relations and less social support if the individual is unable to regulate interactions. Faced with too many unwanted social interactions, people cope by withdrawing and becoming hostile to the presence of others. It is noteworthy that similar generalized coping mechanisms have been reported in city dwellers; city dwellers have been found to be more hostile than country dwellers, even when away from the city itself (Wedmore and Freeman, 1984).

On a final note, a more positive confirmation of the influence of the physical environment on the quality and form of relationships has been provided by a simple intervention study by Baum and Davis (1980). Baum and Davis found that by divid-

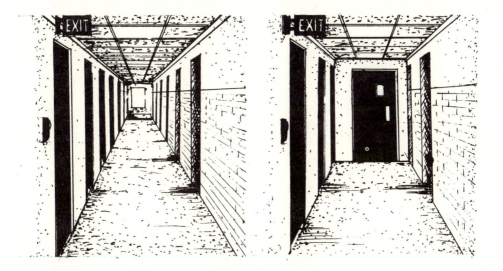

Figure 4.11: *The corridor design before and after invention*

ing the interior space of a corridor dormitory into smaller units, the negative consequences of the design, such as withdrawal and hostility were markedly reduced. This suggests that once we have understood how the environment affects people interact, we can use this knowledge to improve how people support and react to one another.

Conclusion: The Ideal Neighbour and The Ideal Neighbourhood

The overall conclusion of the evidence presented in this and the previous chapters is a relatively simple one – neighbours are in a unique position to either help or hinder each other. The previous two chapters showed that neighbours can be the cause of many chronic and irritating sources of stress such as noise, competition for limited resources, and invasion of privacy. Neighbours are often privy to an individual's comings and goings, and if the individual feels that the neighbours cannot be trusted, the neighbours can become a source of very real concern and even fear. However, the proximity of neighbours also makes them unique in the kinds of social support they can provide. At the very least, good neighbours can watch over one anothers' properties, receive each others' mail (if out), and support each other in issues of mutual local concern (Unger and Wandersman, 1985). If the relationship between neighbours becomes closer, then convenient help becomes available for looking after children or taking children to school, for assistance when ill, for borrowing household goods, for help with household chores, and so on. In some areas, particularly if the population is stable and socially homogeneous, local neighbouring relations may come to form a rich network of friendship and mutual support (Young and Willmott, 1957; Willmott, 1963; Cecil, 1988).

The evidence shows that the probability of positive and supportive neighbouring emerging is strongly influenced by the social and physical characteristics of the environment. Reasonably high levels of social homogeneity, or at least the presence of a *critical mass* of similar others, seems to be a prerequisite for positive neighbouring (or to put this in reverse, high levels of social heterogeneity tend to make supportive patterns of neighbouring less likely). The relevance of social homogeneity to patterns of local social relations and mental health is reflected in the group density effect. As the local concentration of an ethnic, religious or social group falls, the mental health problems of its members tend to rise. However, planners have recognized that they must balance the positive effects of social homogeneity against wider and longer term objectives such as the development of balanced communities and less segregated cities (Gans, 1961). Clearly, there is room for balance and the two sets of goals are not incompatible, the key lying in the scale of division. Planners, in principal, can foster urban mosaics of difference at the neighbourhood level while pursuing balance at the larger scale. Regrettably, empirical evidence suggests that in the past what planners have thought of as neighbourhoods have borne little relation to the much smaller scale of what residents think of as neighbourhoods (Willmott, 1967). It is hoped that things have now changed.

The physical characteristics of the environment also have a significant impact on neighbouring behaviour. For positive and supportive neighbouring relations to develop, environments must allow opportunities for residents to meet. An environment which makes it unpleasant to interact with others, such as a noisy environment, is likely to inhibit the development of positive neighbouring relations. Similarly, residential environments in which residents have little opportunity to meet, or in which their ability to recognize and interact with one another is undermined by the presence of large numbers of outsiders, are also less likely to be characterized by positive neighbouring relations.

Even when an environment is conducive to contact between neighbours, this will not necessarily lead to positive relations. Social contact is not enough. Residents must also be able to decide when, where and how they will interact with their neighbours. As when living in high social densities (see Chapter 3), a critical factor is control and the ability to regulate social interactions. The extent to which the physical environment allows self-regulated social interaction strongly influences the quality of neighbouring relations. If the environment forces residents to interact by channelling them together in ways that they cannot control other than by complete withdrawal (as in the corridor designs described by Baum and Valins or the Pruitt-Igoe project described by Yancey) then the net result tends to be hostility towards neighbours instead of good-will, and the experience of discomfort, a lack of privacy, and ironically, a feeling of isolation. Environments that provide opportunities for social interaction, but which do not force interaction, can lead to very positive and supportive neighbouring relations. Of course, these supportive social relations are only likely to emerge if the residents feel that they have something in common, in other words, if the population is sufficiently homogeneous. Sometimes personalities clash, and when this occurs, people are unlikely to get on whatever the environment.

An important observation can be made at this point. Normally we presume that the subjective experience of isolation (loneliness) must be at one end of a continuum at the other end of which is excessive social interaction. We can now see that this presumption is misleading. When a person is in a situation where he or she is unable to regulate who, when or where they will meet others, he or she is likely to experience both isolation *and* over-stimulation. An example of this is reported by Moore (1975), who found that residents of a development of flats complained more than similar house dwellers of loneliness *and* the lack of privacy. Residents' tensions focused around the use of shared facilities such as laundry rooms and waste disposal. The flat dwellers became inhibited about social interactions – they felt that they either had to avoid their neighbours or be prepared to invite them in (the evidence on the social and mental health consequences of flat dwelling is discussed in further detail in Chapter 5).

Today, the increasing affluence and mobility of the population may, to some extent, have de-emphasized the importance of local ties and neighbouring, although, the claims of social theorists such as Giddens that modernity has destroyed the importance of local ties and embedded affinity to place seems to be somewhat premature (see also Chapters 6 and 7). Perhaps more accurately, increasing affluence and mobility have changed the balance between the potential pros and cons of becoming involved with one's neighbours. The individual's dilemma is captured in Hirsch's (1977) phrase 'the economics of bad neighbouring'. Though in general, the individual may have a great deal to gain from the mutual support and friendship of neighbours, getting involved also risks becoming embroiled in asymmetrical and potentially unpleasant relationships. So if the individual does not *need* to get

Table 4.5: *A model of patterns of neighbouring behaviour*

		Physical environment	
		Undermines regulation	Allows regulation
Social environment	Heterogeneous	Conflict/withdrawal	Low contact
	Homogeneous	Conflict/withdrawal	Supportive relations

involved, then why bother? This attitude becomes expressed in the environment. As Bulmer (1986) put it, for the middle classes 'good fences make good neighbours.'

So what are the neighbours like in the ideal neighbourhood? Perhaps in most affluent areas, the ideal neighbour is simply a familiar stranger who tends his or her own property well but is otherwise notable only for his or her invisibility. In such areas it would be an error to expect to see buffering effects from good neighbours; a good neighbour should simply be one who was not a source of stress. On the other hand, among less affluent and resource-rich populations, a very different pattern would be expected. The ideal neighbouring relationship for those less affluent and able is one that involves real support. These groups must risk bad neighbours, but stand to gain much in return.

Notes

1. Breakdowns by specific disorder are not often reported, though a number of researchers have demonstrated the effect specifically for first admission rates for schizophrenia. However, diagnostic criteria may vary widely (especially in early studies), so conclusions about the differential importance of the effect in specific disorders cannot, at present, be made.
2. The figure of 49 per cent is an extremely low proportion: people are generally extremely reluctant to criticize the area they live in. In the SCPR residential environments data set, 89 per cent of respondents described themselves as satisfied with the area in which they lived.
3. The Pearson correlation between the two variables was a moderate (though highly significant) –.170 [though any correlation between two highly skewed dummy variables is always likely to be fairly low].

Chapter 5

The Environment as Symbol and the Example of the High Rise Flat

Introduction

In the previous chapters the focus has been on the relatively direct and mechanistic effects of the physical environment on behaviour, affect and mental health. In the next two chapters the focus moves away from classical environmental and social psychology towards a focus on the potential influence of *meaning* and *process*. In this chapter we shall also explore the controversy surrounding the relationship between different housing types and mental health. The example of the high-rise flat is used to demonstrate how the symbolic aspects of the environment may affect mental health alongside the more mechanistic consequences of the environment.

The Environment as Symbol

People, especially people in Britain, like to buy their own houses. This is sometimes explained as an economic phenomenon, though this does not take us very far. As soon as one queries what determines a products' exchange value then one soon becomes involved in discussions of use and symbolic value. The issue of interest here is encapsulated in the finding that many people have shown a preference for buying private housing rather than for renting public housing of objectively superior quality and at lower cost (Rapoport, 1982). A survey of 522 owner occupiers and council tenants (conducted in 1986) revealed that, across classes, the overwhelming majority say that they would prefer to own than rent (Saunders, 1989). Similarly, data from the British Social Attitude Surveys shows that, even during the severe recession of the early 1990s, a large majority of the population continued to favour home ownership over renting (Cairncross, 1992). This preference persisted despite a considerable increase in the numbers of people describing home owning as 'a risky investment' (up from 25 per cent in 1986 to 43 per cent in 1991). This overwhelming preference was shared by council tenants, less than one in five of whom said that they would choose to rent from the Local Authority if they could afford to purchase privately. The strong preference among outright homeowners (as opposed to mortgaged owners) exists despite the fact that many of the properties owned by this group are amongst the poorest housing stock and are owned by elderly people who find them very expensive to maintain.

It is difficult, if not impossible, to explain these preferences for ownership in terms of the physical quality of the home. Part of the effect could be explicable in terms of an anticipation of problems with neighbours or amenities, but most researchers see the effect as most readily explained in terms of the symbolic and/or in terms of perceived control (Saunders, 1989). In other words, the problem with renting a house, and especially a council house, has less to do with the objective quality of the house or area *per se*, but more to do with the fact it is *rented* or that it is *council* housing. The desire to own property, and the strong preference of certain property types and forms of tenure, points towards the possibility that the planned environment may be able to influence mental health not only through its function but through the meaning ascribed to it.

There are a number of ways of looking at *meaning* in housing and the environment. First, meaning can be seen through a phenomenological framework, an approach very popular amongst many contemporary schools of architecture. The phenomenological (or semiotic) literature attempts to explore and describe universal experiences of the environment through a linguistic type model (Seamon, 1984; Vesley, 1985). This literature is extremely subjective and does not attempt systematic evaluation. Its difficult and esoteric vocabulary of neologisms has been described as 'virtually unreadable' (Rapoport, 1982: 37). Also, it does not explore the social processes that may give rise to the affective response to a given environment. A second way of looking at meaning in the environment is by examining the meanings assigned to environments through labelling and stigmatization. A third, and closely related, way of looking at meaning is to see it in the context of individual experience, aspiration and past achievement. This stands in contrast to the semiotic approach in that the focus is on explaining individual differences in meaning rather than attempting to capture universal aesthetics. I shall concentrate here on the latter two approaches to the meaning of the built environment.

Labelling

Labelling refers to the ascription of a category or meaning to a person, place or object. As a social and cognitive process, labelling is convenient in that it provides a set of relatively stable expectancies which the individual can use to guide his or her behaviour. The label tends to presume or impute a high degree of consistency to the labelled target, and it is also evaluative in that it typically includes an assignment of valence (positive or negative, good or bad). The labelling process can be seen clearly in the phenomenon of stereotyping, where individuals or groups are classified according to some relatively clear surface characteristic, and then many other characteristics, attitudes and behaviours are presumed to also hold true for that individual or group (Myers, 1990).

It is important to emphasize that the stereotyping or labelling influences not only the person applying the label but also the target, and this latter influence can operate even if the person does not initially share the same set of labels or stereotypes. The labelling clearly affects the behaviour of the labeller as the stereotype or label is used to guide judgments and decisions (Should I employ this person? Should I buy a house in that area?). These judgments can obviously affect the person or area labelled in a direct way (they don't get the job, they can't sell the house), but they can affect the labelled target in subtler ways. The labeller's expectancies can inadvertently promote confirming behaviour and consistency in the target. Hence misleading subjects about the attractiveness of the person they are speaking to, for example, alters not only the behaviour of the subject but also the behaviour and self-image of the uninformed other (Snyder, Tanke and Berscheid, 1977).

When the labelling of an environment is considered, it can be seen as a multi-layered phenomenon. The labelling can occur by residents and by outsiders. People may describe somewhere as a *good* area or a *bad* area. Sometimes the intention of the label may be to convey something about the physical quality of the housing stock or the quality of the amenities, but typically the label also includes a reference to the type of people and behaviour that one would expect to find in the area. A dramatic example of this phenomenon can be seen in the French expression *sarcellite* which refers to social pathology; the term derives from a notorious housing development outside of Paris called Sarcelles (Lefebvre, 1984). The labelling of an area, whether good or bad, can have very dramatic and self-fulfilling effects on that area. Hence the perception that an area is becoming a good area strongly promotes gentrification, and the perception that an area is bad strongly promotes its decay. The occurrence of the process of gentrification is now so familiar as to require little further comment. Of particular interest is how residents actively attempt to maintain or create a positive label and prestige of an area by maintaining its public image and physical appearance and by excluding 'undesirable types' and developments (Newman, 1981). One of the ways in which residents attempt to improve the image of their area is by distorting their cognitive maps of the neighbourhood to include high-status, well-kept areas, and by excluding areas that are seen as less desirable (Rapoport, 1977). Another way is by literally renaming the area, for example, by renaming Battersea as South Chelsea (Chelsea being seen as a better area) or Rochester as Rochester-upon-Medway (to emphasize that the town is on the river). This type of selective distortion is, of course, highly reminiscent of the type of cognitive process employed by people in the maintenance of self-esteem (if we do a task and it turns out well, we attribute it to ourselves; if it turns out badly, we blame it on someone or something else). Another consequence of status maintenance is the NIMBY syndrome: people favour develop-ment but invariably 'Not in my back yard'. The differential success of residents' efforts to maintain the image of their neighbourhood significantly determines the values of their properties and the stability of spatial patterns of social segregation (Firey, 1945).

When residents are not successful in their attempts to maintain the positive image of an area, the value of an area can decline at an extremely fast and self-propagating rate. Newman (1980) illustrated how this occurred to many of the very prestigious private streets of St. Louis, Missouri, due the process of *tipping*. As soon as the fear arose that a street might lose its prestige, perhaps because of the arrival of a single Black family, residents started to move out, thereby causing the value of the properties to fall, which caused further anxiety and prompted further exodus, and so on. Speculators were then able to afford to buy properties, subdivide them into flats for the less affluent, and within a relatively short period of time the nature of the area would change completely.

Within Britain, the dramatic effects of the negative labelling of an area is seen most clearly in the occurrence of so-called *problem estates*. Problem estates arise where a housing estate (typically a council estate) receives a negative image, typically because of the placing of a few high-profile problem families or a disproportionate number of under-15 children on an estate which is easily identifiable as a whole (Department of the Environment, 1981a, b, c). As soon as the estate begins to receive a negative image, potential residents become less likely to apply to live there and, relative to other estates, its waiting list becomes relatively short. This leads to the situation where only those who are relatively desperate are prepared to move onto the estate, such as poor single-parent families, and this exaggerates the unusual demographics and poverty of the population further, and a classic downward spiral is established (Reynolds, 1986).

Yet, as already mentioned, when an estate gets a bad reputation, the degree to which the label refers to the estate *per se*, and the degree to which it refers to the population becomes very unclear. A notorious example is the blaming of slum-dwellers (such as ethnic minorities) for the occurrence of the slum rather than seeing these people as the victims of the slum (Smith, 1988). The question is then, to what extent does the stigmatization of certain estates translate into the stigmatization of the individuals who live on them? Second, to what extent, if at all, does this stigmatization affect the mental health of residents over and above any influence that the physical and social environment may already have?

The first question is easier to answer than the second. Apart from the defining features of problem estates – that people are reluctant to rent or buy housing in them, and that turnover in these estates is very high – qualitative studies clearly show that the residents of problem estates feel that they are stigmatized. Damer (1976), for example, describes a housing estate built in a working-class area of Glasgow called Wine Alley. Local residents resented the fact that the estate was used to rehouse slum clearance tenants from the Gorbals rather than local residents, and this resentment was reflected in the press which sensationalized any misdemeanours of the new residents. Damer found that residents of the estate came to accept the deviant image of the estate as seen by outsiders. Residents retreated 'into the womb of their houses whence they viewed the outside world of their neighbours with fear and suspicion', and residents of the estate blamed its problems on the 'riffraff' that had been dumped there. Indeed, in general, rather than economic deprivation *per se* being the hallmark of problem estates, it is the tension between the majority of the residents and the (perceived) riffraff that tends to distinguish problem estates from others (Reynolds, 1986). Residents internalize the bad name of the estate but they attempt to deal with it by blaming a minority of other residents. However, this strategy tends to be only partially successful as people outside the estate typically do not make the same distinction.[1]

Demonstrating that the negative image of an estate or area can be internalized to the extent that it affects the residents' mental health is more difficult. Rates of mental ill-health vary by tenure, with homeowners and mortgagees having better mental health than those who rent. Home ownership has been found to predict lower levels of depression even after family income has been controlled for (Mirowsky and Ross, 1989). However, this evidence is not conclusive of a causal relationship from ownership to mental health because we cannot be sure of the direction of causation. Also, while it is plausible that the positive effect of home ownership is to do with the symbolic aspect of owning a home, it is also possible that it is to do with other aspects of the environment associated with owner-occupation living such as higher levels of control (see Chapter 6).

A second source of evidence comes from an extensive study by Byrne, *et al.*, (1986) of the relationship between housing conditions and the health of council tenants in Britain. By examining only council tenants, the Byrne, *et al.*, study was able to control for many otherwise compounding factors, including tenure. Byrne, *et al.*, found that even after having controlled for age, physical health, sex and household class, those people who lived in 'difficult to let' housing were significantly more distressed than their peers living in 'good' housing (p.<.001). Furthermore, the authors found that housing type *on its own* was not related to psychological distress, in other words, there was no main effect for housing type (though see later for a discussion of the interactions). Thus, the authors concluded that psychological distress was associated with the area rather than the objective form or quality of the housing.

The evidence presented by Byrne, *et al.*, is strongly consistent with the hypothesis that the reputation of an estate influences mental health. Residents of the estates with poor reputations were certainly very unhappy about living there; 78 per cent expressed a desire to move out of their current accommodation, and 53 per cent had already submitted official applications to the local authority's housing department. However, it is still not possible to isolate the precise cause of the association. It could also have been due to other factors or mediators such as the stress caused by fear of crime or problems with neighbours as well as to stigma *per se.*

In summary, two conclusions are appropriate. First, the labelling of areas as bad is a major cause of the downward spiral of some areas relative to others and of the concentration and compounding of many types of social pathologies as reported in ecological studies (Levine, Miyake and Lee, 1989). In other words, symbolic aspects of the environment act to catalyze and compound other kinds of environmental design problems. Second, labelling and stigmatization may also have a direct effect on the self-image and mental health of residents, though this has yet to be conclusively proven.

Aspiration-achievement Discrepancy

A house may be large or small; as long as the surrounding houses are equally small, it satisfies all social demands for a dwelling. But let a palace arise beside the little house, and it shrinks from a little house into a hut. (Karl Marx, quoted in Myers, 1990: 382)

A second way of looking at the symbolic aspect of an individual's housing environment is by considering the discrepancy between the individual's level of aspiration and his or her perceived level of achievement. The discrepancy is closely related to labelling in as far as achievement tends to be defined through the eyes of others, but it differs in as far as aspiration and achievement are also individual variables. Individuals' aspirations and perceptions of achievement partly result from comparisons to others and partly from comparisons to their own past. When aspirations are higher than perceived achievements, *relative deprivation* is experienced. Research on military personnel during World War II found that levels of satisfaction with rates of promotion were lowest in the parts of the services which had the highest rates of promotions (Merton and Kitt, 1950). Large numbers of promotions led to greater rises in aspirations than it did to feelings of achievement. Similarly, most Americans have been found to believe that even a small increase in their income would make them happier, yet in the 30 years from 1957 to 1987 – during which time real incomes increased by over two-fold – the proportion of Americans describing themselves as 'very happy' actually *fell* (Myers, 1990).

This psychological phenomena has forced sociologists and economists to define wealth and poverty in relative terms (Townsend, 1979).

> By necessaries I understand not only the commodities which are indispensably necessary for the support of life, but what ever the custom of the country renders it indecent for creditable people, even the lowest order, to be without. (Smith, 1776: 351)

Hence, over two-thirds of Americans describe a television set, a clothes dryer and aluminium foil as 'necessities' rather than as a 'luxury you could do without' (*Public Opinion*, 1984) while millions in the third world struggle just to eat.

The evidence suggests that individuals' perceptions of what constitutes *adequate* housing operate in a similarly relativistic way. In a survey of over 2000 households, the Building Research Establishment attempted to establish which features of a house and its surroundings were felt to be the most important in making a home fit to live in (Britten, 1977). Ten items were identified as *basic necessities* by over 70 per cent of households. The ten most frequently identified items were (in descending order): electric lighting, hot water supply, bathroom, refuse disposal, internal toilet, living-room heating, power points, free from damp, ventilation, and daylight. However, the single most important predictor of the factors considered as basic necessities by individual respondents was their own housing experience and the amenities available to them at the present time. Householders' opinions were much more closely related to their own housing experience than to any demographic or sociological variables. Though cause and effect cannot be conclusively determined, this evidence is strongly supportive of an aspiration–achievement model of housing. Once an individual has experienced a given amenity such as hot water, an inside toilet, or a back garden, the amenity becomes seen as a necessity and its absence becomes a source of some irritation or distress. This suggests that the influence of poor environments on mental health may not be a simple function of their absolute quality or level of amenities, but instead may relate to the discrepancy between the individual's image of a good home and the reality of his or her present dwelling.

In terms of mental health, a number of studies have demonstrated the importance of the aspiration–achievement discrepancy. Perhaps the most elegant of these are a series of studies conducted by Kleiner and Parker (1966, 1970) of American Blacks. Kleiner and Parker found that Blacks from the North had consistently higher psychiatric admission rates than Blacks from the South, despite the fact that racism was widely considered to be more blatant and explicit in the South than in the North. Kleiner and Parker found that in Philadelphia, a city which included Black migrants from both North and South, Northern Blacks continued to show substantially higher first psychiatric admission rates. Surveys of northern Blacks showed that they were aspiring to substantially higher goals than southern Blacks, though there was little evidence to suggest that one group was being any more successful than the other. The authors therefore concluded that the reason why the northern Blacks were suffering from higher first psychiatric admission rates and greater levels of dissatisfaction than southern Blacks was due to the substantially greater discrepancy they experienced between their aspirations and their otherwise equivalent achievements. Another example is provided by Brenner (1973) who found that economic recessions had a more serious effect on the mental health of the affluent than those already suffering from poverty.

The aspiration–achievement model stands in some contrast to most classical environmental psychology models which tend to assume that the environment has absolute effects (see Chapters 2 and 3). For example, much of the literature on the effects of density assumed that, in some absolute sense, the higher the level of density, the higher the level of crowding and discomfort that would be experienced. Yet, as later became apparent, in some areas of the world (for example, Hong Kong) people live at densities which would be considered completely appalling in Western industrialized countries, but show little evidence of serious distress (Mitchell, 1971). The simple deduction might have been made that density has no bearing on mental health, but this would certainly be wrong. If someone who had come to see it as normal to have a room of his or her own had to live in a room shared with three or four others, it is very unlikely that he or she would not experience this with some distress. Indeed, where researchers have examined relative changes in density, clear effects have been found (Wener and Keys, 1988; see Chapter 3).

In summary, there seems to be good evidence for the relevance of aspiration–achievement discrepancies in the understanding of the relationship between mental illness and the planned environment. Individuals' experiences advance their aspirations like a ratchet, and today's aspirations become tomorrow's necessities.

The Example of the High-rise Flat

Architecture is the masterly correct and magnificent play of masses brought together in light. (Le Corbusier, 1927; quoted in Short, 1989: 36)

permanent high-rise dwellers are likely to be inadequate, indifferent and coddled . . . we must not go on blindly building these vertical coffins for the premature death of our civilization. (Cappon, 1971: 431)

Whatever the actual evidence concerning the effects of the high-rise on mental health, one thing is certain, *opinions* about the effects of the high-rise are extremely strong. The high-rise flat is the most controversial of modern residential building forms. A number of associations have been reported between different housing types (such as the high-rise flat) and mental ill-health. As we shall see, these associations are difficult to understand without reference to the meaning of the environment to the individual (aspiration–achievement) and label imposed by the context (labelling).

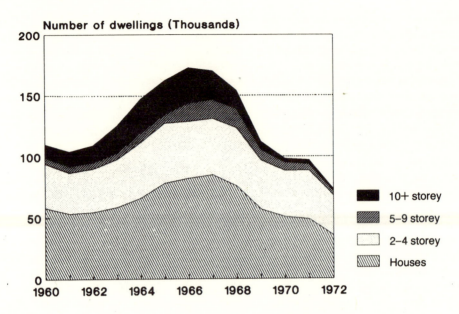

Figure 5.1: *The number of dwellings of different types built from 1960–72 for Local Authorities and New Towns, England and Wales. (Data: Gittus, 1976).*

In Britain, there was a large and relatively sustained period of building after the Second World War to provide more public sector housing. Part of this building programme arose out of the promise of 'homes for heroes' for returning soldiers and from the redevelopment of dwellings damaged during the war. Political pressures for the rapid provision of housing, the development of new system building techniques, and the influential aesthetics of the time led to the building of substantial numbers of high-rise flats in the 1960s. By 1969, over 300000 high-rise flats had been built (Jephcott, 1971).

As high-rise buildings were substantially more expensive to build than equivalent houses (being up to around double the cost per dwelling), they were only viable because of central government subsidies (Gittus, 1976). Under the Housing Subsidies Act of 1956, the basic (60-year) subsidy per new dwelling was £22.05 (about £280 in 1995 pounds or around $410 US dollars) in buildings less than 4-storeys, but this rose to a subsidy per dwelling of £50 (£640) in buildings of 6-storeys or more plus an additional subsidy of £1.75 (£22) per dwelling above the sixth, hence dwellings in a 15-storey building would attract a subsidy of £66 per year (£840 or $1250) – approximately three times that of a normal house.[2] (The storey height in each case referred to the whole building, not to the elevation of the dwelling itself.) Policies changed in 1967 with a revamping of the subsidy system, the introduction of a yardstick blocking subsidies to buildings over a certain unit cost, and the added obligation to conform to the Parker-Morris building standards. The change of heart was reinforced by the partial collapse of the system built flats at Ronan Point on 16 May 1968 which killed two people. The collapse brought extra expenses to local authorities who were obliged to inspect and modify their buildings. The collapse also gave expression to public misgivings about the dangers of high-rise living.

Although the numbers of high-rise flats built after this date shrunk considerably, the debate surrounding them, if anything, increased. Furthermore, though most western governments have now abandoned the building of public high-rise flats, many third-world governments have since begun building them (Farahat and Cebeci, 1982).

In the review that follows, the empirical evidence on the effects of living in flats will be brought together and appraised, and an attempt will be made to interpret the findings in terms of the potential channels of influence described in the preceding literature reviews: environmental stress, social support, and symbolic aspects of the environment.

The Evidence: Does Flat Dwelling Affect Mental Health?

Although there are a large number of articles discussing the influence of flat dwelling on mental health, only a small proportion of these present empirical evidence. The table shows a summary of studies that have attempted to test either the hypothesis that flat dwellers have different levels of mental health to house dwellers or the hypothesis that mental health varies with the height of the dwelling from the ground.

Table 5.1: *Summary of studies on the effects of flat dwelling*

Date	Author	Effect of flat dwelling and summary of result	
1962	Wilner, *et al.*	Positive	Slum-dwellers moved into new flats showed reduced accidents, slight improvement in health and very slight improvement in self-concept (USA)
1967	Fanning	Negative	Army wives and children showed worse mental health in flats than houses. Strong methodology.
1972	DoE	Mixed	'No clear pattern' for differing designs in levels of psychosomatic symptoms.
1974	Bagley	Negative	Demographically similar house dwellers less neurotic and consulted their GPs less often for a 'nervous complaint' than flat dwellers.
1974	Moore	Mixed	Non-significant tendency for Army wives to have higher symptoms and see GP more often, but compounded with other population differences.
1974	Goodman	Negative	Elevated episode rate in 0–4 yr. olds in deck-access flats, higher rates of mental illness in 45–65 yr. olds, and higher rates of illness by height.
1974	Ineichen and Hooper	Mixed	Elevated behaviour problems with children in high-rise, but physical and mental health of wives often even worse among house renters in urban centre.
1974	Richman	Negative	Matched families: higher levels of depression for women in flats but, if anything, worse rates in low rise. However, high-rise dwellers most dissatisfied.
1976	Moore	Negative	Same population as in Moore 1974. Found flat dwellers significantly more neurotic (personality scale) than house dwellers.

Table 5.1 *continued*

1976	Gittus	Negative	Mothers in flats reported significantly more psychosomatic symptoms than those in houses and more problems for the under-5s, especially with more than one.
1977	Gillis	Mixed	Floor level positively associated with psychological strain in women, but negatively associated with strain in men.
1980	Saegert	Negative	Children in 14-storey building were more disturbed than equivalent children in a 3-storey building.
1982	Edwards, *et al.*	Negative	Men living in flats had elevated levels of symptoms (Langner–22) but no significant difference for women. Arguments with partners and children more frequent in flats.
1984	Hannay	Negative	Having controlled for age and sex, those living on the fifth floor or above were found to have significantly more psychiatric symptoms than those living on lower floors or houses.
1986	Byrne, *et al.*	Mixed	No main effect of housing type but strong interaction: levels of psychological distress significantly higher in *bad areas* when high-rises.

The measures of mental ill-health used in the studies vary, but typically they involve the use of some kind of symptom checklist, such as the Langner–22. Concerning flat dwelling, only one of the published studies has reported flat dwellers as having better mental health than house dwellers (Wilner, *et al.*, 1962). Nine studies, however, have reported flat dwellers as suffering from significantly worse mental health than matched house dwellers (Fanning, 1967; Bagley, 1974; Goodman, 1974; Richman, 1974; Moore, 1976; Gittus, 1976; Saegert, 1980; Edwards, *et al.*, 1982; Hannay, 1984). The remaining studies have reported either non-significant differences (DoE, 1972a; Moore, 1974) or more complex or conditional relationships (Ineichen and Hooper, 1974; Gillis, 1977; Byrne et al., 1986).[3]

The problem for researchers is that it is extremely rare that a homogeneous population is randomly sorted between different dwelling types, and this has proved the biggest problem in attempts to resolve the issue. In particular, the widespread belief that flats are unsuitable for young children has meant that the demographic structure of those assigned to flats rather than houses has tended to be very different, few families with young children being put in flats. Furthermore, people are not passive agents – if they are unhappy with their home they vote with their feet. Numerous studies have shown that flat dwellers tend to be less satisfied and more eager to move than house dwellers, and especially if they have children (Richman, 1974; Gittus, 1976; Frank, 1983). A follow-up of the study by Ineichen and Hooper (1974) at 18 months showed that 60 per cent of the flat dwellers had moved compared with only 40 per cent of the house dwellers (Ineichen, 1979). This level of differential movement may well obscure or iron out differences that would otherwise exist (Cook and Morgan, 1982). Differential patterns of movement almost certainly explain the complex and obscure differences that are often found in studies which fail to carefully match comparison groups or to provide adequate controls (DoE, 1972; Ineichen and Hooper, 1974; Kasl *et al.*, 1982).

However, taking the literature as a whole, the impression is given that flat dwelling is associated with slightly poorer mental health than living in a house, at least for families with young children. This was also the conclusion drawn by Kellett (1989) after conducting a similar, though less specific review. The only study which reported a positive effect of flat dwelling involved a comparison with new apartments to the previous slum rather than to equivalent new houses (Wilner, *et al.*, 1962), and the design of the apartments was relatively unusual (see below). Perhaps more importantly, the studies with the best methodologies have been amongst those which have shown the clearest evidence of adverse effects (Fanning, 1967; Richman, 1974; Saegert, 1980). The study by Fanning, for example, involved a comparison between the health of the wives of British servicemen stationed in Germany living either in flats or in houses of equivalent size. All the servicemen were non-commissioned and of the same rank, all were assigned to a house or flat by chance, all shared comparable social facilities, and all were under the care of the same medical practice (which was within walking distance). This study, therefore, represented a near perfect design. Criticisms that have subsequently been made of the study (Ineichen, 1979; Freeman, 1984b) appear to have arisen out of a confusion of Fanning's study with a later attempted replication by Moore (1974) and the comments made by Moore about the problems with compounded differences in his own study. Fanning found that flat dwellers suffered from over double the rate of respiratory disorders, of psychoneurotic disorders, and of vague symptoms for which no diagnosis was made. The author hypothesized that the high rates of these disorders resulted from the confinement of mothers with small children in the flat as they had no private gardens. Evidence for the hypothesis was provided in the finding that the rates of disorder were particularly elevated for mothers aged 20–29, whose first consultation rates of psychoneurotic disorders over a 10-week period were 103.4 for flat dwellers and 38.9 for house dwellers (per 1000 residents). Rates for those aged 30–39, however, were very similar (62.5 versus 60.0).

The evidence on the relationship between mental health and building height is considerably more ambiguous. Once again, differential sorting tends to result in systematic differences in the type of households living at different building heights. Even among populations which are relatively favourable to flats, residents tend to believe that higher flats are unsuitable for young children (Jephcott, 1971; Churchman and Ginsberg, 1984). Certainly in Britain in the last fifteen years, local authorities have tried not to assign high flats to families with children, if only because of public pressure and the damage these children seem able to cause to the buildings.

An adverse effect of height was found by Goodman (1974) who found rates of mental illness among residents of a deck access scheme increased as the access level rose from the ground. Saegert (1980) found that rates of disturbed behaviour in children were higher in a 14 than 3-storey building. However, Richman (1974) found that rates of depression among mothers were, if anything, higher in her sample of low-rise than high-rise flats, though the difference was non-significant and possibly due to the higher levels of mobility of people from the high-rise. The most sophisticated and thorough study of the relationship between dwelling height and mental health, however, is that of Gillis (1977) of public housing projects in Calgary and Edmonton, Canada. All subjects (442) were adults with children living at home.

As the rents of the housing were based on income rather than the property, there was no reason for the normal income based selection to have occurred. Gillis found that for women, higher floor levels were associated with progressively worse mental health, with the exception of the ground floor which was also associated with poor mental health. Yet for men, the reverse pattern was found, higher floor levels being associated with *better* mental health. These relationships were found to remain significant even after controlling for household composition, socio-economic status, demographic characteristics and three plausible intervening factors: confinement, social isolation, and problems with child supervision.

In summary, the evidence from Britain and North America suggests that flat dwellers have slightly higher levels of mental ill-health than matched house dwellers, and especially for women with children. Very few studies have examined the influence on men, though some evidence exists for an adverse effect (Edwards, Booth and Edwards, 1982). However, all studies have been based on less affluent populations (principally because it is only in public housing that residential sorting is not completely compounded with income). It remains very uncertain whether the same effects would be found in affluent populations, first, because these groups can afford to minimize the negative aspects of any given environment, and second, because the meaning of a physically similar environment might be transformed by positive labelling. Concerning the effect of the height of the dwelling from the ground, the evidence suggests a slight negative effect on women with children, with the suggestion of an opposite effect on men.

These conclusions are based upon the assumption that the effect of one flat is very much like the effect of any other flat, and differences in the details of designs are ignored. Clearly, this may not be a fair assumption. Furthermore, the mediators of an effect on mental health may not be the same across all situations. I shall now briefly examine what these mediators might be.

Alternative Interpretations

Environmental stress

A popular belief about developments of flats is that their high density is the cause of many of their problems. However, the population or neighbourhood density of developments of flats rarely exceeds the densities seen in areas of traditional terraced housing. One of the main reasons for building high-rises was the intention to free ground space in otherwise very dense areas, hence the presence of this space means that the average population density of the developments tend to be only moderate.

A more plausible explanation is that problems arise where a large number of people have to share a common entrance, and where the absolute size of developments is very large. When developments become very large, and when large numbers share common entrances, levels of vandalism and turnover increase, and residents feel less safe and less attached to the development (Newman, 1973; Frank, 1983; Lefebvre, 1984; Coleman, 1985). Contrary to popular belief, flats are actually safer than houses in terms of burglary though, as was shown in Chapter 3, this does not mean that levels of fear are any lower. Of course, if residents are relatively affluent, they can afford to minimize the problem of crime (and fear) by paying for doormen and other security and maintenance measures.

Irrespective of income-level, for families with children anxieties are frequently voiced about the possibility that children might fall from balconies (Jephcott, 1971; Churchman and Ginsberg, 1984). Parental anxieties about looking after young children in flats seem to be a cross-national phenomenon (van Vliet, 1983), but there is evidence to suggest that this may have as much to do with the play facilities provided as with the flats themselves. The provision of play facilities for children in flats has tended to be very poor, but there is evidence to suggest that when well-designed play facilities are provided around flats the problems and dissatisfactions associated with flat dwelling can be markedly attenuated (Gittus, 1976; Holahan, 1976; van Vliet, 1983). It is noteworthy that the one study which showed slight positive effects (Wilner, *et al.*, 1962) was of a development of flats which incorporated a shared space on each floor specifically designed for children to play.

Environmentally induced stress, particularly concerning young children and fear of crime, is almost certainly relevant to levels of residential satisfaction in different housing types and is probably relevant to the elevated levels of psychological distress among flat dwellers, but much of the effect may relate to spaces outside the flats rather than within them.

Social support

The idea that flats cause social isolation is probably the most popular explanation of the poorer mental health of flat dwellers both within the academic literature and among the public. A number of studies have shown that (at least for women) flat dwelling is associated with higher levels of loneliness (Richman, 1974; Moore, 1975; Gittus, 1976). However, the popular impression that flat dwellers have smaller social networks and less social contacts has *not* been confirmed. In fact, on average, flat dwellers have been found to have at least as many friends and social contacts as equivalent house dwellers, and often more (Moore, 1975; Frank, 1983; Churchman and Ginsberg, 1984).

These results may seem slightly paradoxical, but they illustrate perfectly the issues described in the chapter on social support and the environment (Chapter 4). Flat dwellers complain far more of the lack of privacy than house dwellers. In terms of intuitive belief, we tend to assume that loneliness must be at one end of a continuum with over-stimulation and the lack of privacy at the other. The residents of large blocks of flats, however, simultaneously complain of both. They tend to feel both lonely *and* lacking in privacy. The critical issue seems to be the lack of the ability to regulate social interaction. Residents must either withdraw into their flats or risk unwanted social interactions in the public spaces outside. In the absence of semi-private spaces which allow for informal interaction without commitment, each social interaction becomes an all or nothing experience. Flat dwellers cannot chat over the garden fence (interacting, but without further intrusion), and they do not know to whom they will be obliged to talk (or ignore) while they wait for the lift, make their way down the stairs or through the shared entrance hall.

It is very likely, therefore, that some of the dissatisfaction and distress that has been found to be associated with flat dwelling relates to patterns of social interaction and support. This means that it should be possible to minimize these problems by careful design such as the avoidance of entrances and lifts shared by very large numbers, and by attempts to provide semi-private spaces which allow for more graded and regulated social interaction. However, even when the effects of social support have been considered, there is evidence to suggest that something still remains to be explained.

Symbol

Although environmental stress and the type of social interaction fostered may account for a large amount of the effects of flat dwelling on satisfaction and mental health, some of the effects reported in the literature do not seem to be reducible to effects of the environment 'as a machine'.

In the study of Canadian public housing by Gillis (1977), floor level was found to be a strong, direct and durable predictor of psychological strain among women, yet a weaker, though as persistent, negative predictor of strain among men. In this study, detailed information was also gathered about a large number of possible mediators of the effects including levels of confinement, activity outside the home, social isolation, and problems with child supervision, as well as background socio-economic, household, and demographic variables. Yet controlling for all these variables did not eliminate the effects of floor height, though many of the variables had independent effects of their own. The resilience of the effects of floor height on psychological strain led Gillis to postulate that the effects must result from 'the *aesthetics* rather than the function of design' (p. 427) Gillis suggested that the disjunction between residents' actual and idealized environments was affecting their mental health rather than any functional consequence of height.

> The high rise may merely be a constant and dramatic reminder to women that they fail to occupy a single, detached house, an important goal to the occupants of traditional wife-mother status roles (Gillis, 1977: 427–8).

Men on the other hand:

> may be attracted to high-rise living, seeing it as symbolic of upward social mobility (rent in high-rise apartments is frequently a direct correlate of floor level) and from a man's perspective, the 'good life' (Gillis, 1977: 427).

Clearly, these gendered and culturally specific aspirations may not hold across all populations or across time, but they indicate the potential importance of ascribed meaning in housing related outcomes. In a separate study, also of Canadian public housing, Edwards, *et al.*, (1982) proposed a similar symbolic explanation for their finding that apartment living was associated with adverse effects on family relations and higher levels of marital discord even after controlling for age, education and socio-economic differences. The authors suggested that the effects seemed to have been related to the unfulfilled preferences of the residents and their resulting dissatisfaction. Combining the results of the two studies one could postulate that the higher levels of marital discord found in apartment dwellers could have resulted specifically from the contrasting gender-specific differences in aesthetic preferences described by Gillis. Perhaps when these studies are replicated in the future the findings will be somewhat different reflecting changed values, but as they stand, the results provide support for the aspiration–achievement model proposed earlier in the chapter.

Finally, symbolic effects may account for findings such as that reported by Byrne, *et al.*, (1986) who found that although high-rise flats had no main effect on mental health, they did have a highly significant interaction with area. In *good* areas of public housing, high-rises were not associated with mental health problems, but in *bad* or difficult to let areas high-rises were associated with extremely poor mental health. This effect may have resulted from some kind of complex selection effect, but an alternative (though related) explanation is that the effect resulted from a labelling process. The literal prominence of the high-rise makes it a form that is especially susceptible to labelling. If an area gets a bad reputation, which the difficult to let areas obviously had, then almost inevitably the easy to identify high-rises would have become the target of the most severe stigmatization.

Summary

In this chapter it has been shown that symbolic aspects of the environment are also implicated in the relationship between mental health and the planned environment. Residential environments can become labelled or stigmatized, and these labels have a significant impact on the areas labelled and on the residents who live in them. Secondly, the personal meanings of environments can be very important. An individual's aspirations and expectancies have a major effect on their judgments about the quality and acceptability of their home. Even if a home appears good by some absolute external standard, if it fails to match the individual's aspirations it will lead to disappointment and dissatisfaction. Finally, the issue was illustrated by an examination of the evidence on the relationship between flat dwelling and mental health. It was found that the evidence does suggest some adverse effects of flat dwelling on mental health, at least in public sector housing. The effects were found to be mediated not only to the relatively direct, mechanistic influences of the environment, but also by the symbolic aspects of the environment.

Notes

1   For example, a number of residents on a problem estate interviewed for some of my own research (the Eastlake estate, see Chapter 7) graphically described how people outside the estate would become reserved or even hostile when they realized that they were speaking to someone from the notorious Eastlake estate.

2   Data on the relative purchasing power of the 1956 and 1995 pound are based on extrapolations derived from Social Trends (1994).

3   One could argue, here as elsewhere, that there might exist many studies which showed no evidence of a relationship between flat dwelling and mental ill-health, but that they have never been published due to the reluctance of journals to publish non-significant results. However, if no relationship exists and the positive findings reported here all arose by chance, one would still have to explain the reason why more of these chance results were not of positive results in the *opposite* direction, in other words, of flat dwellers having significantly better mental health.

Appendix

C.1: *The scale used by Bryne*, et al *(1986) was*:

1) Are you affected by

       a) depression or weeping so that you can't face your work or mix with people?
       b) being unable to concentrate?
       c) sleeping badly
       d) feeling that it's too much effort to do anything?
       e) feeling helpless and overwhelmed?

2) Do you have trouble with your nerves?

The index of psychological distress was the sum of all *yes* responses.

Chapter 6

The Planning Process and Mental Health

Introduction – The Planning Process

The potential relevance of the planning process to mental health is two-fold. First, it can have an *indirect* effect on mental health as a preceding cause of many of the aspects of the environment already described as potentially relevant to mental health in earlier chapters such as pollution, density, traffic, fear of crime, or the relations between neighbours (all of which have been shown to be affected by design features). However, it was reasonable to discuss these aspects of the environment without close reference to the planning process that may have helped create them. Generally, the planning process is not a unique cause of these environmental problems and would not have explained further variance in levels of distress.[1] In other words, the causal relevance of the planning process could be considered as independent from the final effects. Second, the planning process may have a *direct* effect on mental health. Sometimes the planning process cannot be separated from its outcome as the process itself is implicated in how the event or environment is experienced. Perhaps the clearest instance of this is the effect of relocation and slum clearance, which is explored below. This discussion is followed by a more general consideration of the importance of resident participation in the planning process. The possible conflict between the aesthetics of designers and residents is discussed. Finally, a study is presented of the impact of a series of planning decisions on the 2000 residents of a New Town housing estate unexpectedly threatened with demolition.

Relocation and Slum Clearance

In Chapter 1, the literature on the mental health of New Town residents was reviewed and the findings were found to be complex and contradictory. Much to the disappointment of the planners and politicians involved, moving people out of slums into new and relatively high quality housing estates did not necessarily lead to high levels of satisfaction and sometimes appeared to result in elevated rates of mental ill-health and the so-called *New Town blues* (Taylor, 1938; Martin, Brotherston and Chave, 1957; Higgins, 1984). One of the main reasons for the disappointing findings was identified as the elevated rates of distress caused by the move rather than the new environment *per se*. The most recent arrivals to new estates were found to be suffering from the highest rates of neuroses (Bagley, 1974) though a number of studies suggested that this elevation was a relatively temporary effect (Young and Willmott, 1957; Clout, 1962; Willmott 1967; Kasl, 1974).

Having completed the literature reviews of the previous chapters, we can see that it is unlikely that much of the variation in mental health associated with the new towns and estates resulted from higher levels of classical environmental stress as, in general, the new housing was of better quality than the old, with the possible exception of the availability of some amenities. In terms of classical environmental stress, one would have expected the residents of the new towns to have had better mental health (see Chapter 2). More plausibly, it can be argued that the disruption of social networks due to the move to a new area undermined social support and took away many positive sources of stimulation and satisfaction (see Chapter 4). As one of the housewives who moved out of Bethnal Green to a new semi-detached house outside London described: 'When I first came, I cried for weeks, it was so lonely.' (Young and Willmott, 1957: 122). Clearly, the disruption and loss of social networks was, for many, a major cause of distress, and was the reason why a sizeable minority of migrants attempted to move back to the slums which they had left, despite the fact that this involved moving back to housing of a much poorer physical standard.[2]

An extremely important factor which divides housing developments into the successful and unsuccessful, at least in terms of mental health, is the extent to which the relocation was voluntary (Kasl, 1974). In the years 1955 to 1975, around three million people were rehoused in Britain alone as part of the redevelopment and slum clearance programs (Freeman, 1984b). The extent of choice offered to people varied, but often the choice was relatively constrained. In Bethnal Green, for example, residents were offered the choice between a house on an estate and a flat in the city. Moving to a house implied moving away from kin, but then against this, flats were widely disliked for their lack of a garden and their communal facilities.

> 'I was between two thorns,' said one of our informants still in the borough, 'I didn't want a flat but I didn't want to leave Bethnal Green' (Young and Willmott, 1957: 127).

In general, studies which have examined housing where the population actively chose to move have shown much more positive results (for example, Wilner, *et al.*, 1962; Taylor and Chave, 1964). Where rehousing is clearly involuntary, such as sometimes in the case of the institutional transfer of the elderly, the effects can be very negative. In the United States, a literature review of the evidence on involuntary relocation led Kasl (1974) to conclude that the evidence was 'clearly sufficient to mount an attack on the way in which the federal and local governments have managed this social problem' (p. 9).

However, perhaps the most infamous and dramatic example of the consequences of forced relocation was the redevelopment of a part of Boston which had been known as the West End. The story of life in the West End and the fight to prevent its redevelopment is graphically described in a book by the planner Herbert Gans, *The Urban Villagers* (1962). The West End was an area which had been occupied by successive waves of immigrants, but, by the time demolition was proposed, it had become a primarily Italian, Jewish and Polish area. In 1910, the population of the West End had been around 23 000, but this gradually fell as a result of decreasing family size among the descendants of immigrant groups, and as a result of the gradual reduction in the number of dwellings as the hospital expanded and as deteriorated buildings became vacant. The population of the area in 1950 was about 12 000. In 1951 it was announced that the area would be redeveloped. In 1953 the area was declared a slum, and between 1958 and 1960 it was torn down under the federal renewal program. The 7000 people (in 2800 households) still living in the West End in 1957 were dispersed all over the metropolitan area, and a luxury housing complex built on the site. The reason given for the demolition was the physically poor condition of many of the buildings and the narrow and awkward streets that comprised the area.

Yet despite the physically poor quality of the buildings, a survey of 500 West End households showed that the vast majority (78 per cent) said that they liked their apartments (Hartman, 1963). Furthermore, most of those who lived there were actually relatively affluent and could easily have afforded to have lived elsewhere, a fact confirmed by the finding that many of those forced to leave moved to relatively expensive areas of the city. As Hartman later concluded, 'people do not live only in houses':

> The experience of social and personal satisfaction in the local area markedly limits the effect of objective housing quality on attitudes towards the apartment. Only in the absence of these meaningful experiences does the objective physical quality of the dwelling become an important determinant of housing satisfaction (Hartman, 1963: 162).

Or as Gans concluded, a physical slum does not imply a social slum (Gans, 1962).

Nonetheless, the West End was demolished and the population dispersed. In a follow-up study, Fried (1963) attempted to establish how the ex-West Enders were doing in their new environments, most of which were of higher physical quality than those they had left. He found that among a sample of 250 women, 20 per cent reported a period of depression lasting from between six months and two years, and a further 26 per cent were still depressed over two years after the demolition. Altogether, 46 per cent of women and 38 per cent of men appeared to have suffered 'severe grief reactions'.[3] These results could not have arisen out of a bias in the selection of respondents as the sample was a follow-up of a set of random interviews *before* demolition, of which 92 per cent of the women were recontacted and 87 per cent of the men. Only a small minority expressed no sadness at the demolition, and many were extremely distressed:

> 'I felt like my heart was taken out of me', 'I felt as though I had lost everything'. 'I always felt I had to go home to the West End and even now I feel like crying when I pass by', 'Something of me went with the West End', 'I felt like taking the gaspipe' (Fried, 1963: 151).

In answer to the question, 'How did you feel when you saw or heard that the

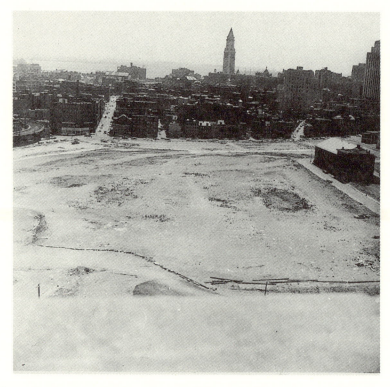

Figure 6.1: *The West End of Boston after demolition, reproduced with permission of Herbert J. Gans.*

building you had lived in was torn down?', 54 per cent of the women and 46 per cent of the men reported severely depressed or disturbed reactions, 27 per cent of the women and 23 per cent of the men reported moderately depressed or ambivalent feelings, and 19 per cent of the women and 23 per cent of the men reported indifferent or satisfied reactions.

The story of the West End is one of the most dramatic in planning history, but is probably not unique (it was well documented presumably because of the large concentration of academic institutions nearby.) The demolition was strongly opposed by the majority of residents, and the fact that the demolition and rehousing was against their wishes seems to be central in the understanding of why the impact on their mental health was so bad. Unsurprisingly, those residents who reported the highest levels of satisfaction with living in the West End before the demolition were the ones who exhibited the most severe grief reactions afterwards.[4]

The demolition of the West End provides a relatively clear example of the personal costs of the involuntary relocation of residents for the purpose of slum clearance. Widespread criticism of involuntary slum clearance programs has led to today's emphasis on refurbishment rather than demolition (Malpass and Murie, 1987). However, the extent to which residents are excluded or involved in major planning decisions and the relationship of this involvement to mental health remains as a major issue, and it is to this that the discussion now turns.

Resident Participation in the Planning Process

There are two principal arguments for having resident involvement in planning decisions. The first is that without consultation, the decisions that are taken are more likely to produce unsuitable designs for the residents. These poorly designed environments could then lead to the types of problems described in Chapters 2, 3 and 4, and thereby affect mental health. They could also lead to dissatisfaction and resentment if the resulting designs clash with the aesthetic preferences of the residents, even if they perform their function adequately (see Chapter 5). As the functional problems that can arise from poor planning decisions have already been discussed in earlier chapters, I shall concentrate here on the likelihood of aesthetic clashes arising.

The second argument for involving residents in planning decisions is that the act of exclusion *per se* may have a negative impact on mental health, regardless of the decision itself.

Conflicts in Aesthetics

Despite occasional attempts to inform architects of the aesthetic preferences of the general public (Raven, 1967a,b; Cooper Marcus and Sarkissian, 1986), architects are infamous in popular culture for the ugliness of many of their designs (Prince of Wales, 1989). Architects have also been accused of overdesign, and the modern movement of being 'an attack on users meaning', for not recognizing residents' preferences for *what-nots* (Rapoport, 1982: 22). Residents like to personalize their homes by adding extra details such as brass door knockers or particular light fittings (what-nots), but architects have often attempted to offset this tendency by pre-designing these details and by using materials that are as indestructible as possible (such as concrete and industrial ceramics or polymers).

Empirical work has confirmed the popular suspicion that the aesthetic tastes of architects differ markedly from those of the general population. As part of a project exploring *mere exposure* effects (the tendency to like things the more they are seen) and the hypothesis that exposure effects would be influenced by levels of expertise, an early piece of my own research involved comparing the aesthetic preferences of architecture students and non-architecture students (Halpern, 1987). Subjects were shown photographs of unfamiliar people and buildings (with varying frequencies) and were asked to rate each in terms of attractiveness. One of the findings of this research was that although correlation between the architects' and non-architects' ratings of the attractiveness of people was extremely high, the correlation between their ratings of the attractiveness of buildings was low and non-significant. This was despite the fact that the within-group correlations remained very high. In other words, the architects all agreed with one another as to which buildings were attractive, and the *non*-architects all agreed with one another as to which buildings were attractive, but there was almost no correspondence between the two sets of preferences.

Differences in the aesthetic preferences of architects have since been confirmed in a study comparing the preferences of practising architects to those of other professionals (Devlin and Nasar, 1989). Subjects were shown photographs of single

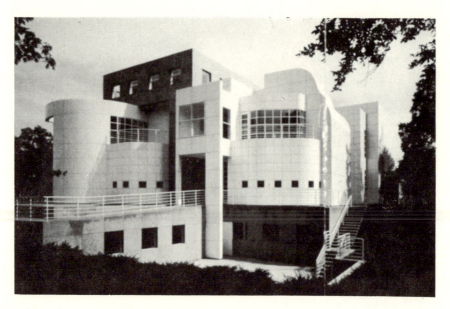

Figure 6.2: *The consistently least popular of 12 buildings shown to non-architect students, proved to be the most and second-most popular among two groups of architect students. (Halpern 1987)*

family dwellings taken either from architectural journals or from more popular magazines (for example, *House and Garden*). The style of the former were referred to as *high* and the latter as *popular*. Photographs were chosen to exclude people, cars and other objects. Very marked differences were found between the architects and the other professionals. While the architects rated the high designs as more pleasant and relaxing than the popular designs, the reverse pattern was found for the other professionals who found the popular designs more pleasant and relaxing than the high designs. The architects also found the high designs more meaningful, clear and coherent than the popular designs, while again, the exact reverse pattern was found for the other professionals.

A clue to the development of the aesthetic differences can be seen in the study of the students (Halpern, 1987). The students were presented with a series of four abstract line drawings taken from the Welsh preference test, and asked to rank them in order of preference. This task discriminated very clearly between the two groups of students, architects showing a strong tendency to prefer the more complex and asymmetrical designs, while the non-architects (and the general population) showed the reverse preference. The results suggested that the architects had a general preference for complexity and asymmetry in designs, a phenomenon not surprising given the current ethos in design (see Venturi, 1977, *Complexity and Contradiction in Architecture*). Furthermore, a closer analysis of the preferences of the architecture students showed that their divergence from the norm became more marked the longer they had been studying architecture; the difference between first-year architects and the norm was relatively small (though still significant) but became markedly stronger among later year students. This result suggests that the normal training of architects fosters the development of divergent aesthetic preferences from the general population giving rise to a *designer's paradox*. If an architect designs a building that he or she really likes, the chances are that the general population will dislike it for the same reasons that the architect finds it attractive.

A series of studies by Darke (1984a,b,c) has shown that architects are not generally aware of, or do not want to recognize, the possibility that their under-standing of what constitutes good housing may not be shared by the residents. Darke interviewed the architects of six public housing schemes in London to establish what assumptions they held about the users of the estates and what attempts the architects had made to validate their assumptions. Somewhat alarmingly, Darke found that the architects held generalized, imprecise, and stereotyped views of the residents, and made no distinction between their own aesthetic preferences and those of residents. The most strongly articulated social objective of the architects was the encouragement of social contact, while factors such as providing individuality and privacy (about which household surveys show residents to be far more concerned; Britten, 1977) were given less emphasis. The architects made almost no attempts to validate their impressions, either before or after the completion of their projects.

Of course, none of these results prove that because architects are poorly informed of the preferences of the public, the residents of the estates designed by them suffered from anything more than perceived ugliness, and to date, nobody has proven that the experience of ugliness *per se* can affect mental health. However, we saw in the previous chapter that the mental health of residents was adversely affected by a mismatch between the aesthetic aspirations of the resident with that of the actuality of the design (Gillis, 1977). These studies also show that the differences in aesthetic preferences of architects make it much more likely that the types of design problem described in earlier chapters will arise. Yet, perhaps the most important factor is the sense of frustration that residents must experience in the face of planning and design decisions imposed on them by people who are not aware of or interested in their own views.

Lack of Control

If architects and planners impose their preferences on residents, and particularly if the preferences of the residents are very different, then residents are likely to feel themselves as powerless, frustrated and without control over their environment. The feelings of powerlessness and frustration which result from the exclusion of residents from the decision-making process (either from the original design or the ongoing management of their environment) could have a negative impact on residents' mental health even if the resulting environment is of an objectively excellent physical quality.

The importance of participation in the planning process has been emphasized by Rohe (1985) who argued that 'both the product and the process of city planning can influence mental health.' He has suggested that participation in the planning and decision process can benefit mental health in two ways. First, participation brings with it a sense of control, and second, participation fosters social interaction and support among residents. The evidence for the second assertion is the finding of a strong positive association between levels of participation in local voluntary groups and levels of informal social interaction. Rohe suggests, therefore, that it should be standard practice to incorporate neighbourhood improvement councils as part of the normal planning process.

The relevance of lack of control and powerlessness has been strongly emphasized in the more general psychological literature on mild psychopathology and depression (Seligman, 1975; Pearlin, *et al.*, 1981; Meyer and Salmon, 1984), with recent literature suggesting that there may exist an optimum level of control for positive mental health (Mirowsky and Ross, 1989). Unfortunately, hard empirical evidence specifically on the mental health benefits of residents' involvement in the decision process (about their environment) is relatively rare. We saw above that there is strong evidence of the adverse effects of forced relocation on mental health, but obviously, this is an extreme example of a lack of control over the decision process and is also compounded with the move and demolition itself. More modestly, however, a cross-sectional survey by Kasl, *et al.*, (1982) of a sample of 337 female residents from various parts of Waterbury, Connecticut, showed that, after controlling for socio-demographic and background variables, evaluations of residential management explained significant variance in levels of mental health. Negative evaluations of styles of management were associated with higher levels of depression (Zung scale) and higher anomia. In fact, Kasl, *et al.*, found that style of management was one of their best residential predictors of mental health and concluded that 'the area of management relations is the most promising direction to move in order to enlarge the explanatory variance of Housing Index and Neighbourhood Conditions' (Kasl, 1982: 26). Of course, the finding does not rule out the possibility that negative evaluations of management styles were simply a symptom rather than a cause of poorer mental health, though it must then be explained why this variable *in particular* was susceptible to bias.

Research by Power (1984) supports the causal relevance of management styles in favourable residential outcomes, though no direct information on mental health was gathered. Power found that the introduction of tenant involvement and local-based management into the running of difficult-to-let-estates led to lower rates of crime and vandalism even in the absence of physical alterations. It is noteworthy that in recent years the Department of the Environment, on the basis of its own evidence, has strongly emphasized the importance of management style and resident involvement in the running of local authority estates. Resident involvement is now supposed to be a central element in all types of estate action and improvement in Britain, though inevitably, many of the old obstacles to resident participation persist – the reluctance to relinquish power, the lack of public finances, and the dependence on developers (Fagence, 1977).

Case Study – Demolition!

In order to demonstrate conclusively the relevance of the planning process *per se* to mental health, it must be shown that a planning decision can have an impact on residents' mental health even in the absence of actual physical changes on the environment. The following study was designed to document such an effect.

The Southgate estate (totalling 1300 dwellings) was an example of the architectural style described as *brutalism* and was composed of a combination of massive concrete blocks of maisonettes and flats with walkways 15 to 20 ft off the ground and row houses built of plastic which residents called *legoland.* Southgate was the source of many jibes in the local area, and even in architectural textbooks it had been described as resembling *a prison* (Cooper Marcus and Sarkissian, 1986: 53). The estate had proven expensive to run (its components were generally non-standard) and its social profile was appalling; a 1985 Cheshire County Council report found that on a composite scale of six indicators of social disadvantage, the Southgate estate was by far the worst of the 207 areas into which the County was divided.

On 21 February 1989, the decision was announced to demolish the Southgate housing estate. Letters were sent by the Development Corporation to all the estate's 2000 residents informing them of the decision to demolish the estate. Given the estate's physical appearance and reputation, one might have expected that everyone would have been glad about the announcement, but it soon became clear that this was not the case. The next eight weeks saw a period of vigorous resident activity and protest with meetings attracting in excess of 500 residents a time. The protests culminated in an apparently successful meeting with the Under Secretary of State (14 April 1989), jubilantly reflected in the local newspaper – 'Southgate Saved – Devco [the Development Corporation] forced to abandon demolition'. However, the jubilation was short-lived, as within four weeks the original decision to demolish was re-confirmed. Despite a belated offer of monetary compensation, residents' protests continued.

This series of events on Southgate was reminiscent of some of the notorious planning blunders of the 1950s and 1960s where planners mistakenly assumed that the physical deterioration of an estate implied a corresponding social decay of the community (see above). Residents were not fighting to save the original design but were fighting against the dispersal of their community; they wanted new or refurbished housing, but *on Southgate.* The surprise decision to totally demolish the estate had dismissed alternative plans for the estate's refurbishment which had been prepared by a local housing association in consultation with the estate's 2000 residents. The decision-making process concerning the estate's future lacked almost any consultation with the residents, and the entire affair was clumsily and insensitively handled by the Development Corporation.

The purpose of my study was to establish whether the announcement, and the events that followed it, had any demonstrable effects on the physical and mental health of the residents. The study design was retrospective, longitudinal and based on two principal measures: general practitioner consultations by the resident population and psychiatric community nurse visits to pre-existing patients living on the estate. Some of the results concerning general practitioner consultations have already been reported (Halpern and Reid, 1992) but are supplemented here by other previously unpublished data.

General practitioner consultations

The Southgate estate and the surrounding area were served by two general practices in a shared health centre just outside the Southgate estate (the two practices combined had nine doctors serving a total of 17000 patients). Virtually all Southgate residents were registered with one or the other of the two practices. Residents' consultation rates were found by a check of the old appointment sheets of the two practices for the first six months of 1989 and, for a comparison period, the first six months of 1988 (the total number of consultations for the two periods was around 60000 – a long haul). Each consultation was classified according to the patient's home address as either Southgate or non-Southgate. The weekly number of Southgate patients (S), and the weekly number of non-Southgate patients (NS), were thus compiled. This was done for both the first six months of 1989 (the critical period) and the first six months of 1988 (the control period). The weekly numbers of Southgate resident consultations were then expressed as a ratio of non-Southgate resident consultations. The advantage of using a ratio (or relative consultation rate) was that it would control for spurious fluctuations in the absolute numbers of patients seen in any given week. For example, seasonal variations in consultations would cause fluctuations in the absolute numbers of Southgate and other patients seen, but it should leave the ratio relatively unaffected (though see below). Similarly, if one or two of the two practices' nine doctors happened to be away in any given week, then this would be expected to result in a fall in the absolute numbers of patients seen, but not in the ratio. Hence the use of the ratio (S/NS) provided an unbiased estimate of the relative rate of Southgate residents' general practitioner consultations over the period studied – it provided a good measure of *estate specific* variation.

However, it could still have been argued that some estate-specific, seasonal variation might occur. For example, it could have been argued that there might have been an interaction between the time of year and the consultation rate of an estate's population, for example, due to the relative affluence of residents (the poorer Southgate residents being less able to heat their homes in winter). Similarly, differences in the demographic structure of an estate's population might cause some estate specific variance. If an estate had an unusually large (or small) number of children or elderly people, and if these groups were differentially affected by seasonal variations in rates of illness, then this could introduce estate-specific seasonal variations. This was controlled for by comparing the relative consultation rates to those in the same week in the previous year.

One final correction had to be made, and that was for any change in the size of the base-line population. An examination of the housing records revealed that there had been a gradual fall in the population of Southgate from January 1989 onwards, (no new residents were housed on the estate after this date). This was clearly very important as, potentially, it could mask any change in the rates that occurred over the period. The exact numbers of occupied units on the estate in any given week (U_i) were derived from records kept by the Housing Association, which was responsible for the day-to-day management of the estate. This allowed the calculation of an adjustment factor (U_{base}/U_i), where U_{base} was the baseline number of units occupied during the previous year. Account was taken of the delays involved in patients failing to register changes in address by off-setting the value of U_i by a period of three weeks. This correction factor was calculated on the basis of information from the practice administrators. This led to a final formula of:

$$\frac{(S_1/NS_1)}{(S_2/NS_2)} \cdot \frac{U_{base}}{U_i}$$

The critical question was, having taken account of all the above, was this ratio higher during the time when the demolition of the estate was expected than when no demolition was expected. The dates of the total demolition announcement, the apparent reprieve, and re-confirmation of the original decision were verified from filed documents and from micro-fiches of the local newspapers held in the local library. Each week of the first six months of 1989 was coded as either demolition expected (=1) or demolition not expected (=0).

Psychiatric consultations

An attempt was made to compile similar statistics for psychiatric consultations. Southgate is very near to the local general hospital which provides a psychiatric out-patient service. However, unlike for appointments for a general practitioner, it is not normal for a psychiatric out-patient's address to be written down with the appointment record as there are fewer patients involved and it is unlikely that two patients have the same name. This meant that patients' addresses had to be checked from other records, but as many had left the area, this was often not possible. As home addresses could not be reliably identified, area specific rates of psychiatric out-patient attendances could not be accurately calculated and these data had to be abandoned.

It was possible, however, to examine fluctuations in rates of psychiatric community nurse visits to the estate, as the nurses kept diaries listing the names and addresses of patients visited. The diaries made it possible to compare the rates of visits to the estate during the weeks before and after the demolition announcement. Data were not available for the previous year or for other areas, so the comparison was between the rates of visits during the times when the demolition was expected and the rates during the times when the demolition was not expected. As the total number of patients visited was quite small, this comparison served to identify how the events surrounding the demolition announcement affected those people with pre-existing psychiatric problems who lived on Southgate. Clearly, this group was not representative of the general Southgate population but was of considerable interest nonetheless.[5]

Results – The Impact of the Announcements on Residents

Changes in general practitioner consultation rates

In the period prior to the demolition announcement, the odds ratio was consistently less than one, but rose shortly after the announcement (Fig. 6.3). The ratio fell in week 15, the week of the apparently successful resident meeting with the Under Secretary or State (14 April). By week 18, when it started to become clear that the original decision to demolish the estate was going to be confirmed, the odds ratio began to climb again.

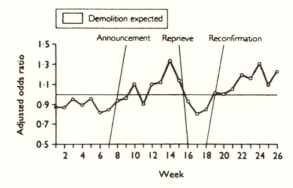

Figure 6.3: *The weekly adjusted odds ratio of general practitioner consultations for Southgate residents to non-Southgate residents during the period when demolition of the estate was announced.*

A t-test was applied to test the null hypothesis that the odds ratio during the periods following the demolition announcements (mean = 1.12, sd. = 0.12) was no higher than during the periods when the demolition was not expected (mean = 0.877, sd. = 0.05). For clarity, the two weeks within which the events fell midweek (8 and 19) were excluded from this analysis. The t-test was highly significant (t = 5.94, df = 22, p.<.001). Significance was maintained even if the adjustment for the fall in the size of the Southgate population was removed (t = 3.70, p.<.01), which is remarkable considering that the Southgate population fell by nearly 30 per cent over the period.

The impact on patients with pre-existing psychiatric problems

Although data were not available on fluctuations in rates of psychiatric out-patient

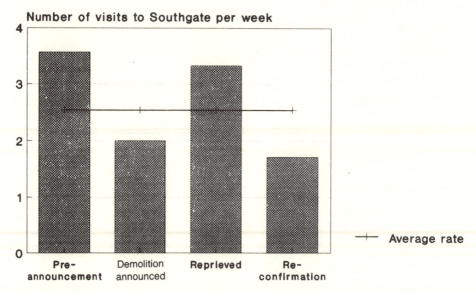

Figure 6.4: *Community psychiatric nurse visits over the period of the demolition announcements*

consultations, data were gathered on rates of psychiatric community nurse visits to the estate. The pattern of psychiatric community nurse visits to the estate was exactly the reverse of that for the general practitioner consultation rates. It was found that during the periods following the demolition announcements, rates of visits to the estate were lower than during periods when the demolition was not expected. Use of the chi-squared test confirmed that the difference between the rates of visits at times when the demolition was expected and when it was not expected was statistically significant (chi-squared = 5.56, df = 1; $p < .02$ [two tailed]; Yates correction applied).

Interpreting the Changes in Consultation Rates

The results showed an estate-specific variation; during the times when demolition was expected, and the future of the Southgate estate looked bleak, Southgate residents' general practitioner consultations increased significantly. The results are comparable to those which have shown an elevation in the rates of medical consultations of workers threatened with redundancy even before the redundancy has occurred (Beale and Nethercott, 1988). The study is unusual in that it was possible to accurately and externally verify the timing and occurrence of the events and the direction of causation was constrained. There is no way in which the changes in consultation rates could have caused the announcement! However, a number of interpretations of the effect were possible.

First, residents could have gone to see their doctors simply to have had someone to talk to about what was happening on the estate. Second, the announcements on the estate could have led to an increase in the *reporting* of illness. Third, the announcements could have led to an increased manifestation of *psychosomatic* symptoms or illness. Fourth, the announcements could have led to an increase in the occurrence of *physical* illness as a result of the stress.

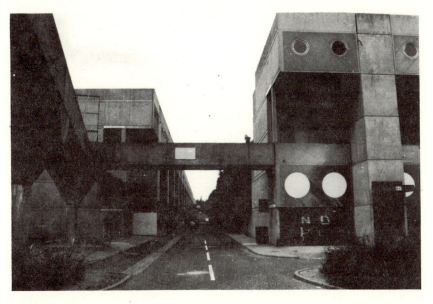

Figure 6.5: *The Southgate estate*

Informal discussions with the general practitioners suggested no evidence for the first interpretation, that Southgate residents were consulting just to talk about the estate. This interpretation also seems unlikely given that residents had ready access to other more appropriate sources of information and support, such as the Housing Association who managed the estate and to the estate's Residents Association (both of which had offices on the estate).

An attempt was made to discriminate between the latter three interpretations by an examination of a sub-sample of the medical records of patients who consulted during the periods of marked excess and shortfall. However, by the time the study was conducted, a considerable proportion of the medical records were missing, due to the large number of residents who had left the area. Of those records which remained, the elevation in rates was found for all types of disorders and not just for psychological and psychosomatic symptoms. Which of the latter three interpretations was most accurate, therefore, had to be left somewhat open. A realistic understanding would probably have to include aspects of all three – they are not, of course, incompatible. Researchers who have attempted to divide the types of complaints seen by general practitioners into psychological and non-psychological disorders have found it extremely difficult and have typically been forced to conclude that no clear line can be drawn between the two (Kessel, 1960; Shepherd, *et al.*, 1966; Higgins, 1984). General practitioners tend to classify between a quarter and a third of their patients as suffering from psychiatric symptoms, but there is also a large amount of *hidden psychiatric morbidity* which is unrecognized by family doctors (Goldberg and Blackwell, 1970; Goldberg and Huxley,1980). It is plausible that for some people the extra stress made an existing complaint less tolerable, for some it led to psychosomatic complaints, and for others it led to more physical complaints and illness. The interrelationship between the last two possibilities is strongly underlined by recent work showing that stress can lead to substantial reductions in the efficiency in the immune system (Perez, 1988; Kennedy, Kiecolt-Glaser and Glaser, 1990) indicating how the psychological component of stress can lead to a non-psychological disorder.

However, while the prospect of demolition had a negative impact on the health and well-being of most Southgate residents, the evidence suggested that it led to a fall in the occurrence of psychiatric problems for those with pre-existing psychiatric conditions who lived on the estate. How can this discrepancy be explained? Informal discussions with the community psychiatric nurses suggested that their patients on the estate were not integrated into the community and had no desire to stay on the estate. The psychiatrically impaired tend to have little choice in their housing and must take whatever is available; that is why there were a disproportionate number of ex-patients on Southgate in the first place. The nurses' comments made it clear that at least some of the patients had never really wanted to live on the estate and were delighted at the prospect of being paid to leave. For them, the demolition announcement represented a lucky break, and was certainly nothing to protest about.

In sum, the announcements of the intention to totally demolish and not rebuild the Southgate estate led to a significant increase in the frequency with which residents went to see their doctors. The increase in consultations appeared to be for both psychological and physical disorders. The pattern of results strongly suggest that the stress caused by the demolition announcements and the prospective break-up of the community had an adverse effect on both the physical and mental health of many of the residents. Having controlled for overall levels of consultations, the number of doctors available in any given week, with seasonal and other spurious fluctuations, it can be estimated that on average there were around 20 per cent more Southgate patients being seen by their general practitioners during the periods following the demolition announcements than during the periods when the estate was thought to be safe (in other words, approximately 30 more Southgate patients per week went to see their doctors on top of a mean of about 160 Southgate and 850 non-Southgate patients per week).

However, the demolition announcements were experienced in a different way by the few residents on the estate with pre-existing psychiatric problems, as they were happy to leave and were pleased about the idea of being paid for doing so. This was reflected in a fall in the level of community psychiatric nurse visits to residents with pre-existing psychiatric problems.

Epilogue

In the end, the vigour of the residents' campaign was not enough to prevent the demolition of most of the estate but was successful in preventing the demolition of the *legoland houses* (though they may still be demolished in the future). The Department of the Environment was pressured into agreeing to finance the building of 130 conventional houses on Southgate, though the rest of the site was still expected to be sold commercially. I understand from the ex-chair of the residents' association that the houses have been four to five times oversubscribed.

Summary

In this chapter, evidence has been presented to show how the planning process, as well as its physical outcomes, is relevant to the mental health of residents. The most dramatic and notorious examples of the impact of the planning process on mental health come from the slum clearance programs of the 1950s and 1960s. However, in these instances it is difficult to separate the impact of the planning process from the eventual outcomes and destroyed social networks that followed from the planning decisions.

Other kinds of evidence also suggest that the planning process can adversely affect mental health. Architects and planners often do not share the aesthetic preferences of the residents that they design for, and yet community architecture in the form of resident participation in the design process remains relatively rare. It is also important for residents to be involved in the management of their dwellings. When a management style makes residents feel that decisions about their residential environments are not under their control, the decisions are more likely to be unpopular and the residents are likely to feel frustrated and powerless.

The relevance of the planning process to mental health was illustrated by the case study of Southgate, an estate unexpectedly threatened with demolition and its residents with separation. Even in the absence of any physical changes to the estate, the announcements made by the Development Corporation, both positive and negative, had a direct impact on the residents' physical and mental health.

In the 1950s and 1960s, the publication of studies on the social consequences of demolition programmes in Britain (Young and Willmott, 1957) and America (Gans, 1962; Fried, 1963) forced an awareness among planners and politicians that areas that they saw as physical slums might not be perceived as slums by those who lived there, and that slow to form social structures can often be more important to residents than the physical forms that contain them. Although there is some evidence of a recent revival of interest in the relationship between the physical quality of housing and health (Lowry, 1991), there is a very real danger that as the experimental housing designs of the 1960s and 1970s come to look tired and out-dated, the painfully learnt lessons of the 50s and 60s – that a physical slum does not imply a social slum – will have to be learnt again. Planners and policymakers alike must recognize the importance of the planning and communication *process* as well as its product. Regrettably, as we have seen, unpopular planning decisions imposed against the wishes of residents and without consultation did not end with the sixties and still occur today.

Notes

1   Clearly, most aetiologies involve complex chains of causality, and what is seen as a 'cause' and what is seen as mediating agent will vary depending upon our mental framework. If many people die from cholera after flooding in the rainy season, what should be understood as 'the cause'? Was the cause of the epidemic the micro-organism, the heavy rainfall, or the poor sewage and water supply systems which became so easily mixed?
2   From the opening of Greenleigh (the new estate studied by Young and Willmott, 1957) in the late-40s until early 1956, 26 per cent of the tenants who had gone there moved away again, most of them returning to the East End. The removal figures for many other London County Council estates were even higher.
3   The responses to the question 'Would you describe how you felt?' were graded from minimal grief through to severe or marked grief. Cross-tabulating responses to other related questions, it was found that those who were classified as suffering severe grief almost invariably were found to have suffered severe grief by any of the other criteria used, but many who were categorized as suffering minimal grief were still found to be extremely dissatisfied or unhappy on other items. This evidence supports the validity of the measure of *grief*, suggesting that, if anything, it may have led to conservative estimates of residents' distress.
4   This finding is also important in that it demonstrates that the effects were not simply due to a neurotic sub-group of the population who tended to express severe dissatisfaction whatever their circumstances.
5   The patients were mainly suffering from schizophrenia or were people with a history of drug abuse.

Chapter 7

Improving Mental Health Through the Environment: A Case Study

Introduction

In the previous chapters, a large amount of evidence has been examined concerning the relationship between mental health and the environment. This evidence suggested that the environment can have quite significant effects on people's behaviour and mental health. The environment can be source of stress causing irritation and annoyance (Chapters 2 and 3), it can affect the quality and supportiveness of the relationships between people (Chapter 4) and it can affect people through the meanings that are ascribed to it (Chapter 5). Finally, we saw how the planning process itself can affect people's mental health and well-being (Chapter 6).

An implication of this evidence is that, by improving the environment and the way it is managed, we should be able to improve people's mental health. Perhaps some readers will feel that this is obvious – surely if we improve the quality of a poor environment, the residents' mental health would benefit? However, the answer to this question is hotly contested. Many psychologists have come to suspect that mental health, and even happiness, are actually *traits* rather than something that depends on the world outside. In other words, the people who tend to be happy and in good mental health tend to be like that whatever their circumstances, while those who tend to be unhappy or have neurotic symptoms tend to be similarly unhappy wherever they are and whatever they are doing. A slight refinement of this somewhat pessimistic model of humanity is that happiness and mental health depend on relative circumstances. In other words, our satisfactions and disappointments depend on the environment to a limited extent, but only relative to everyone else's environment. When most people have got only an outside toilet, but ours is inside, then we are happy and satisfied. However, when everyone else has got several inside toilets and we still have only one, then we are unhappy and dissatisfied. As we saw in Chapter 5, there is some evidence to support this hypothesis. Unfortunately, the implication of this view is that we can never improve the overall level of people's happiness or mental health because if we improve one person's environment, he or she may be happier, but the person next door will be less so! This hypothesis implies that there is no point improving everyone's environment, because if satisfaction and happiness is relative then no one will be any more satisfied or happy than before.

This issue can provoke considerable angst and concern among well-meaning psychologists, architects, planners and even policymakers. As one slightly demoralized architect explained to me with a sigh, 'We don't believe in progress in architecture any more; there's only fashion.' Is there a way forward? Fortunately, the issue of what determines happiness and mental health is an empirically addressable question and not just a philosophical one. If the literatures that we have reviewed in the previous chapters are correct, then it ought to be possible to improve the mental health of a group of people by improving the quality of their environment – if we do it correctly. This seems, in retrospect, like an obvious thing to test, but surprisingly, very few people have tried to do so. The physical environment is often altered, but it is very rare for anyone to evaluate the impact of such alterations on mental health.

A Comparison to Environmental Criminology

The situation is similar to that in environmental criminology a few years ago. At that time, there was a considerable amount of evidence suggesting that the design of the environment affected the occurrence of crime and the fear of crime, but evaluations of the impact of alterations to the environment on crime and fear were rare. It was also believed that the styles of management and response of the official agencies and the behaviour of neighbours in watching over one another's properties could affect crime. On the basis of these beliefs, policymakers became interested in the idea that it might be possible to reduce crime and fear through environmental interventions. The idea emerged of formally encouraging *neighbourhood watch* schemes and of training police staff to look at the designs of new (and old) developments to see whether the designs could be altered to reduce levels of crime.

Unsure of the strength of the evidence, many people remained sceptical about the prospects of reducing crime through such seemingly peripheral methods. Much of the evidence concerning the relationship between the environment and crime was in the form of simple associations from cross-sectional studies and, as we have seen in earlier chapters, such associations do not demonstrate causality. What was needed was a carefully constructed test of whether an environmental intervention, based on the evidence from environmental criminology, would actually lead to a reduction in crime. This led to the commissioning of the watershed study, The Kirkholt Burglary Prevention Project (Forrester, Chatterton and Pease, 1988).

Having agreed that such a study should be done, the composition of the study still had to be decided. In such situations, the researchers (and policymakers) have two options. They can either attempt a series of specific interventions where only one type of alteration is tried at a time, or they can attempt a full intervention, as would occur in practice. In methodological terms, the former possibility is clearly superior as it allows researchers to isolate the effect of one particular type of change, for example, the effects of *target hardening* schemes alone (such as putting better locks on doors) as opposed to the effects of neighbourhood watch schemes (residents watching over each others' homes) or target reduction schemes (such as removing electricity meters that take cash). However, if you do not have the opportunity to do many different studies, then the most important question is whether or not a realistic, multi-factor intervention works. The dilemma was discussed in the report following the Kirkholt project.

One of the most valuable lessons to be learned from earlier work is that the adoption of a *series* of measures is likely to have much greater impact than simply taking one or two steps. Methodologically this is less attractive because it is scarcely ever practicable to tease out the relative contributions to crime prevention of the various measures and the interactions between them. A crime prevention package of four elements contains fifteen possible ways of achieving its impact. We were persuaded that a programme involving just one of the changes we had in mind would be less likely to have an effect than an initiative comprising a package of measures. We realised the cost of this decision. We would be unable to say precisely how the combination had worked. As long as there was an effect, we would be content! (Forrester, *et al.*,1988: 11–12).

The Kirkholt project proved to be a considerable success. Following the environmental and related changes, the burglary rate on the estate more than halved from around 1 in 4 houses being burgled per year to less than 1 in 8 after the intervention. Furthermore, there was no evidence for the occurrence of displacement, in other words, there was no parallel increase in burglaries elsewhere or in other types of related crime. The study demonstrated that environmental interventions could be used to reduce crime (though the researchers were, of course, 'unable to say precisely how the combination had worked').

Returning to the issue of mental health and the present study, a similar dilemma existed about the design of the study and a similar conclusion was reached. As has been seen, a large amount of evidence suggests that the environment can affect mental health, just as a large amount of evidence suggested that the environment could affect levels of crime and fear. The implication of this literature is that, if we identified a group of people with poor mental health living in an environment suffering from design-related problems, then we should be able to improve the mental health of these people by altering and improving the environment. This is what the study presented below attempted to test.

Design and Methodology of the Intervention Study

The basic idea behind the study was very simple. A housing estate was identified which had design-related problems but that was scheduled for refurbishment. Residents were to be interviewed at different stages of the changes, preferably both before and after the changes had occurred. If the environmental alterations were successful, then this should be reflected in residents' attitudes towards the estate, and if the conclusions drawn in earlier chapters were correct, in improved residents' mental health. There are many advantages to such a methodological design. Not least among these is that an intervention study as this does not uproot people from their social networks and thereby compound the environmental improvements with disrupted social networks (as in the New Town studies). Also, the longitudinal component to the study enables the issue of selection to be checked.

A search was conducted to identify a potentially suitable problem housing estate, in other words, an estate that was due for refurbishment and the problems of which appeared to relate to its design. In Britain, since the mid-1980s, the Department of the

Environment (DoE) has provided special funding for problem estates (the Estate Action Programme) so it was relatively straightforward to identify a selection of such estates. An estate was sought which was scheduled for partial or phased improvements, such that different aspects of the refurbishment could be distinguished. Also, the eventual improvements to the estate had to be sufficiently extensive to provide a reasonable test of the hypothesis that improvements to the environment could improve residents' mental health – a coat of paint would be unlikely to be enough. A housing estate called Eastlake was identified as meeting all the necessary criteria, and detailed preparatory work for the study began in the Spring of 1989.

Initially, sufficient money had been allocated to Eastlake to refurbish part, but not all, of the estate. One part of the estate was to be fully refurbished as soon as possible, but the remainder was to remain unchanged until funding became available. As soon as this initial funding was confirmed and consultations with the residents in the test area began, interviews were conducted on the estate. The structure and content of the interviews is described below. As it turned out, around two years after these first interviews were conducted and shortly after the refurbishment of the first part of the estate had been completed, the council succeeded in securing further funding in order to extend the refurbishment to the other areas of the estate. These funding arrangements meant that one area of the estate was refurbished three years in advance of the other areas, although before the refurbishment had begun, the housing across the estate was of identical design and the residents were drawn from the same population (the council waiting list) and were randomly placed across the estate. This phasing of the refurbishment works enabled comparisons to be made between areas that had initially been the same but now differed in the extent to which they had been refurbished. Comparisons were also possible across time, as residents were re-interviewed three years after the works began. Hence for a period of a few years, areas of the Eastlake estate could be distinguished according to their stage of refurbishment, though at the outset they were of identical design. Residents on the estate were interviewed on two occasions separated by a period of three years. When the residents were first interviewed, most of the estate was unchanged (stage 1), but in one area (Green Close) the residents had just been informed about the intended refurbishment of their homes and some minor improvements had begun (stage 2). When residents were re-interviewed three years later, the refurbishment of Green Close had been completed (stage 3) and the remaining areas had just been consulted about the refurbishment of their areas, in other words, these areas were then in the same situation that Green Close had been three years earlier (stage 2). Both waves of interviews were conducted at the same time of year (autumn) in order to control for seasonal fluctuations.

The research was coordinated with the local authority which was responsible for the management of the housing, but it was made clear to residents that the study itself was being conducted by researchers from the University of Cambridge and that all information and responses would remain confidential and no individual data would be passed on to the council. Interviews were conducted in the area marked for early improvements (Green Close) and in other non-adjacent areas of the estate characterized by identical housing in similar spatial arrangements. In order to reduce variation in the sample, and also because there were a large number of female single-parent families on the estate, it was decided to interview the oldest female in the household. This was also thought desirable as it was typically women who spent the

Table 7.1: *The stages of development of the Eastlake estate*

	Wave 1	Wave 2 (Three years later)
Green Close	Minor improvements; expectancy of full refurbishment (Stage 2)	Fully refurbished (Stage 3)
Other areas	No change (Stage 1)	Minor improvements; expectancy of full refurbishment (Stage 2)

most time in the residential home environment on Eastlake and who would therefore be most affected by living conditions on the estate. Where there were no women in the household, the oldest male was interviewed. This only happened on a few occasions and these latter data have been excluded from the current analysis.

Residents in these areas were sent a letter informing them about the survey and letting them know that an interviewer would be calling at their address to interview them over the next few days. The letter explained that the survey was examining opinions and concerns about Eastlake, neighbourhood patterns, fear of crime and health. Pre-paid self-addressed envelopes were provided for residents who wished to specify a time for the interviewer to call or to decline to be interviewed. The interview itself began by asking basic questions about the respondent (date of birth, employment status, and so on) but then moved directly to a short, 14-item self-completion questionnaire on mental health (the Hospital Anxiety and Depression scale, or HAD; Zigmond and Snaith, 1983). This scale was introduced as being a check-list on general health. The rationale behind asking respondents to complete the HAD at the beginning of the interview was to avoid their answers being affected by their responses to the questions about the estate that followed later in the interview. Respondents were also asked to complete the 10-item Rosenberg self-esteem questionnaire (Rosenberg, 1962). Once these two scales had been completed, the interview turned to questions about the residents' living arrangements and about the estate. Information was gathered about how long the resident had lived at their present address and about how far away their previous home had been. A series of attitudinal questions were then asked about the residents' experiences of living on the estate, such as the extent to which they were bothered by different types of noise or other problems, and about their level of concern about issues such as safety from traffic, burglary or attack. These were coded on 7-point Likert scales. Detailed questions were also asked about relationships with neighbours, involvement with and attitudes towards the Residents' Association and the Council, and about their views on the likely effectiveness of council-run changes to the estate.

In total, the structured interview generally took between 20 and 25 minutes to complete, though often the interviews continued beyond the end of the structured questions. The qualitative information gathered after the structured interview provided a valuable extra source of information about the estate and about the residents' relationships with one another.

In the first wave of the study, interviews were conducted with 55 Eastlake residents, these being divided approximately equally between the Green Close or stage 2 area (n=26) and the other or stage 1 areas of the estate (n=29). In the second wave of the study, conducted three years after the first, 62 residents were interviewed, with a similar split between the Green Close area, by then in stage 3 (n=27) and the other areas, by then in stage 2 (n=35). The total number of completed interviews conducted was therefore 117. Exactly the same areas of the estate were sampled in the second as the first wave of the study. Considerable efforts were made to re-interview the residents in the same houses as in wave 1. Of course, in some cases, the original residents had moved out during the preceding three years. Also, having used the same sampling frame in both waves, there were inevitably some houses at which residents were successfully interviewed in one wave but not the other. In total, 65 per cent of houses where interviews were conducted in the first wave of interviews were reinterviewed in the second wave (N=36), and of these, 75 per cent were the same residents as in wave 1 (N=27).

The response rate for those sampled was between 60 to 70 per cent, and this remained fairly constant throughout the study. Most of the shortfall was due to households with whom no contact was established despite repeated visits to the house (up to ten visits were made). Conversations with neighbours suggested that the bulk of those with whom contact was not made were working couples without school-age children. This implies such people may have been under-represented in the sample and that non-working women with children (a high-risk group in terms of mental ill-health) and retired respondents may have been over-represented. These sampling details were not a source of serious concern as the comparisons were to be made between groups that had been sampled in the same manner, and subsequent checks confirmed that the relative composition of the groups did not differ significantly over the samples (see below).

About the Eastlake Estate and its People

Sometimes when you walk onto a problem estate, you feel as though you have walked onto a battle-zone. For example, when I first visited the Southgate estate in Runcorn (see Chapter 6) it felt as though I had wandered into a scene from one of those gloomy futuristic science fiction movies – like *Bladerunner* or *Batman* – with burnt out cars, a network of suspended overhead walkways, broken glass everywhere and with massive dark and stained concrete buildings looming over everything. Eastlake however, was very different. Its housing was relatively conventional, consisting mostly of two-storey row houses with sloping roofs and built primarily of brick. It also had seemingly pleasant communal green areas and many trees. Signs of its problem status could certainly be found – graffiti on the walls, broken windows, dismantled cars on blocks, shops with permanent security grills – but still, the estate appeared to have much to recommend it. So what was wrong with Eastlake?

The Estate had come to the attention of the local authority because of its emerging unpopularity. The estate was situated in one of Britain's New Towns, but despite a severe housing shortage in the area, the estate had become very unpopular. This was reflected in the length of the waiting list to get onto the estate – a few months compared to the average of many years. The shortage of housing ensured that there were relatively few voids, but the unpopularity of the estate meant that there was a real danger of it becoming a sink area where only the desperate would go. The police had also become concerned about the estate which was developing a reputation as a relatively high crime area in an otherwise generally safe city.

The Design of the Estate

The Eastlake estate, built in the late sixties and early seventies, consisted of 712 dwellings: 493 two- and three-bedroom houses, plus 219 one-bedroom flats. The most immediately striking feature of the estate was its *Radburn layout*. A Radburn design is one in which access by car is via dead-end roads that run behind the dwellings such that the fronts of the houses face onto a pedestrian-only area. This design was intended to segregate the pedestrian from the car, providing safety from traffic and a quiet and pleasant interior to the estate. The net result can be thought of as something like an inside-out cul-de-sac.

Unfortunately, as has occurred with similar designs elsewhere, human behaviour confounded the designers' original good intentions. It must have been hoped that residents' use of the footpaths, shielded from traffic and confident of their children's safety, would foster positive social relations and a natural sense of community and neighbourliness. The reality proved somewhat different, and the estate was characterized by a strong sense of distrust and uneasiness. Many residents were uneasy about the use of the public footpaths and hardly used their front doors at all. Increasing numbers of residents simply parked their cars as close to their back gates as possible, avoiding the use of their garages and the alleyways that led from the roads to the footpaths at the front. In addition, many residents kept large dogs in their back yards in an effort to discourage unwanted visitors. The alleyways were a particular point of concern both to the police and to the residents. Residents feared the alleyways' poorly lit and unseen corners and the police despaired of the network of escape routes that they provided to offenders. The areas of garages were similarly distrusted; many residents refused to use them while the police found them difficult to patrol and suspected their role in the storage of stolen goods.

However, as suggested by the immediate appearance of the estate, the basic quality of the housing stock was quite good. The houses were reasonably spacious two-storey row-houses (see plates), alternating between two and three bedroom units. The flats were low-rise 12-unit dwellings and were spread throughout the estate. All houses had their own enclosed back gardens and a garage available either immediately at the back of the house or in a block of garages close by. There was a public house (a drinking establishment) and a few shops at the centre of the estate, and a local council housing office had been set up in two converted houses. The pub, however, did have a reputation (apparently justified) of being a violent place and had had a rapid succession of landlords. As one resident explained, 'The floor show is a fight every night.' Similarly, it was noteworthy that the security grills on the shops were never taken down. Nonetheless, the council operated a policy of rapid repairs, and graffiti was removed as soon as possible thus helping to maintain the estate's generally clean appearance. Eastlake was therefore in fairly reasonable condition for a problem estate and though unpopular, still had few vacancies, though largely due to the shortage of housing that has been common in the New Towns as the second generation emerges.

The People

As mentioned earlier, where possible, the oldest woman in the household was interviewed. The average age of the women interviewed was 40.5 years old and did not vary significantly or systematically across areas or stages of redevelopment (42.4 in stage 1; 39.8 in stage 2; 40.2 in stage 3). The average length of residence at their present address was 8.2 years, which again did not vary significantly across areas or stages of development (8.6 years in stage 1; 7.7 in stage 2; 9.0 in stage 3). The average number of children under 14-years-old was 1.4, the proportion who worked was 37 per cent, and the average reported household income was in the range of £97–134 per week (none of which varied significantly by area, wave or stage of development). The latter figure was substantially below the national average: the median real weekly income of a two-child household in 1988 was estimated at £176.4, the figure for the lowest decile point being £118.5 (Central Statistical Office, 1990).

The residents did not fall into a uniform group. Cluster analysis confirmed the general impression of the housing managers that two relatively distinct groups lived on the estate. The majority of the residents were young families with children, many of whom had moved to the estate relatively recently and often in a state of some desperation. There was a minority of residents, however, who were substantially older and who had lived on the estate for considerably longer. (The correlation between age and length of residence was .78, p.<.001). This older subgroup clearly corresponded to the remnants of the estate's earlier population, in other words, those who had moved onto the estate when it was relatively new and when the New Town had just been completed. Older, longer-term residents also differed from the younger residents in that they tended to have originally moved from further away and, unsurprisingly, were less likely to have children under 14-years-old living at home.

The Intervention

The intervention program was originally to be a pilot project focusing on the houses and road on one particular part of the estate (Green Close). The remaining areas were initially to remain unchanged. However, during the course of the study, further money was raised so that by the time the residents were re-interviewed for a second time, the areas outside of Green Close were in the same situation as Green Close three years before.

Residents in the pilot area were sent an information pack explaining the proposed changes, offering further choices and encouraging residents' comments and suggestions. This consultation phase had already begun when the first wave of interviews were conducted.

During the course of the refurbishment of the estate, the council were to work closely with the police and with the DoE guidelines on estate design. The police were particularly concerned that the surveillablity of the estate should improve and especially that areas of car parking should be made clearly visible to residents. The police were also encouraging the replacement of the windows with higher security designs. The council were under pressure, because of the DoE guidelines to listen to and consult with the residents. Hence, for example, some of the residents had made repeated complaints about the dangers of speeding cars, and this led directly to proposed changes to the road surface and the addition of speed ramps. Similarly, the council were committed to involve the residents in each stage of the planning process

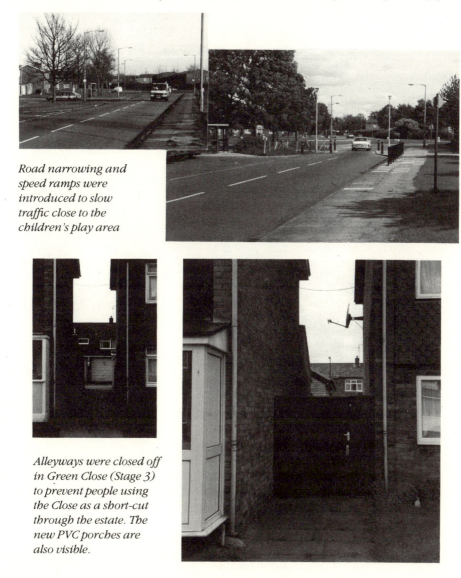

Road narrowing and speed ramps were introduced to slow traffic close to the children's play area

Alleyways were closed off in Green Close (Stage 3) to prevent people using the Close as a short-cut through the estate. The new PVC porches are also visible.

Figure 7.3 (a): *The Eastlake estate before and after the intervention*

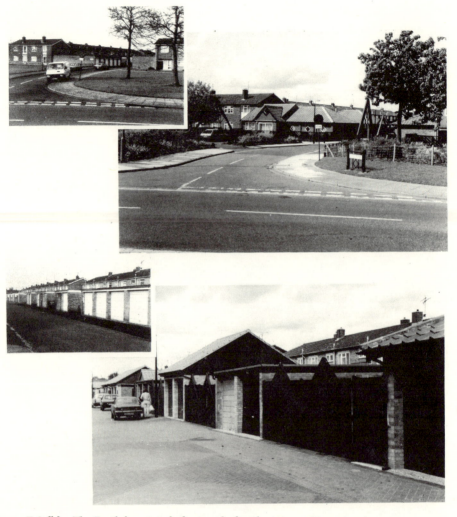

Figure 7.3 (b): *The Eastlake estate before and after the intervention*

and to give residents an opportunity to express their own views about the changes. All in all, the expected cost per dwelling for the full refurbishment was to be between £10000 and £15000.

Stage 1 of the Development

Stage 1 simply refers to the situation before any alterations had taken place. This was the situation that applied to all the areas outside of Green Close during the first wave of interviews and was as described above. In this stage of the development, routine repairs and maintenance was occurring, but there was no systematic upgrading of the estate. In essence, the houses and areas in stage 1 were unchanged, except for wear and tear, from when the estate was first constructed: no systematic changes had occurred to the estate in around 20 years and, in as far as anyone knew, no such changes were about to occur.

Stage 2 of the Development

By stage 2 of the development, two things had occurred. Minor improvements had been made to the areas concerned and residents were being briefed and consulted about a series of far more extensive changes.

The main, and most visible of the minor improvements that distinguished houses in stage 2 from stage 1 was the addition of new PVC porches and front doors. The old wooden porches and doors, dating from when the estate had been built 20 years earlier, had become increasingly leaky and shoddy in appearance. These improvements to porches and doors were done to the Green Close houses by the time of the first interviews and to the rest of the estate by the time of the second interviews.

Perhaps more significantly, however, by stage 2 of the development the residents had been informed that the houses in their area were scheduled for more extensive changes and the residents had been involved in a consultation exercise with the local council about the details of these future improvements. Hence, although there were only minor physical differences between the houses in stage 2 to those in stage 1, there was a large difference between the residents in the extent to which they were in contact with the council and in the extent that they were expecting future improvements to their area.

The future changes that residents in stage 2 had been led to expect included both internal and external works. Hence, when interviews were first conducted among the Green Close residents, the residents were informed that the council was considering the resurfacing of the road, perhaps in brick (to signify it as private), the introduction of measures to slow traffic, the provision of more convenient parking spaces, the re-building and re-siting of garages, the fencing in of ambiguous semi-private space and the closing of the alleyways. The internal works that were being considered included the replacement of windows and locks with double-glazed, higher security types, the refitting of old kitchens with modern fitted units, and the refurbishing of bathrooms. Three years later, residents on the other parts of the estate were told that they could now expect a similar package of measures. In the light of the council's experiences with Green Close, the exact details of the package differed slightly but still contained the same main elements such as the closure of alleyways, the introduction of speed control measures, the replacement of all windows with double-glazed, higher security types and the replacement of old bathrooms and kitchens (the latter to be done on a needs-basis). The few differences in the new programme tended to reflect the residents' wishes, such as the prioritizing of play areas for the under-fives instead of the rebuilding of garages.

The only other minor difference between the areas in stage 2 in the second wave of interviews compared to those in stage 2 at the first wave (Green Close), was that the main play area for the estate had been improved in the intervening period. Clearly, this benefited all the residents on the estate, not just one group. The play area, which lay on the other side of the ring road surrounding the estate, had been modernized and new facilities added. Perhaps more significantly, the road that children had to cross to get to the play area was narrowed and a speed ramp added. The intention of this was to restore parents' confidence that it was safe for their children to go to the play area by themselves. In previous years the play area had become little used and had simply become an area for older teenagers to gather. It was hoped that the improvements to the play area would lead to the re-colonization of the area by younger children and also thereby reduce the problems associated with large numbers of children playing games outside people's houses.

In sum, residents in Green Close when first interviewed, and residents on the rest of the estate when interviewed three years later, were in essentially the same situation. They had received minor improvements to their houses (notably the addition of new porches) and had been consulted by the council about future improvements. Although the minor physical changes were modest, they appeared to be positive. The improved doors and porches were intended to make the houses warmer, more secure, and more attractive in appearance. More importantly, the consultations by the council should have made the residents feel more positive about the council, the estate and about their own power over their residential environment. Even in the absence of more extensive physical changes, this process of consultation may have had a positive effect on residents (see Chapter 6). The process could also have had a beneficial effect if it indirectly encouraged positive contacts between residents (see Chapter 4). Finally, the improvements to the play area and the access to it should have made the estate a better place for children and reduced the concerns of their parents and the irritation to residents of children playing in front of their houses.

Stage 3 of the Development

Stage 3 of the development refers to the stage after the full refurbishment had been completed. This was the situation in Green Close when the residents were re-interviewed three years after the start of the study. Perhaps inevitably, the building work on the estate had taken longer than originally intended. The contractors were changed three times during the work and the council suffered financial problems, both of which resulted in considerable delays in the project.[1] Nonetheless, the building work was completed by November 1991, though this was around a year later than the original target date. (The second set of interviews were conducted in September 1992, just under a year after the refurbishment of the Close was completed.)

Most of the changes as planned in September 1989 were eventually built. In terms of the external works, the road at the centre of Green Close (which had been the source of so much resident concern) was narrowed and re-faced with red brick to denote to drivers that they were entering a private area. Ramps were built into the road in order to slow speeding vehicles. New larger garages were built at the back of residents' gardens (unless residents requested not to have the new garage) though curiously, the old separate block of garages was not demolished. Residents were provided with an area of hard-standing alongside the garage on which a car could be parked and new higher and stronger back gates and fences were built. New lighting was installed and the area in front of Green Close was planted and a sculpture added. The nearby flats were provided with garages, and extra parking was built near the end of Green Close for visitors. These new parking areas were landscaped and surrounded by low planting, and height barriers matching the sculpture were built to prevent lorries using the parking. The alleyways that cut between the houses were blocked off, though keys were given to the residents who lived immediately adjacent to the alleys for their own use. Finally, a bungalow for the disabled was built on a piece of spare ground at the end of Green Close and a small garden fenced off for its resident's use.

Internal building works had also been done though the details of the work varied from house-to-house. All the houses had new double-glazed PVC higher security windows added, and central heating was installed in any houses that did not already have it. The new kitchens and bathrooms, however, were only installed in some of the houses (around half) as it was found that these cost substantially more than expected. Instead of replacing all the kitchens and bathrooms, the council decided to replace these according to need.

In short, there were substantial changes to the houses and the design of the Close as a result of the refurbishment. These changes involved both internal and external works and closely followed the changes offered to residents in stage 2. On the basis of the literature reviewed in the earlier chapters of this book, there was good reason to think that these changes were positive. The internal changes should have made life more pleasant and may have improved pride in living in the houses. The new double-glazed windows may only have had a limited effect on noise levels (see Chapter 2) but should have increased security and made the houses physically warmer. The improvements to the access road and to the back areas of the houses should have made the road safer for children by slowing speeding traffic. The safer arrangements for parking cars should have reduced annoyance from blockages and reduced concerns about car theft and damage, and the improved lighting should have reduced fear. Finally, the closure of the alleyways that allowed people from outside the Close to use it as a short cut should have reduced the numbers of strangers in the Close. This should have further reduced levels of fear and made it more likely for a positive and friendly atmosphere to emerge.

Summary – The Three Phases of the Development

In summary, the development work on the estate could be divided into three distinct phases. In the sections that follow, these will be used as a shorthand to refer to the multiple changes that had taken place on the estate.

Stage 1

No change and no expectancy of change. (Areas outside of Green Close during the first wave of interviews).

Stage 2

Minor changes plus the expectancy of further change. (Green Close during the first wave interviews and other areas of the estate during wave 2). The minor changes included the replacement of old leaky wooden porches and front doors with new PVC porches and front doors. The improvements also included the upgrading of the play area and the safer road crossing to it for all areas of the estate by wave 2. Most important, this stage covered the period during which there was the expectancy of further change derived from the consultations with the council and the information passed on through the residents' association.

Stage 3

The full refurbishment. (Green Close during wave 2). The refurbishment included the replacement of windows with double-glazed higher security PVC designs, the re-surfacing and re-styling of access roads including speed ramps, landscaping, improved lighting and hard-standing for cars by the backs of houses, the replacement of garages at backs of houses with higher quality and larger design, the landscaping of waste ground and the provision of extra parking, the enclosure of gardens for flats, the closure of the alleyways, and the installation of central heating (where not already installed) and the replacement of kitchens and bathrooms (on a needs-priority basis).

There were reasons why each of the changes should have improved the living conditions on the estate. We shall now examine how these changes *were* received and whether or not they did have a positive effect on living conditions on the estate and on residents' mental health.

The Impact of the Changes on Residents' Attitudes, Fears and Concerns

Residents were asked a series of questions about their attitudes towards living on the estate, towards the council, and about their fears and concerns that might be connected to estate living. These ranged from relatively specific questions assessing, for example, the extent to which residents were bothered by particular types of noise or were concerned about particular forms of crime, to relatively global questions assessing residents' general feelings about how safe the area was or how good the area was in which to bring up children.

Responses to questions were, for the most part, on Likert scales (1 to 7) such that residents could either pick a number, for example *5* or *7*, or could pick a description, for example *safe* or *very safe*. The statistical significance of changes were calculated by comparing the means of residents' responses to each question (formally by stage) as calculated from their responses on the Likert scales (1 to 7) or, for simple *yes* or *no* responses, to the average numbers responding one way or the other.

Attitudes Towards the Council and the Potential of the Changes to Improve the Estate

Attitudes towards the council and the changes became progressively and significantly more positive through the stages of the refurbishment. When asked, 'Is the council interested in your view?' 55 per cent of residents in stage 1 had said that the council were *not at all* or *not very* interested. This fell to 31 per cent in stage 2 and to 25 per cent in stage 3. This shift was consistent with the fact that the council consulted the residents in some detail over the proposed changes during stage 2 and actually carried out the changes in stage 3.

More specifically concerning the changes, residents were asked, 'You may have heard that the council are hoping to get some changes done to the estate. From your experience, how much difference do you think that any such changes will make?'[2] Among the residents living in the unchanged and unconsulted stage 1 areas, less than half – 43 per cent – said that any such changes would *improve* or *greatly improve* the estate. Many of these residents tended to respond by making a comment such as, 'I don't think it would make any difference – it's the people.' However, once residents had been consulted about the changes, they seemed to be impressed; 75 per cent of residents after being consulted (stage 2) said that the changes would *improve* or *greatly improve* the estate, and this rose to 85 per cent once the changes had actually been completed (stage 3). Similarly, the proportion of residents who were sceptical about the impact of the changes fell sharply. In stage 1, 43 per cent of residents thought that any changes done by the council to the estate would make *absolutely no difference* or *almost no difference* to the estate, but by stage 2 this proportion had fallen to 23 per cent and by stage 3 had fallen to just 11 per cent. This shift in attitudes was statistically significant.

The direction of these changes were encouraging as they suggested that the council's proposals were being reasonably well received. In fact, the strength of the difference between those who had been consulted and the remainder was strong enough to be discernible (and statistically significant) even after the first wave of interviews and before any major physical alterations had taken place.

Specific Fears and Concerns

There was a reduction in several types of minor concerns as the refurbishment proceeded, though many of these trends were not statistically significant. Concerning noise, for example, 59 per cent of residents in stage 1 said that they were sometimes bothered by noise, the most common complaints being about noise from children followed by noise from traffic. The overall proportion who were sometimes bothered by noise fell to 50 per cent in stages 2 and 3, but this was not statistically significant. For most types of noise, such as being able to hear noise from inside adjacent homes or from children, there were almost no significant changes in complaints over the stages of the development. This was unsurprising given that none of the changes (with the possible exception of the double glazing) were designed to reduce noise.

Prior to the changes, there were fairly high levels of concern about traffic on the estate. Concerns were especially high in Green Close, though there was nothing obvious about the plans to suggest that it was actually any more dangerous than other areas on the estate. In fact, the concern about traffic was particularly surprising given that the design of the estate, a Radburn layout, is specifically intended to separate cars from pedestrians (see above). Nonetheless, it had provoked residents to sign a petition requesting speed ramps a couple of years earlier, and was repeatedly mentioned in interviews. Some of the residents even referred to the incident of a young boy, about 6-years-old, who was fatally rundown on the Close some three years previously.

In order to pursue the possibility that certain parts of the estate might be more dangerous concerning traffic than others, access was obtained to County Council Department of Transportation records on traffic accidents (the department holds computerized records of surveyors' accident reports). A print-out of all accidents to have occurred on Eastlake from 1981 to 1989 proved something of a surprise. Not only was the accident rate very low, no trace could be found of any accident resembling the one described by the Green Close residents. The only fatality that had occurred on Eastlake roads over this period was that of a bus conductor who fell out of the back of his own bus going around the round-about that leads onto the estate. The anomaly was sufficiently intriguing to merit further investigation. A second search was conducted, this time looking for any fatal accident that might have occurred in the whole of the Upton area. An accident was identified that exactly matched the description, but it had occurred on a nearby estate, not on Eastlake. The puzzle was finally solved when one of the housing officials recalled a transfer from that estate shortly after the date of the accident identified by the computer search. What appeared to have happened is that the family that had suffered the accident had moved to the estate (to Green Close) shortly after the accident. Rumour had got out about the accident, but in a garbled form. By a process of Chinese whispers the residents came to believe that the accident had actually occurred in Green Close.

Anyhow, whatever their original cause, the focus of residents' concerns was that cars were often driven at speed up the dead-end roads that ran behind the houses, and that children emerging from the alleyways or playing around the back streets were likely to be hit. Following the refurbishment, there was a sharp fall in levels of concern about traffic on Green Close. The proportion of residents in Green Close who were *very concerned* about safety from traffic fell from 65 per cent before the refurbishment (stage 2) to 39 per cent afterwards (stage 3), while the proportion remained approximately constant in the other parts of the estate (stage 1 to stage 2). Similarly, there was a fall in the level of complaints about traffic noise in Green Close after the full refurbishment. Before the refurbishment (stage 2), 54 per cent of residents said they were sometimes or often bothered by traffic noise, but after the refurbishment (stage 3) this fell to 27 per cent. These reductions suggested that the road narrowing scheme and the speed ramps were effective, at least in as far as they reduced the high levels of concern of the Green Close residents. However, as the levels of concern about traffic and traffic-noise were so high in Green Close prior to the refurbishment, even with the reduction in levels of concern, the post-refurbishment levels were only slightly lower than in the other areas of the estate.

Concerning privacy, there were considerable numbers of complaints about the presence of people in the communal areas outside the fronts of homes, the most common of which concerned children playing directly outside of residents' home, people coming too close to the front of homes, and dogs. Most houses had no barriers to mark their front gardens and hence children and passers-by tended to make no distinction between these and the communal green areas. There were modest falls over the course of the refurbishment in the proportions of people complaining about people coming too close to their homes, being bothered by passers-by looking into their homes or by stray dogs, but these were not statistically significant. However, residents appeared to become more aware of the issue insofar as they became more eager to have segregated front gardens. In stage 1, 48 per cent of residents said they felt it was important to have one's own front garden, but this rose to 69 per cent in stage 2 and 77 per cent in stage 3.[3]

One of the main hopes of the council, and indeed the police, was that the improvements to the estate would lead to reductions in crime and fear. Residents were not explicitly asked about their victimization experiences, but they were asked about their fears and concerns about particular forms of crime – burglary, car theft or damage, vandalism and attack, as well as safety from traffic (see above). All types of concern were lower in stage 3 than in stage 1, though not all of the differences attained statistical significance. Also, there was a slight tendency for some types of concern to rise in stage 2. The strongest overall changes were in concerns about attack and about car theft or damage. The proportion of residents who were *very concerned* about attack fell from 48 per cent in stage 1 and 50 per cent in stage 2 to 35 per cent in stage 3, and the proportion of residents who were *very concerned* about car theft or damage fell from 30 per cent in stage 1 and 32 per cent in stage 2 to just 12 per cent in stage 3. Most of the change was therefore due to the reduction in concerns among residents following the full refurbishment. For example, the proportion of Green Close residents who described themselves as *very concerned* about car theft or damage fell from 37 per cent before the refurbishment (stage 2) to 12 per cent afterwards, while the same proportion on the other areas of the estate remained constant at around 30 per cent. This reduction in fear appeared to relate specifically to the physical alterations to the Close.

The situation concerning the changes in the perceived safety of the estate was captured in residents' responses to the more general question. On balance, how safe would you describe this area to be?' In stage 1, before any improvements or consultations had occurred, only 41 per cent of the residents described the estate as *safe* or *very safe*. In stage 2, after the residents had been consulted, this proportion fell slightly to 34 per cent, suggesting that levels of concern had, if anything, increased. This slight fall might partly have been accounted for by the rumours of unsafety that seemed common among the Green Close residents in stage 2, but it is noteworthy that even in the other parts of the estate there was an increase in concerns about safety following the consultations with the council. This suggests that the occurrence of the consultations themselves may have raised residents' concerns. However, by stage 3, when the physical alterations had been completed, the proportion of residents describing the estate as *safe* or *very safe* had risen sharply to 81 per cent. Hence the actual physical alterations appeared to have more than overcome any increases in residents' concerns about safety following the consultation exercises.

General Attitudes Towards the Estate

As we have seen, the pattern of changes among residents' specific concerns and fears was complex, but where change had occurred, it was generally in a positive direction. In order to check this overall impression, it is helpful to examine residents' more global attitudes towards the Eastlake estate.

After being asked the more detailed questions about the estate, residents were asked, 'So, do you think it's [Eastlake] a good place to bring up kids?' This was an important question because it touched on most of the minor concerns that residents seemed to have, and also because one of the main intentions behind the original design and the latest alterations was to make the estate *child friendly*. Most of the respondents had young or school-age children and had thought about the issue at some length. The minority of older residents who did not have young children were asked to think about this question as if they were being asked to advise someone with children who was considering moving onto the estate.

Before any alterations or consultations had taken place in their area (stage 1), only 22 per cent of residents described Eastlake as being a *good* or *very good* place to bring up children. A much larger proportion – 59 per cent – described the area as being either a *bad* or *very bad* area in which to bring up children. This was a very damning comment on an estate which was supposed to have been designed to be child friendly. Some of the residents' reasons for not recommending the area were relatively clear, such as the lack of play areas and the dangers from traffic. As mentioned earlier, the main play area for the estate was located on the outside of the ring-road which surrounded the estate. The intention of this had presumably been to separate the noise and ball-play of the children from the residents, but as parents were reluctant to allow their children to cross the ring-road by themselves, few younger children used it. Of course, this had meant that the play area tended to be used by older children and teenagers, and the presence of these youngsters made parents even less happy about letting their children out to play there. Other reasons that residents gave were more nebulous and were to do with the social atmosphere on the estate and the widespread perception that the other residents on the estate were not to be trusted or represented a potentially bad influence on their children (see below). However, as the development progressed residents' views became more positive. By stage 2, 34 per cent of residents described the area as a *good* or *very good* area to bring up children (compared with 22 per cent in stage 1), and this proportion rose further to 52 per cent in stage 3. Similarly, the proportion describing the estate as a *bad* or *very bad* area to bring up children fell from 59 per cent in stage 1, to 30 per cent in stage 2 and to 11 per cent in stage 3. This shift in residents' attitudes to the bringing up of children on the estate was highly statistically significant and appeared to capture the general feeling among residents that the estate was improving.

Finally, it is interesting to note that despite residents' clear views that the changes to the estate were improving it, they continued to describe the external image of the estate as very poor. Residents were asked, 'What do you think that others (people outside the estate) think about Eastlake, in other words, how would they rate it (on a scale of 1 to 7) as a place?' In stage 1, 59 per cent of residents said that people outside the estate thought of it as *terrible* (or *1*, the lowest point on the scale); none chose *excellent* and only 7 per cent chose anything above the mid-point. A number of residents also spontaneously described experiencing prejudice on the part of outsiders once they realized that they were speaking to someone from Eastlake. As one resident explained, people think of Eastlake as being *the lowest of the low*. As the changes to the estate unfolded, there was a slight improvement in residents' perceptions of the external image of the estate. By stage 2, the proportion describing the external image of the estate as *terrible* fell to 48 per cent and in stage 3 it fell to 44 per cent. However, this difference was not statistically significant and the external image of the estate continued to be seen as very bad. This suggests that residents' own perceptions that the estate was improving were based on the nature of the changes themselves rather than on a perception that the changes had improved the external reputation of the estate.

The Social Atmosphere of the Estate

In Chapter 4, it was shown how the social atmosphere of an area and the quality of the relationships between the residents could be influenced by the design of the environment. In some cases the social atmosphere of an area or building had become so bad that the decision was taken to demolish the entire structure (for example, the Pruitt-Igoe project) or to convert it to non-residential uses (for example, the double-loaded dormitories at Sarah Lawrence College). Also, there was evidence to suggest that a universal characteristic of so-called *problem estates* is the level of social distrust between residents (Reynolds, 1986). As we shall see, Eastlake was no exception.

Quantitative Measures of Neighbour Involvement

There were a number of questions and measures in the Eastlake interviews designed to explore the quantity and quality of the relationships between residents. The more quantitative or factual questions explored issues such as the number of visits residents received from neighbours (other Eastlake residents), the proportion of other residents they felt able to recognize on their Close, and the levels of involvement in the Residents' Association. Other more qualitative questions (though also coded to give quantitative data) attempted to explore the relationships between neighbours; these are described later.

One measure of residents' involvement with one another was derived from the question, 'Concerning your neighbours, i.e. those on Eastlake, in the last six months how many have stopped by?' In stage 1, the average number of neighbours reported visiting was around 6, but this average is deceptive in that the number of visits varied greatly between residents and the distribution of answers was very skewed. Around a third of residents (31 per cent) reported having received no visits at all from neighbours in the past six months, and over half (59 per cent) reported having only one, or less, neighbours visit. A number of the residents reported having just one regular visitor, perhaps a relative who lived on the estate, while having almost no contact at all with the other residents. However, a small minority of residents reported very high levels of visits from neighbours: around 1 in 6 (17 per cent) of the residents reported having 20 or more different neighbours visit in the previous six months. These people were who Festinger, *et al.*, (1950) would have called *sociometric stars*. One couple in their sixties reported having around 40 different neighbours visit over the period. This claim was supported by the fact that they had several visits even during the course of the interview – 'The door is always open', this popular resident explained, 'and you, dear, are you sure you won't have another cup of tea?' As the development progressed, the number of people who were totally isolated from their neighbours fell. By stage 2, the proportion of residents who had received no visits from neighbours in the previous six months had fallen from 31 per cent to 21 per cent, and by stage 3 it had fallen to 15 per cent. The overall average level of visits, however, did not change as the small number of people who received very large numbers of visits fell slightly. This indicates that the visiting behaviour became more evenly spread across the residents.

A second way of quantitatively examining residents' relations to one another was derived from the question, 'Would you be able to recognize your neighbours who live on this block by sight?' The proportion reporting being able to recognize most or all of their neighbours rose from 55 per cent in stage 1, to 59 per cent in stage 2 and to 74 per cent in stage 3. Clearly, most of the shift coincided with the full refurbishment rather than with the more minor changes and the consultations of stage 2, and it is tempting to think that the increase was largely the result of the closure of the alleyways and the consequent exclusion of strangers from the Close.

The third simple measure of resident involvement with one another comes from a series of questions about involvement in the Residents' Association. The level of knowledge about and involvement in the Residents' Association increased significantly as the development progressed. In stage 1, 72 per cent of residents had heard of the Residents' Association, but this had risen to 81 per cent in stage 2 and to 96 per cent in stage 3. In stage 1, only 3 per cent (1 person) had attended any Residents' Association meetings, but by stage 2 this had risen to 14 per cent and to 19 per cent in stage 3. Similarly, the proportion of people who read the Association's newsletter and the proportion who knew somebody who attended meetings also increased.

Rohe (1985), among others, has argued that a major reason for encouraging residents' involvement in the management of housing through structures such as Residents' Associations is that this can lead to more positive relationships between neighbours. The simple data presented above is consistent with that hypothesis, though they are not, by themselves, conclusive. It is difficult to know whether the increasing strength of the Residents' Association was the cause of the reduced isolation of residents or whether it was the consequence of such contacts.

More seriously, there are limitations to how much can be established from simple quantitative measures about the quality of the relationships between residents. For example, let us consider a simple factual question about how many people visit a particular resident. Some residents said that they did receive occasional visits from neighbours but indicated that they were still deeply suspicious of them fearing, for example, that these visitors might just be checking out what they possessed so that they could come back and steal it. Others indicated that they did not go into one another's homes but this did not necessarily imply that they were on poor terms with their neighbours. In order to assess the quality of the relationships between residents more carefully, it is necessary to turn to more detailed and qualitative questions.

Qualitative Measures of Neighbour Relations

The common way of assessing the quality of a person's relationships with others – their social support – is to ask people about the helpfulness of others in particular situations, especially in situations of need. Before the improvements to the estate had begun (stage 1), the general impression given by many residents was that although some of their neighbours might help if asked, they themselves would be reluctant or wary to ever ask for such help. Overall, the impression was given of a high level of distrust between the residents, though without any clear focus. Again and again, the same expression would arise. 'Well, we just keep ourselves to ourselves.' As one young mother put it, 'I know it sounds an awful thing to say, but I just don't get involved. It's the only way to be here. I didn't understand when people said this before I came here.'

The comments of many residents were reminiscent of those reported by Yancey (1971) of the infamous and ill-fated Pruitt-Igoe project in St. Louis (see Chapter 4). Typically, residents would just talk vaguely about the problem with *the people* on the estate. Yet the curious thing about this situation was that while many people reported being wary of the other residents, it was very unclear who exactly the *bad uns* were. Wherever you were, the problem people and areas tended to be seen as somewhere else on the estate. 'We're lucky living on the outside (of the estate) – it's much worse in the middle.' Yet a woman living in the area to which she was referring similarly explained 'We're lucky in this bit; in other streets there's quite a bit of riffraff.' The few neighbours that residents did have some contact with were seen as the exceptions rather than the rule. This is a similar phenomenon to that described by Reynolds in her in-depth study of a large problem estate (Reynolds, 1986) and seems to be typical among problem estates.

In order to assess the quality of the relationships between neighbours more systematically, residents were asked to imagine a series of situations and to rate how helpful they would expect their neighbours to be in each situation. For example, the first situation was, 'If you were ill and needed helping out with shopping etc,' and residents had to rate how helpful and supportive their neighbours (any non-household members who lived on Eastlake estate) would be in this situation. Ratings were made on a seven point scale ranging from *very unhelpful* (1) to *very helpful* (7). In the first wave of interviews, residents were also asked to rate how helpful three other groups of people would be in each situation – their partners and other resident household members, their friends and relatives (not living on Eastlake), and official sources of support such as religious, council, police or medical personnel. This latter information about non-neighbours was not gathered in the second wave of interviews as it was not essential and considerably extended the interview. The seven situations included: being ill; being bored; needing help with the children at short notice (if the respondent had children); needing someone to talk to; coming home to find they had been burgled and their home a mess; wanting to borrow some household items (for example, some tools or foodstuff); and needing to borrow some cash. These items were designed to tap the kinds of social support that might be derived from neighbours and were developed especially for the study. If an item was inapplicable (for example, due to the absence of children) it was coded as *n/a* or system-missing. If the respondent said that they simply would not approach the person or group in that situation (for example, would not go to neighbours to borrow cash), this was coded as a *3* (unhelpful). An overall social support scale was calculated by summating residents' ratings of helpfulness from six of the seven situations – the item concerning help for children was excluded from the composite scale as this item did not apply to about one-third of respondents.

The helpfulness of each group – household members, neighbours, and so on – was highly correlated across situations. Summating the helpfulness of each group across situations showed that, in the situations presented, average levels of support were greatest from within the household, followed by support from friends and relatives outside the estate, then from neighbours, and lastly, from official sources. Support from officials was very much less important than support from other sources. The mean score for household social support would have been higher still except for the fact that a number of interviewees lived alone or with only a young child leading to a clear bi-modal distribution to the levels of household social support. While the

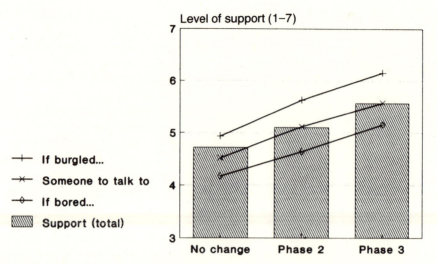

Figure 7.1: *Social support from neighbours by phase of redevelopment*

level of estimated support from neighbours, friends and relatives, and officials were significantly correlated, these were unrelated to the level of support from within the household. This suggests that the level of support from outside the home was independent of that from within. The social support scale showed that there was a clear increase in the perceived supportiveness of neighbours as the refurbishment of the estate proceeded, average supportiveness rising from 4.7 in stage 1, to 5.1 in stage 2 and 5.6 in stage 3 ($r=.20$, $p<.05$). In all seven of the situations, the reported supportiveness of neighbours increased with the stage of the refurbishment. This trend was statistically significant at the .05 level for three out of the seven situations, though the pattern was similar throughout. The three situations showing the strongest effects were, in descending order of strength, the helpfulness of neighbours in the event of coming home to find that you had been burgled (35 per cent said *very helpful* in stage 1 compared with 65 per cent in stage 3), of being bored and wanting to do something (17 per cent said *very helpful* in stage 1 compared with 35 per cent in stage 3), and of needing someone to talk to (28 per cent said *very helpful* in stage 1 compared with 46 per cent in stage 3).

The improved relations between residents was also reflected in their responses to a general question about friendliness: 'So on balance, on a scale of 1 to 7, how friendly an area would you describe this as?' In stage 1, only 7 per cent of residents described the area as *very friendly*, but by stage 2 this had risen to 18 per cent and by stage 3 to 26 per cent. The overall shift in residents' responses to this question showed the same level of positive change to that of the more specific social support scale ($r=.20$, $p.<.05$), and indeed, the two measures were closely related ($r=.49$, $p<.001$).

In sum, the changes to the estate appeared to have brought with them significant improvements in the social atmosphere of the estate. Before the refurbishment or consultations had begun, the estate had a very depressing social atmosphere. Although there were a few people on the estate in stage 1 who were extremely sociable, most residents led extremely private and withdrawn lives. For some, their fear of the other residents led to complete withdrawal: 'I daren't let my kids out, I have never known an estate as bad as this one.' For most, however, it simply led to caution and to keeping themselves to themselves. Possibly as a result of the increased contact between the residents fostered by the consultation process, the situation appeared to have markedly improved by stage 2, and by stage 3 the difference was very striking. Again, it is difficult to say exactly what aspect of the physical changes or consultation process led to this marked improvement, but it seems likely that a combination of factors acted to reverse the vicious cycle of withdrawal and distrust between neighbours. The prospect of the changes, the ongoing consultation process and strengthened Residents' Association gave residents an excuse to talk to one another and thereby broke down the level of distrust. In stage 3, the physical alterations (notably the closure of alleyways) reduced the presence of strangers and enhanced the ability of residents to recognize their neighbours (the association between the social support scale and the ability to recognize neighbours was high, r=.52, p<.001).

Finally, perhaps the simple fact that the estate was visibly improving gave residents greater confidence in the estate and the people who lived on it and enabled them to see beyond the stereotype of the estate as a place forgotten by the council full only of *riffraff* and trouble. When residents actually spoke to their neighbours they discovered that they weren't such monsters after all and that, at least for the most part, they were people very much like themselves and with the same needs, hopes and fears.

The Impact on Residents' Mental Health

As mentioned earlier, a standard mental health measure was administered to all respondents. These scales were designed to measure anxiety and depression (the Hospital Anxiety and Depression Scale or HAD) and self-esteem (the Rosenberg Self-Esteem Scale). The internal consistency of the scales was good, and the associations between the three scales were high (around r=0.7, though clearly the associations between the self-esteem scale and the other two were in the negative direction).[4]

The Relationship between Mental Health and the Population Characteristics

When interviewing commenced on the estate, the immediately striking aspect of the mental health data was how high the scores were, in other words, the residents appeared to be in extremely poor mental health. In stage 1, the average combined score on the HAD was 13.6, and the average scores on the anxiety and depression sub-scales were 8.2 and 5.5 respectively. Zigmond and Snaith (1983), the original designers of the scale, tested the HAD on clinical and other populations and developed suggested cut-off points for the assessment of severity. They estimated that a cut-off point of 8–9 (on each scale) would catch most cases, while a more conservative cut-off of 10–11 would catch only *highly probable* cases. The cut-off point chosen depends on the number of false positives acceptable, but either way, it was clear that a sizeable proportion of the Eastlake population in the unaltered areas

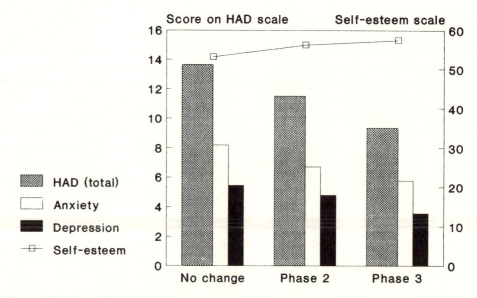

Figure 7.2: *Mental health of residents by phases of redevelopment*

of the estate would be classified as cases even if the more conservative cut-off point were used. This was especially true of the anxiety scale: 57 per cent of the residents in stage 1 would have been classed as cases if the 8+ cut-off was used, and 32 per cent would have been classed as cases if the conservative 11+ cut-off was used. The proportions suffering from depression were somewhat lower but were still very high: 25 per cent would have been classed as cases if the 8+ cut-off was used and 7 per cent would have been classed as cases if the 11+ cut-off was used.

These very high figures become more comprehensible once it is recalled that subjects were from a high-risk population for mental ill-health: female, poor, and with children, as well as living in a grim area with a poor social atmosphere. Both by selection and by causation, high rates of anxiety and depression were to be expected.

The mental health measures were compared to individual demographic variables. This provided a useful check on the validity of the measures as well as being of interest in itself. As expected from previous work (Brown and Harris, 1978; Mirowsky and Ross, 1989) significantly higher levels of symptoms and lower levels of self-esteem were found among those with a larger number of children under the age of

Table 7.2: *Correlations between the mental health scales and the background variables*

	Anxiety	Depression	HAD (total)	Self-esteem
Age	−.34 ***	−.21 *	−.30 **	.29 **
Length of residence	−.28 **	−.10 ns	−.21 *	.27 **
Number of children < 14 years	.19 *	.19 *	.21 *	−.30 **
Income	−.29 **	−.27 **	−.31 **	.32 ***

(N = 112; * = p < .05, ** = p < .01, *** = p < .001)

14 and with lower incomes. Age also showed a negative association with symptom levels, older people having slightly better mental health. Closer examination reveals that this association derived principally from the superior mental health of the older subgroup of long-term residents described earlier. It was noteworthy that these associations were much stronger in the current data than those found in the secondary data analysis of the SCPR data set reported earlier in the book (Chapter 2). This appeared to reflect the more sensitive measures used in the Eastlake survey.

The relationship of age to symptoms was clearly related to position in the life cycle and especially to the having of young children. However, it may also have related to the more positive attitude that older residents had towards their situation and to living on Eastlake. A number of the older women interviewed spoke of the very harsh conditions they had lived in before they moved to the estate. They had memories of pre-slum clearance London housing with which to compare Eastlake and this appeared to be reflected in their more positive attitudes towards the council and in their more positive rating of the estate's image in general.

Changes in Residents' Mental Health Across the Stages of the Refurbishment

Before the alterations to the estate began, the average resident's mental health was clearly extremely poor: 57 per cent of residents had levels of symptoms reaching the probable case criteria for anxiety on the HAD (average score =8.2) and 25 per cent had levels reaching the probable case criteria for depression (average score =5.5). However, as the refurbishment of the estate proceeded, residents' mental health steadily improved. Residents' average scores on the HAD fell from 13.6 in stage 1, to 11.5 in stage 2 and to 9.3 in stage 3 (r=−.22, p<.05; or between stage 1 and 3, F=6.85, p<.05). Average scores on the anxiety section of the HAD fell from 8.2 in stage 1, to 6.7 in stage 2 and to 5.8 in stage 3 (r=.−.21, p<.05; F=6.64, p<.05), while average scores on the depression section fell slightly more slowly, but still significantly, from 5.4 in stage 1, to 4.9 in stage 2 and to 3.6 in stage 3 (r=−.18, p<.05; F=4.29, p<.05). Levels of self-esteem, as measured by the Rosenberg scale rose over the stages of the

Table 7.3: *Percentage of residents reaching 'caseness' across the three stages of the development*

	Cut-off	Stage 1 No change (N = 28)	Stage 2 Partial change (N = 57)	Stage 3 Complete (N = 27)
Anxiety	Probable (8+)	57.1	45.6	22.2
		(16)	(26)	(6)
	Very probable (11+)	32.1	14.0	7.4
		(9)	(8)	(2)
Depression	Probable (8+)	25.0	21.2	3.7
		(7)	(12)	(1)
	Very probable (11+)	7.4	5.3	0
		(2)	(3)	(0)

refurbishment from 53.1 in stage 1, to 56.2 in stage 2 and 57.5 in stage 3, but this was not significant at the .05 level (r=.13, p<.1; F=2.02).

Translating these results into *probable* or *very probable* cases illustrates the scale of the improvement in residents' mental health. For anxiety, the proportion of probable cases fell from 57 per cent in stage 1 to 22 per cent in stage 3, and the proportion of very probable cases fell from 32 per cent to 7 per cent. For depression, the proportion of probable cases fell from 25 per cent in stage 1 to 4 per cent in stage 3, and the proportion of very probable cases fell from 7 per cent to none. In sum, there was a substantial and statistically significant pattern of progressively improving residents' mental health as the improvements to the estate proceeded.

The pattern of differences across the stages of the refurbishment was not the result of overall differences between the two test areas. When the two areas of study (Green Close and the other areas) were in the same stage of refurbishment (stage 2; Green Close in wave 1 and the other areas in wave 2), the mental health of the residents in the two areas were very similar. For example, the mean HAD score of the Green Close residents when in stage 2 was 11.7 (compared to 9.3 when the same area was in stage 3) and the mean HAD score of the other areas' residents when in the same stage, though three years later, was very similar at 11.4 (compared to 13.6 when in stage 1). Clearly, the critical factor was the stage of refurbishment rather than the area *per se*.

As there was a longitudinal component to the study, it was also possible to check whether the improvements in mental health were happening within individuals as well as across groups. Checks were run to identify the same individuals living in the same houses (by using the home address and the date of birth) so that their mental health before the interventions could be compared with their mental health afterwards. This is called a within-pairs comparison. Just over half of the residents who were interviewed at wave 1 were re-interviewed at wave 2. Hence the sample size for the comparisons was relatively small (N=27), but this was partly offset by the improved sensitivity of the within-pairs comparison. The average mental health at wave 1 of those successfully re-interviewed was very similar to those not re-interviewed, suggesting that those who were re-interviewed were not atypical in terms of mental health (average HAD score at wave 1 of those re-interviewed was 12.9 compared with 12.4 for those not re-interviewed). The within-pairs comparisons showed that there was a reasonably high degree of consistency in the residents' mental health over the three years, in other words, the people with the best and worst mental health tended to be the same in both wave 1 and 2 (the correlations across waves for the mental health measures varied between .43 and .51). More importantly, the within-pairs comparisons revealed a similar pattern of change over time to that shown by the between groups comparisons. Residents showed falls in levels of anxiety, depression and an increase in levels of self-esteem. As in the between groups comparisons, levels of anxiety showed the strongest falls over time (t=2.5, p<.01). The fall in the total HAD scores was also statistically significant but the changes in depression and self-esteem, though showing the same pattern, were not statistically significant in the smaller within-pairs comparisons. The falls tended to be slightly sharper in the Green Close residents than in the other areas of the estate, in other words, from stage 2 to stage 3 (10.6 to 8.7 on the HAD) as compared with from stage 1 to stage 2 (11.5 to 10.6 on the HAD) but, as in the between groups comparisons, the average mental health scores of the two groups when both in stage 2 were very similar (10.6 on the HAD).

Interpreting the Changes in Mental Health

There were clearly substantial improvements in residents' mental health coinciding with the residents' consultations with the Council and with the physical changes to the estate. The improvements in mental health were most marked for anxiety which showed substantial falls over the three years. The improvements in mental health could not simply be attributed to a selection effect – to people with worse mental health leaving or people with better mental health moving in – as the within-pairs analysis (where the individuals concerned stay the same) showed similar evidence of improvements in residents' mental health.

Similarly, the improvements in mental health could not be attributed to changes in the background characteristics of the population, such as a change in the average age of the residents or in the average number of children under 14 years per household. Statistical controlling for age, length of residence, number of children under 14, employment status and income, although explaining a significant amount of variation in mental health (for anxiety, for example, multiple R=.34) such statistical controls did not attenuate the size of the improvements in mental health associated with the stages of the refurbishment. This was because the basic demographic and social characteristics of the Eastlake population did not vary much across areas of the estate nor across the time of the study.

Clearly, any plausible explanation of the improvement in residents' mental health has to make reference to the improvements on the estate. A series of multiple regressions were employed in order to see whether any of the reported changes in the estate would explain the improvement in residents' mental health. Having first controlled for the effects of background social and demographic differences, a forward-entry stepwise regression was employed. It was found that, for anxiety, once residents' concerns about crime and their ratings of how good the area was considered (in terms of bringing up children) were controlled for, then the stage of development no longer significantly predicted residents' mental health. A similar result was found for depression; once residents' concerns about privacy (children playing outside, people outside the home) and how good the area was considered for bringing up children, the stage of development no longer significantly predicted residents' levels of depression. These results strongly support the hypothesis that it was the changes, or at least residents' perceptions of these changes, that mediated residents' improved mental health.

Of course, many of the residents' perceptions were closely related to one another. Hence, for example, people who rated the area as a good place to bring up children were also more likely to describe the area as safe (r=.56, p.<.001), to rate the reputation of the area as positive (r=.51, p.<.001) and to describe the area as friendly (r=.44, p.<.001). This makes it very difficult, as suggested in the introduction, to identify exactly which aspect of the environmental and management changes led to the improvements in mental health. In reality, it is likely that it was a combination of the factors that led to the marked improvements in mental health. In stage 2 of the development, the promise of the changes to the estate by the council combined with the fact that some minor improvements had already taken place, made residents feel positive about the future of the estate and the council's commitment to improving it. The prospect of changes also acted as a positive force to bring residents into contact with one another and these contacts began to break down the atmosphere of distrust.

The mental health of residents improved still further following the full refurbishment of Green Close, suggesting that the more extensive physical changes led to greater benefits than the hope of change alone could deliver. The closing off of alleyways to reduce the presence of strangers, the improved layout of the access road to allow cars to be safely parked at the backs of houses, the improved lighting to reduce fear, the new windows and locks to reduce the risk of burglary and reduce heat loss, the replacement of old kitchens and bathrooms – all of these improvements probably had positive effects on residents' mental health, and it is not possible to conclusively separate their effects. What we can say is that the overall impact of the package of changes was extremely positive and that this change for the better appeared to mediate substantial improvements in residents' previously poor mental health.

Discussion and Summary

The Eastlake study provides positive evidence that, at least in some important instances, mental health can be improved through an environmental intervention. Of course, the situation on Eastlake before the intervention was particularly bad, but the situation was not *that* unusual. Even in the UK, there are many problem housing estates like Eastlake, and this is reflected in the fact that many millions of pounds have to be spent through the DoE's Estate Action Programme every year. Similarly, although some detailed aspects of Eastlake's problems and the subsequent solutions might not apply elsewhere, the main themes of Eastlake's problems are probably typical of many problem estates. These main themes included the estate's unpopularity, the widespread fear of crime, the atmosphere of distrust, the withdrawal of the residents and the common view, both among residents and outsiders, that the estate was a bad place, especially for the raising of children.

The methodology used in the present study, rather like that of the famous Kirkholt project in environmental criminology, demonstrates that the intervention worked. However, it does not allow us to separate out the individual contributions of different aspects of the intervention. In reality, the various aspects of the intervention probably acted to reinforce one another. Hence, the minor improvements and the consultations with the council that had occurred by stage 2 probably had a more positive impact as a combination than they would have done individually. The fact that some minor improvements had already occurred when the council asked residents for their views on a series of future changes probably made the residents take the consultations far more seriously than they otherwise would have done. Similarly, the minor changes took on a greater significance in the context of the consultations because they came to symbolize the start of a series of positive changes to the estate rather than being seen as a one-off alteration. As one resident said, 'They've done those new porches, haven't they? That's got to mean something, hasn't it?' The full refurbishment had a further positive impact on the estate, although once again, it was not possible to separate the effects of the different aspects of the full refurbishment on mental health. It seems likely that certain changes in residents' concerns and attitudes were the result of specific alterations, for example, the reduction in concerns about traffic seemed to relate to the introduction of speed ramps and road narrowing, and the reduction in concerns about car theft and damage seemed to relate to the new garages, areas of hard-standing and gates. However, it is difficult to know which aspects of the changes led to less specific improvements such as in the social atmosphere of the estate as manifested in both quantitative measures (such as the proportion of neighbours recognized or the level of involvement in the residents' association) and qualitative measures (such as the social support scale or the rated friendliness of the area). This type of more general attitudinal and behavioural change did not relate in a simple way to any one aspect of the physical changes on the estate. True, the closure of the alleyways may have encouraged residents to use the area in front of the houses more and thereby made it easier for them to recognize and get to know one another, but this alone seems unable to account for the breadth of the change (nor the change that had occurred by stage 2). Perhaps the occurrence of change itself was important as it brought residents together and gave them something to discuss. Perhaps the cosmetic changes to the area were equally important in that they encouraged residents to reappraise the estate and those who lived on it. Perhaps all these things contributed to the shift. The same applies for the improvements in mental health; there were many aspects to the changes on the estate, and any or all of these many have contributed to the improvements in residents' mental health. In short, the Eastlake study shows that a well-balanced package of improvements to a problem housing estate can improve the situation and the residents' mental health, but we will have to wait for future studies before we can say with certainty exactly which changes lead to which effects.

Finally, it should be stressed that it would be wrong to conclude from the success of the intervention described in this study that all aspects of mental ill-health among all people could be improved by environmental interventions. Mental ill-health is an extremely complex and multi-faceted phenomenon, and even within a single individual, psychiatric or psychological symptoms can have many determinants. A very wide range of genetic, individual and social factors have been shown to affect mental health, and the exact influence of each of these factors on different types of mental illness varies. Even in the present study, the effects of the environmental changes seemed greater on one type of mental symptom than another (anxiety rather than depression). Clearly, the environment is just one of many factors that can affect mental health, but nonetheless, it *is* a factor, and it can be a very important one among those living on society's problem estates.

Notes

1   As the project was financed by the DoE and not the council itself, the project was never in serious danger of cancellation but the administrative chaos caused by the crises meant that the project was delayed nonetheless.

2   The wording of the question to those in stage 3 was slightly altered to take account of their altered circumstances, 'Concerning the changes that the council have made: how much difference would you say that the changes have made to the estate?'

3   Since the study was completed, a council worker told me that they are now considering offering to fence in residents' front gardens.

4   During interviewing, it was noticed that question 11 of the HAD – 'I feel restless as if I have to be on the move: very much indeed . . . not at all?' – was answered affirmatively by a few subjects but in a *positive* sense. However, despite this the item continued to be generally associated with the other anxiety items (r=.5, p<.001) and this item was left in for the analyses, not least in order to maintain comparability with other studies.

Appendix

Table D.1: *Correlations between background measures (N = 112 except where stated otherwise)*

	Age	Residence	Distance
Age	.		
Length of residence	.78 ***	.	
Distance from previous home	.41 ***	.42 ***	.
Number of children < 14 yrs	−.59 ***	−.49 ***	−.27 **
Income	−.09 ns	.04 ns	−.11 ns

[** = p < .01, *** = p < .001]

Table D.2: *Correlations between the mental health measures*

	Anxiety	Depression	HAD
Anxiety	.		
Depression	.66	.	
HAD (tot.)	.92	.91	.
Self-esteem (Rosenberg)	−.68	−.72	−.77

[All p < .001]

Table D.3: *Pair-wise correlation matrix*

	Anxiety	Depression	Self-esteem
Age	−.37 **	−.25 *	.21
Length of residence	−.31 *	−.18	.13
Distance from previous home	−.00	−.12	.01
Children < 14 yrs	.31 *	.36 **	−.38 **
Household income	−.19	−.29 *	.32 *

[Minimum N = 50; * = p < .05, ** = p < .01]

Table D.4: *Summary statistics of the social support subscales*

	Mean	Median	s.d.
SSH (House)	5.51	6.3	4.3
SSN (Neighbours)	4.92	5.3	2.5
SSF (Friends)	5.42	6.2	3.1
SSO (Official)	2.84	2.6	2.4
SSSum	18.64		

Table D.5: *Correlation matrix for Social Support subscales*

	SSH	SSN	SSF	SSO
SSH	.			
SSN	.02	.		
SSF	−.02	.41 **	.	
SSO	.01	.33 **	.38 **	.
SSSum	.47 **	.69 **	.65 **	.63 **

[N = 53; ** p < .01]

Chapter 8

Mental Health and the Built Environment: Conclusions

Is There a Causal Relationship between Mental Illness and the Built Environment?

This book has explored the relationship between mental illness and the built environment. Early research revealed strong associations between aspects of the environment and mental illness but was not able to establish the direction of causality of this relationship (Chapter 1).

In an effort to resolve the issues more clearly, all of the available literature on the relevant topics was reviewed. We have explored the possibility that the built environment might be able to affect mental health through four channels of influence: environmental stress (Chapters 2 and 3), social support (Chapter 4), meaning and symbol (Chapter 5) and the planning process (Chapter 6). The existing literatures were supplemented by a series of new studies and analyses. The re-analysis of a large data set containing objective measures of respondents' residential environments supplemented and extended the existing literatures on environmental stress and social support. A series of multivariate analyses demonstrated that there were significant associations between the objective environmental measures and residents' mental health, and that these associations could not be attributed to background variables such as age, sex and income. Another study demonstrated how the planning process can affect mental (and physical) health, even in the absence of physical change (Chapter 6). It was shown that general practitioner consultations by the residents of a housing estate fluctuated according to the decisions taken by planners and politicians about the estate's future. A final test study examined the effects of the refurbishment of a problem estate and explored the issue of whether mental health could be improved through an environmental intervention (Chapter 7). It was found that, across the stages of the refurbishment, problems associated with the estate were perceived to be reduced and residents' mental health substantially improved, the strongest reduction being found in levels of anxiety (as measured by the Hospital Anxiety and Depression scale). These differences were found for both between-group and within-subject comparisons.

The results from the literature reviews and the new studies provided many insights into the social and behavioural consequences of the environment and, more specifically, provided clear evidence of the environment's ability to causally affect mental health. Each of the new studies, though based on differing methodologies and exploring different aspects of the planned environment, demonstrated that the null hypothesis – that the built environment does not affect mental health – should be rejected. The built environment is causally implicated in the aetiology of mental illness, and especially in the types of mild psychiatric and somatic symptoms that are common in the community.

How does the Environment Affect Mental Health?

Following the structure established through the book, four channels of environmental influence may be distinguished, there being evidence that each of them can affect mental health to some extent.

Environmental stress

The most direct way in which the planned environment can affect mental health is by acting as a source of stress. Environmental stress, such as pollution, noise, heat, certain weather conditions, and high social densities can lead to negative mental states (irritation and annoyance). The types of environmental stress which lead to psychiatric or somatic symptoms as opposed to just irritation tend either (a) to be difficult for the individual to identify as the source of their irritation (for example, pollution); (b) to involve chronic difficulties in social regulation (for example, sharing living space with unrelated others); or (c) to involve personal threat (for example, high density prison living, the fear of crime). In these instances the source of stress affects not only mood but also tends to compromise patterns of coping behaviour.

Social support: the mixed blessing of neighbours

The hypothesis was explored that neighbours could have a positive influence on mental health by providing support and assistance to one another. The close proximity of neighbours means that they can be a very convenient source of support and assistance if neighbouring relations are good, but their proximity also means that they can be a major source of irritation, annoyance and even fear if these relations turn sour. The physical environment can be very important in determining the form and character of neighbouring relations. Positive neighbouring relations are less likely to develop where large numbers of strangers are present and where residents are forced into social interactions which they cannot regulate. The continuing presence of large numbers of strangers makes it less likely that residents will get to know or recognize one another, and this leads to less friendly neighbouring relations, greater fear of crime and more concerns about the safety of children. The effects of many environmental stressors, such as noise, density and fear, may also be partly mediated by the way in which they affect the social relations between neighbours.

Conclusions

Symbolic aspects of the environment

There is suggestive evidence that symbolic aspects of the environment can affect mental health. First, social labelling can have dramatic effects on the environment; residential sorting is strongly influenced by the labelling process such that labels often become self-fulfilling prophesies. It seems probable that this process of labelling also has an effect on the mental health of residents living in the labelled area, but the direct link to mental health has yet to be conclusively proven. A second way in which symbolic aspects of the environment may affect mental health is through discrepancies between individuals' aspirations and their perceived achievements, and the evidence on this is more convincing. The wider literature on relative deprivation suggests that an individual's aspirations and achievements are seen in comparison to those of others and relative to the individual's own past experience. Although there is little evidence to suggest that such aspiration achievements have a *net* effect (across the entire population) on mental health, there is evidence to suggest that the higher levels of mental illness associated with certain groups and certain building types (notably the high-rise) partly may result from such discrepancies. Further research is needed on the mental health effects of symbolic aspects of the environment before firmer conclusions can be drawn.

The planning process

Mental health can also be affected by the planning process itself. If residents are unable to participate in the decisions concerning their own environment, then not only is it more likely that the decisions taken will be unpopular, it is also likely that residents will experience a sense of powerlessness and frustration. The adverse consequences of the planning process was notoriously illustrated by the negative impact on residents of forced relocation resulting from slum clearance programmes but, of course, much of this negative impact resulted from social dislocation rather than the planning process itself. However, the case study of Southgate (Chapter 6) illustrated that even in the absence of physical change, the planning process can have dramatic and negative impact on the mental health of residents. In this respect, it will be interesting to see whether future research will find any improvements in residents' mental health associated with the empowerment of residents through the spread of housing associations (self-management).

If There is an Effect, then How Large is it?

Although the work presented here has shown that the planned environment has at least *some* effect on mental health, it is difficult to put an exact figure on how large this effect is. The amount of variance in mental illness explained by any given variable depends partly on the causal relevance of the variable, but also partly on the level of variance of that (and other) variables in the sampled population. For example, it has been reported that students' grades at school are a poor predictor of the classes of degree attained at university (A-level grades appear to account for little of the variance in classes of degree). However, it would be quite incorrect to deduce from this finding that grades at school bear little relation to the ability to get a good grade at university.

There is very little variance in the grades of the students at university (the sampled population), and this substantially diminishes their predictive power (Cronbach, 1990). If students with a fuller range of A-level grades (or SATs) were allowed to go to university, the total variance in classes of degree explained by grades would increase. Similarly, the amount of variance in mental illness accounted for by environmental variables will depend on how varied the subjects' environments are; if a group of people live in very similar environments, then the environment cannot explain much variation in mental health even if it is causally very important. The amount of variance accounted for is also likely to depend on the outcome measure used.

Bearing these serious qualifications in mind, it is possible to translate the strength of the associations reported in this book between various objective measures of the environment (such as noise, traffic flow, density) and symptom levels into estimates of how much of the variance in mental health was accounted for by the environment. After partialling out the effects of background variables (such as age, sex and income), most of the objective variables were found to account for around 1 to 5 per cent of the variance found in the mental health of subjects living in normal residential environments. However, as indicated above, this figure may seriously underestimate the *potential* importance of the environment on mental health (a) because of the lack of variation in the quality of many people's environments and (b) because of limitations in the measures employed. Environmental *perceptions* account for substantially more variance in levels of symptom levels than objective measures of the environment, but part of this excess is due to the more negative perceptions of individuals suffering from mental illness. This was illustrated by showing that even having controlled for an objective level of an environmental variable (for example, traffic flow or density), significant associations were still found between subjects' symptom levels and their perceived level of the variable.

A second way of appraising the potential influence of the environment over mental health is to examine a situation where the environment is altered and then estimate the net difference in residents' mental health over the course of the change. This can be done using the results from the Eastlake study (Chapter 7). If we compare the average symptom score (between groups) on the Hospital Anxiety and Depression Scale before the environmental intervention with afterwards, we find that the level of symptoms fell by nearly a third (32 per cent). It can be argued that this figure may have been affected by selection effects, but this was controlled for by the use of within-pairs comparisons. The within-pairs comparison showed that there was a fall of around a quarter (24 per cent) in the average level of symptoms coinciding with the environmental intervention. This was clearly a very substantial effect. Furthermore, the most severely affected residents (those with the highest symptom scores) tended to be the ones who were most positively affected by the improvements on the estate so that the fall in the number of residents reaching 'caseness' was even greater.

In principle, the implication of the present findings are that the total level of mental ill-health in the population could be significantly reduced by environmental manipulations. Whether these effects are considered large enough to have policy or clinical implications depends on a broader cost-benefit analysis than can be attempted here. However, given that the impact of the environment may be especially strong on those with the poorest mental health and living in the worst conditions, the key strategy would be to target interventions on those people and areas.

Conclusions

Why has it Taken so long to Establish Clear Evidence of a Causal Relationship between Mental Illness and the Planned Environment?

In retrospect, we can see that there are a number of reasons why much previous research failed to find clear evidence of a causal relationship between mental illness and the planned environment.

The small size of the effect

Many previous researchers have made the a priori assumption that the influence of the environment on mental health must be very large. As we have seen, this is not the case, although the effect can still be quite substantial in some instances. The failure to demonstrate a large effect of the environment on mental health may have led some researchers to prematurely conclude that there was *no* effect.

The influence of selection

The occurrence of selection – the social and spatial sorting of individuals according to their preferences and abilities – has greatly complicated attempts to establish the causal relationship between mental illness and the environment. The causal inter-pretations of the results of very large numbers of studies (especially within psychiatric geography) are undermined by their failure to address adequately the influence of selection.

The problem of response bias

The occurrence of response bias – the tendency of individuals' perceptions of the environment to be distorted by their mental state – has similarly complicated attempts to establish causality. Where studies have not included objective independent measures of the environmental variables, the causal directions of the associations are difficult to establish. Unfortunately, such oversights are very common.

Poorly specified models

Much previous work on the relationship between mental health and the built environment has lacked coherent theoretical models to guide the research. Different aspects of the environment and context, some of which have opposing effects, have often been confused and compounded. This type of research (ecological studies, the New Town studies) has frequently led to results which were difficult or impossible to interpret. Narrower research strategies (such as those within environmental psychol-ogy) have not always escaped this problem either; variables have often been selected on the basis of ease of measurement rather than as the result of theoretical insight. Even if research is directed towards a specific variable, if it is based on a poorly specified theoretical model it remains very likely that the results that follow will seem contradictory and confused. For example, the effects of density seem confused and contradictory until one realizes that it is not a unitary concept, that its effects may not be linear (living alone may be as problematic as living at high density) and that its effects may depend on other factors often not measured (such as group orientation).

Partialling fallacy

It is possible that some researchers have underestimated the importance of the planned environment as a result of the *partialling fallacy*. If the influence of a variable strongly associated with the environment is statistically controlled for (such as income), then the amount of variance accounted for by the environment will appear to be sharply reduced or even eliminated. However, the possibility must be considered that the environment may have been a significant mediator of the control variable's influence; the environment might have been one of the reasons *why* the control variable had an effect.

Fragmentation

Finally, a major obstacle to progress has been the fragmentation of knowledge across disciplines. The present work has drawn on research from within psychiatry, social psychology, psychiatric geography, architecture and planning, sociology, criminology and environmental psychology. Sadly, it remains surprisingly rare for researchers within different disciplines to refer to each other's work, and this has obscured many over-arching themes and insights.

Further Questions to be Answered by Future Research

This book has, I hope, helped to re-open the door to the study of the relationship between mental health and the built environment. It has shown that the environment can causally effect the types of mild to moderate psychopathology commonly found in the community. However, many questions remain unanswered. Do specific aspects of the environment and context affect some types of disorder more than others? To what extent can symbolic aspects of the environment have a direct effect on mental health? Are there national differences and trends across time in mental health that relate to changes in the environment?

Also, there are choices that individuals make about their environments which may not be reducible to an analysis of mental health or well-being. People often seek activities, places and life-styles that do not appear to be optimum for their mental (or physical) health: contentment is not the only aim in people's lives. Furthermore, even if we could specify which types of environment would be best for people *on average*, it is unlikely that this environment would be the best for everyone individually. As they say, one person's heaven is another person's hell. A great deal of research will have to be done before we can begin to answer (or predict) why one person prefers one particular environment relative to another person. There is clearly plenty of research left to be done.

Broader Implications

There are some implications which extend beyond the concerns of environmental psychologists. First, the study of the relationship between the planned environment and mental illness gives us important clues as to the nature of mental illness in general. Second, the study of the mental, social and behavioural consequences of design provides invaluable feedback for planners. Decisions *do* have to be made and it is entirely appropriate that mental, social and behavioural consequences be considered.

What the Research Tells us about Mental Illness

Understanding how the built environment can foster mental illness (in the form of mild psychopathology) gives us clues as to the aetiology of mental illness in general. In Chapter 1, a brief typology of distress was presented. It was argued that we can only understand the nature of mental illness and its relationship to mental health by considering the individual's well-being in terms of two separate dimensions: state and process, where *process* refers to the individual's ability to cope and adapt across time.

We can now see that one way in which the environmental context can affect mental health is by affecting the individual's mental state: in other words, by inducing frustration, irritation, fear or annoyance (i.e. by moving individuals along the horizontal axis of Figure 8.1). For most people, environmentally induced annoyance or irritation is not enough to lead to psychosomatic symptoms or illness. It is only among individuals who were already predisposed towards mental illness because of their style of coping or personality (neurotic, sensitive, or low hardiness) that an environmentally induced negative mood might lead to disorder. In these individuals it could be argued that the environment – the concern about children getting run over or about crime or whatever – was merely the trigger, or even rationalization, for the illness behaviour: the pathology can be argued to be largely within the individual's style of coping.

Can the environment affect individuals' coping abilities, i.e., move individuals

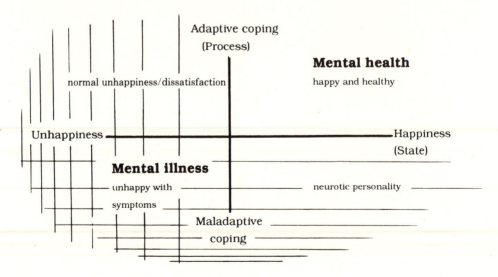

Figure 8.1: *A typology of distress and well-being*

along the vertical axis of Figure 8.1? If the model is correct, then an aspect of the environment that undermines or derails an individual's normal coping mechanisms would be expected to lead to pathology. Evidence was found for this in Chapters 2 and 3. It appears that aetiologically transparent stressors (such as noise), though inducing annoyance, cause only limited psychopathological symptoms. However, it was found that certain less obvious stressors (such as pollution and heat) lead to annoyance *and* psychopathological symptoms. It was suggested that individuals' lack of insight into the cause of their irritation leads them to mis-attribute the cause of their mental state and to employ inappropriate coping mechanisms. This results in failed coping and leads to further stress and frustration. This hypothesis, that individuals' own understanding of aetiology can be critical in the development of psychopathology, should be investigated further in future research.

The environment can also affect individuals' coping behaviour in another way. If an environment leads the individual to physically and socially withdraw, then this precludes certain types of coping behaviour. A social environment characterized by hostility and distrust, and one which makes it difficult for an individual to experience positive and supportive social relations, undermines many normal patterns of adaptive behaviour. If you live in an environment where you feel that you cannot let your children play outside, where you cannot conveniently drop in on a friend for a chat when you feel bored, or where you feel you cannot invite anyone into the house because they will come back to steal the video, the range of adaptive behaviour available to you is reduced. Factors such as knowing that you *could* turn to your neighbour if you had to and that your children *can* play outside without danger increase the range of adaptive options available to you.

These simple observations imply a somewhat different way of looking at coping behaviour and mental illness. They suggest that an individual's ability to cope, and even the nature of mental illness, is not located only in the individual but depends also on the environment and context. This view could be compared to that expressed in contemporary understandings about what it means to be disabled. An individual's disablement is argued to be as much a function of the environment as it is the individual; an individual in a wheelchair only becomes disabled when confronted with environments without wheelchair access. Similarly, perhaps as we develop a better understanding of the aetiology of everyday distress we will conclude that a great deal of mental illness is as much located in the context as in the individual. Having children might be less of a risk factor if there were places for them to play, crime might not be such a source of fear if you felt you could trust your neighbours, and living alone might not be such a problem if you felt you had someone to turn to.

One thing is certain, the more closely we study mental illness, the less random the pattern appears. The planned environment is just one small part of this complex pattern.

What the Research tells Planners

The research presented reminds us that the environment matters – that the design of houses, developments and cities have significant and demonstrable effects on the behaviour and well-being of the people who live in them. Perhaps this is obvious, but then sometimes it is worth reminding ourselves of the obvious lest it become lost under the tide of fashion or invisible through familiarity. Beyond this general but important point, a number of more specific insights can be gleaned.

Some of the findings of the research presented in this book will come as no surprise to planners, architects and policymakers. Various kinds of environmental stress are experienced as unpleasant by most people most of the time. These include air pollution, extreme temperatures, noise, high density, and crime. However, the impact of such stressors depend on a range of social factors such that it is extremely difficult to draw up simple guidelines about what is and is not an acceptable level of the stressor. For example, the impact of density depends on the nature of the relationships between the people involved. There is no evidence that a lack of space *per se* affects mental health, but having to share space with people with whom one does not have a cooperative relationship can lead to very negative outcomes.

Interestingly, the negative impact of an environmental stressor may not relate directly to the level of people's complaints about it. There appear to be certain types of environmental stress which may lead to negative outcomes in terms of mood and mental health (such as air pollution) but which people find it quite difficult to identify. Of course, where possible planners should seek to reduce the levels of such stressors, but when this is not immediately possible, consideration should be given to increasing the information available about the source of stress so that people can attempt to cope in more appropriately adaptive ways.

On the specific issue of crime, it is now very clear that the design of the environment can have a large impact on the occurrence of burglaries, attacks and vandalism, and these insights should be employed on a routine basis in design. However, two supplementary points should be stressed. First, the environmental factors that affect levels of fear of crime are not always the same ones that affect crime itself, and there may even be occasions where the two are in tension. For example, cohesive communities may be able to reduce levels of crime, yet the gossip between residents that spreads rumours of specific incidents in cohesive communities can be a major source of fear. Clearly, it may be important to supplement certain types of environmental interventions with specific public information campaigns. Second, there may sometimes be tensions between environmental interventions aimed at reducing the fear of residents with those aimed at reducing the fear of visitors to an area. For example, the presence of large numbers of strangers generally increases levels of fear among residents in the area, yet to the visitors (the strangers) the presence of larger numbers of 'eyes on the street' decreases fear. These tensions must be borne in mind by planners hoping to use environmental interventions to reduce crime and fear of crime.

One of the central themes we have encountered is that the ability to control the environment is of great importance. The negative impact of environmental stressors is greatly reduced when people feel that they have control over them. Similarly, the impact and quality of people's relationships with their neighbours is critically mediated by the extent to which they are able to regulate their interactions with them. Environments which encourage and facilitate social contacts between neighbours will not necessarily lead to positive social relations between neighbours. If residents are unable to regulate these contacts, then relations are likely to turn sour and residents will experience hostility to their neighbours and, ironically, often withdrawal and loneliness. The existence of semi-public spaces used by a restricted number of residents are important in this respect, but such spaces must be designed in such a way as to allow residents to choose whether or not to use them. The issue of control also extends into how the environment is managed and maintained. The management and planning of the environment must be an open process in which residents feel they are involved. Planners must seek to avoid imposing their views of how the environment should be upon residents, however well-intentioned this may be. The involvement of residents is important not only because of the acceptability of final decisions – planners and architects have been shown to have aesthetic tastes that differ markedly from those of most of the community – but also because the process of involvement itself is important.

In terms of the structure and balance of communities, the evidence on mental health clearly illustrates the tensions that planners must accommodate, but the evidence also offers some clues to the possible solutions. On the one hand, homogeneous neighbourhoods in terms of social class, ethnicity, demographic profile and land use appear to offer significant benefits on the local level in terms of the relationships between neighbours and residents' mental health. People who come from similar backgrounds and who have similar levels of resources tend to get on better with one another than those who do not. Similarly, the mixing of different land uses (notably, commercial and residential) tends to weaken the quality of neighbouring relations, this tends to be associated with worse mental health at the local level. On the other hand, there are wider and longer term social and mental health penalties associated with socially or functionally segregated neighbourhoods. Spatial patterns of social or ethnic segregation can lead to uneven distributions of resources and larger scale patterns of social conflict, and large scale divisions of areas by land use lead to widespread commuting and the spoiling of *corridor* areas by excessive traffic, all of which are reflected in poorer mental health. Clearly, the role of the planner is essential in attempting to balance these tensions, the critical issue being scale and the meshing of contrasting but complementary areas and populations. The adverse consequences of social and functional divisions arise as the scale of these divisions increases, while the positive benefits of limited local homogeneities tend to arise on very small scales. The difficult goal of planners must be to encourage communities that are socially and functionally balanced at the medium scale, while simultaneously allowing and encouraging the emergence of socially and culturally distinctive neighbourhoods at the immediate and very local scale (the micro-level).

Planners, architects and policymakers have an extremely difficult but interesting and exciting role. We have seen that the environment can have very significant effects over people's behaviour and mental health, yet we have also seen that it can be disastrous for particular planning decisions to be imposed upon the community. We will always need planners, architects and policymakers to develop ideas, designs and initiatives, and to create, inspire and challenge. Yet their role also must be to inform rather than to specify, to arbitrate rather than to impose, and to offer options rather than prescriptions. In this way we will create environments for the well-being of all.

References

ABEY-WICKRAMA, I., A'BROOK, M.F., GATTONI, F.E.G. and HERRIDGE, C.F. (1969) 'Mental hospital admissions and aircraft noise', *Lancet*, **II**, pp. 1275–7.

ADAMOPOULOU, A., GARYFALLOS, G., BOURAS, N. and KOULOUMAS, G. (1990) 'Mental health and primary care in ethnic groups', *International Journal of Psychiatry*, **36**, 4, pp. 244–51.

AIELLO, J.R., BAUM, A. and GORMLEY, F. (1981) 'Social determinants of crowding stress', *Journal of Personality and Social Psychology Bulletin*, **7**, pp. 643–4.

ALTMAN, I. and CHEMERS, M.M. (1984) *Culture and Environment*, Monterey, CA: Brooks & Cole Publishing.

AMERIGO, M. and ARAGONES, J.I. (1990) 'Residential satisfaction in council housing', *Journal of Environment Psychology*, **10**, pp. 313–25.

ANTUNES, G., GORDON, C., GAITZ, M. and SCOTT, J. (1974) 'Ethnicity, socioeconomic status and the etiology of psychological distress', *Sociology and Social Research*, **58**, pp. 361–8.

APPLEYARD, D. and LINTELL, M. (1972) 'The environmental quality of city streets: The residents' viewpoint', *Journal of the American Institute of Planners*, **38**, pp. 84–101.

ARCHITECTURAL FORUM (1951) *Slum Surgery in St.Louis*, April, pp. 128–136.

ARGYLE, M. (1987) *The Psychology of Happiness*, London: Methuen.

ARGYLE, M. (1992) *The Social Psychology of Everyday Life*, London: Routledge.

BABA, Y. and AUSTIN, D.M. (1989) 'Neighbourhood environmental satisfaction, victimization, and social participation as determinants of perceived neighbourhood safety', *Environment and Behavior*, **21**, 6, pp. 763–80.

BAGLEY, C. (1971) 'The social aetiology of schizophrenia in immigrant groups', *International Journal of Social Psychology*, **17**, pp. 292–304.

BAGLEY, C. (1974) 'The built environment as an influence on personality and social behaviour: A spatial study', in Cantor, D. and Lee, T. (Eds) *Psychology and the Built Environment*, London: Architectural Press.

BALDWIN, J. and BOTTOMS, A.E. (1976) *The Urban Criminal*, London: Tavistock.

BANKS, J.K. and GANNON, L.R. (1988) 'The influence of hardiness on the relationship between stressors and psychosomatic symptomatology', *American Journal of Community Psychology*, **16**, 1, pp. 25–37.

BARKER, S.M. and TARNOPOLSKY, A. (1978) 'Assessing bias in surveys of symptoms attributed to noise', *Journal of Sound and Vibration*, **59**, pp. 349–54.

BARON, R.A. (1990) 'Environmentally induced positive affect: Its impact on self-efficacy, task performance, negotiation, and conflict', *Journal of Applied Social Psychology*, **20**, 5, pp. 368–84.

BARON, R.M., MANDEL, D.R., ADAMS, C.A. and GRIFFEN, L.M. (1976) 'Effects of social density in university residential environments', *Journal of Personality and Social Psychology*, **34**, pp. 434–46.

BARRERA, M., SANDLER, I.N. and RAMSAY, T.B. (1981) 'Preliminary development of a scale of social support: Studies on college students', *American Journal of Community Psychology*, **9**, pp. 435–47.

BASTLIN NORMOYLE, J. and FOLEY, J.M. (1988) 'The defensible space model of fear and elderly public housing residents', *Environment and Behaviour*, **20**, 1, pp. 50–74.

BAUM, A. and DAVIS, G.E. (1980) 'Reducing the stress of high density living: An architectural intervention', *Journal of Personality and Social Psychology*, **38**, pp. 471–81.

BAUM A. and GREENBERG, C.I. (1975) 'Waiting for a crowd: The behavioural and perceptual effects of anticipated crowding', *Journal of Personality and Social Psychology*, **32**, pp. 667–71.

BAUM, A. and PAULUS, P.B. (1987) 'Crowding', in Stokels, D. and Altman, I. (Eds) *Handbook of Environmental Psychology*, Chichester: Wiley.

BAUM, A. and VALINS, S. (1977) *Architecture and Social Behaviour: Psychosocial Studies of Social Density*. Hillsdale, NJ: Lawrence Erlbaum Associates.

BAUM, A. and VALINS, S. (1979) 'Architectural mediation of residential density and control: Crowding and the regulation of social contact', *Advances in Experimental Social Psychology*, **12**, pp. 131–75.

BAUM, A., AIELLO, J. and DAVIS, G. (1979) 'Neighbourhood determinants of stress symptom perception', Paper presented at the meeting of the *American Psychological Association*, NY: reported in FLEMMING, R., BAUM, A. and SINGER, J.E. (1985).

BAUM, A., SINGER, J.E. and BAUM, C.S. (1982) 'Stress and the environment', in Evans, G.W. (Ed.) *Environmental Stress*, Cambridge: Cambridge University Press.

BAUMER, T.L. (1985) 'Testing a general model of fear of crime: Data from a national sample', *Journal of Research in Crime and Delinquency*, **22**, 5, pp. 239–55.

BEALE, N. and NETHERCOTT, S. (1988) 'Certified sickness absence in industrial employees threatened with redundancy', *British Medical Journal*, **296**, pp. 1508–10.

BELL, P.A. and FUSCO, M.E. (1989) 'Heat and violence in the Dallas field data: Linearity, Curvilinearity, and heteroscedasticity', *Journal of Applied Social Psychology*, **19**, 17, pp. 1479–82.

BELL, P.A. and GREENE, T.C. (1982) 'Thermal stress: Physiological, comfort, performance, and social effects of hot and cold environments', in Evans, G.W. (Ed.) *Environmental Stress*, Cambridge: Cambridge University Press.

BELL, W. (1958) 'The utility of the Shevky typology for the design of urban sub-area studies', *Journal of Social Psychology*, **67**, pp. 71–83.

BETHLEHEM, D.W. (1985) *A Social Psychology of Prejudice*, Bekenham: Croom Helm.

BEVIS, C. and NUTTER, J.B. (1977) 'Changing street layouts to reduce residential burglary', Presented at the American Society of Criminology, Cited in Mayo, J.M. (1979) *Environment and Behavior*, **11**, 3, pp. 375–97.

BILTON, T., BONNETT, K., JONES, P., STANWORTH, M., SHEARD, K. and WEBSTER, A. (1987) *Introductory Sociology*, Basingstoke: Macmillan.

BIRTCHNELL, J., MASTERS, N. and DEAHL, M. (1988) 'Depression and the physical environment: A study of young women on a London housing estate', *British Journal of Psychiatry*, **153**, pp. 56–64.

BLAKE, R.R., RHEAD, C.C., WEDGE, B. and MOUTON, J.S. (1956) 'Housing architecture and social interaction', *Sociometry*, **19**, pp. 133–9.

BONNES, M., BONAIUTO, M. and ERLOLOANI, A.P. (1991) 'Crowding and residential satisfaction in the urban environment: A contextual approach', *Environment and Behaviour*, **23**, 5, pp. 531–52.

BOOTH, A. (1976) *Urban Crowding and its Consequences*, New York: Praeger.

BOOTZIN, R.R., HERMAN, C.P. and NICASSIO, P. (1976) 'The power of suggestion: Another examination of misattribution and insomnia', *Journal of Personality and Social Psychology*, **34**, 4, pp. 673–9.

Box, S., Hale, C. and Andrews, G. (1988) 'Explaining fear of crime', *British Journal of Criminology*, **28**, 3, pp. 340–56.

Bracey, H.E. (1964) *Neighbours: On New Estates and Subdivisions in England and USA*, London: Routledge & Kegan Paul.

Bradburn, N.M. (1969) *The structure of psychological well-being*, Chicago, IL: Aldine.

Brain, P. (1984) 'Human aggression and the physical environment', in Freeman, H.L. (Ed.) *Mental Health and the Environment*, London: Churchill Livingstone.

Brenner, M.H. (1973) *Mental Illness and the Economy*, Cambridge, MA: Harvard University Press.

Briere, J., Downes, A. and Spensley, J. (1983) 'Summer in the city: Urban weather conditions and psychiatric emergency-room visits', *Journal of Abnormal Psychology*, **92**, pp. 77–80.

Bristol Victim Support Scheme (BVSS) (1975) 'Summary of the first six months work of the Bristol Support Scheme', Cited in Maguire, M. (1982) *Burglary in a Dwelling*, London: Heinemann.

Britten, J.R. (1977) 'What is a satisfactory house? A report of some households' views'. Building Research Establishment Current Paper.

Broadbent, D. (1972) 'Individual differences in annoyance by noise', *Sound*, **6**, pp. 56–61.

Bronzaft, A.L. (1993) 'Architects, engineers and planners as anti-noise advocates', *Journal of Architectural and Planning Research*, **10**, 2 pp. 146–59.

Bronzaft, A.L. and McCarthy, D.P. (1975) 'The effects of elevated train noise on reading ability', *Environment and Behaviour*, **7**, pp. 517–27.

Brown, B.B. and Altman, I. (1983) 'Territoriality, defensible space, and residential burglary: An environmental analysis', *Journal of Environmental Psychology*, **3**, pp. 203–20.

Brown, G.W. and Harris, T. (1978) *Social Origins of Depression*. London: Tavistock.

Brown, G.W. and Prudo, R. (1981) 'Psychiatric disorder in a rural and an urban population: 1. aetiology of depression', *Psychological Medicine*, **11**, pp. 581–99.

Brownell, A. and Shumaker, S.A. (1984) 'Social support: An introduction to a complex phenomenon', *Journal of Social Issues*, **40**, pp. 1–9.

Bullinger, M. (1989) 'Psychological effects of air pollution on healthy residents – a time-series approach. *Journal of Environmental Psychology*, **9**, pp. 103–18.

Bulmer, M. (1986) *Neighbours: The Work of Philip Abrams*. Cambridge: Cambridge University Press.

Burke, A.W. (1984) Racism and psychological disturbance among West Indians in Britain. *International Journal of Social Psychiatry*, **30**, pp. 50–68.

Byrne, D. and Buehler, J.A. (1955) 'A note on the influence of propinquity upon acquaintanceships', *Journal of Abnormal and Clinical Psychology*, **51**, pp. 147–8.

Byrne, D.S., Harrison, S.P., Keithley, J. and McCarthy, P. (1986) *Housing and Health: The Relationship Between Housing Conditions and the Health of Council Tenants*. Aldershot, Hants: Gower.

Cairncross, F. (1992) 'The Influence of the Recession', in Jowell, R., Brook, L., Prior, G. and Taylor, B. (Eds) *British Social Attitudes, the 9th Report*, Aldershot: Dartmouth.

Cairns, E. (1988) 'Social class, psychological well-being and minority status in Northern Ireland', *International Journal of Social Psychiatry*, **35**, 3, pp. 231–36.

Calhoun, J.B. (1962) 'Population density and social pathology', *Scientific American*, **206**, pp. 139–48.

Calhoun, J.B. (1973) 'Death squared: The explosive growth and demise of a mouse population', *Proceedings of the Royal Society of Medicine*, **66**, pp. 80–8.

Campbell, A., Converse, P.E. and Rogers, W.L. (1976) *The Quality of American Life*, New York: Sage.

Campbell, D.E. and Beets, J.L. (1981) 'Human response to naturally occurring weather phenomena: effects of wind speed and direction', Unpublished manuscript, Arcata,CA: Humboldt State University.

CANTER, D. and DONALD, I. (1987) 'Environmental psychology in the UK', in Stokols, D. and Altman, I. (Eds) *Handbook of Environmental Psychology*. Chichester: Wiley.

CAPLAN, R.D., COBB, S., FRENCH, J.R.P., VAN HARRISON, R. and PINEAU, S.R. (1975) 'Job demands and worker health, US Department of Health, Education and Welfare, HEW (NIOSH) Publication No. 75–160. Washington, DC: GPO.

CAPLOW, T. and FORMAN, R. (1950) 'Neighbourhood interaction in a homogeneous community', *American Sociology Review*, **15**, pp. 357–66.

CAPPON, D. (1971) 'Mental health and the high-rise', *Canadian Journal of Public Health*, **6**, pp. 426–31.

CASPI, A., BOLGER, N. and ECKENRODE, J. (1987) 'Linking person and context in the daily stress process', *Journal of Personality and Social Psychology*, **52**, 1, pp. 184–95.

CATTELL, R.B. (1965) *The Scientific Analysis of Personality*, Harmondsworth, Penguin Books.

CECIL, R. (1988) 'Studying informal welfare', Unpublished paper.

CEDERLÖF, R., FRIBERG, L., HAMMARFORS, P., HOLMQUIST, S.E. and KAJLAND, A. (1961) 'Studier över ljundnivaer och hygieniska olagenheter av trafikbuller samt förslag till atgarder', *Nordisk Hygienisk Tidskrift*, **42**, pp. 101–92.

CENTRAL STATISTICAL OFFICE (1990) *Social Trends 20*, London: HMSO.

CENTRAL STATISTICAL OFFICE (1992) *Social Trends 22*, London: HMSO.

CHO, S.K. (1985) 'The labour process and capital mobility: The limits of the new international division of labour', *Politics and Society*, **14**, pp. 185–222.

CHOWNS, R.H. (1970) 'Mental-hospital admissions and aircraft noise', *Lancet*, **1**, p. 467.

CHRISTIAN, J.J. (1955) 'Effects of population size on the adrenal galnds and reproductive organs of male mice in populations of fixed size', *The American Journal of Physiology*, **182**, pp. 292–300.

CHRISTIAN, J.J. (1963) 'Pathology of overpopulation', *Military Medicine*, **128**, pp. 571–603.

CHURCHMAN, A. and GINSBURG, Y. (1984) 'The image and experience of high-rise housing in Israel, *Journal of Environmental Psychology*, **4**, pp. 27–41.

CLEMENTE, F. and KLEIMAN, M.B. (1977) 'Fear of crime in the United States: A multivariate analysis', *Social Forces*, **56**, 2, pp. 519–31.

CLOUT, I. (1962) 'Psychiatric illness in a new town practice', *Lancet*, **I**, pp. 683–5.

COCHRANE, R. (1979) 'A comparative study of the adjustment of Irish, Indian and Pakistani immigrants to England', The Mahesh Desai Memorial Lecture of the British Psychological Society.

COCHRANE, R. (1983) *The Social Creation of Mental Illneess*, London: Longman.

COCHRANE, R. and BAL, S.S. (1987) 'Migration and schizophrenia: An examination of five hypotheses', *Social Psychiatry*, **22**, pp. 181–91.

COCHRANE, R. and BAL, S.S. (1988) 'Ethnic density is unrelated to incidence of schizophrenia', *British Journal of Psychiatry*, **153**, pp. 363–66.

COCHRANE, R. and BAL, S.S. (1989) 'Mental hospital admission rates of immigrants to England: A comparison of 1971 and 1981', *Social Psychiatry and Psychiatric Epidemology*, **24**, pp. 2–11.

COCHRANE, R. and STOPES-ROE, M. (1981) 'Psychological symptom levels in Indian immigrants to England – a comparison with native English' *Psychological Medicine*, **11**, pp. 319–327.

COHEN, A. (1969) 'Effects of noise on psychological state, *Noise as a Public Health Hazard*, Report No. 4, Washington, DC: American Speech and Hearing Association.

COHEN, S. and HOBERMAN, H.M. (1983) 'Positive life events and social supports as buffers of life change events', *Journal of Applied Social Psychology*, **13**, pp. 99–125.

COHEN, S. and SYME, L. (Eds) (1985) *Social Support and Health*, New York: Academic.

COHEN, S. and WEINSTEIN, N. (1982) 'Non-auditory effects of noise on behaviour and health', in Evans, G.W. (Ed.) *Environmental Stress*, Cambridge: Cambridge University Press.

References

Cohen, S. and Wills, T.A. (1985) 'Stress, social support, and the buffering hypothesis', *Psychology Bulletin*, **98**, pp. 310–57.

Cohen, S., Glass, D.C. and Singer, J.E. (1973) 'Apartment noise, auditory discrimination, and reading ability in children', *Journal of Experimental Social Psychology*, **9**, pp. 407–22.

Cohen, S., Evans, G.W., Krantz, D.S. and Stokols, D. (1980) 'Physiological, motivational and cognitive effects of aircraft noise on children: Moving from the laboratory to the field', *American Psychologist*, **35**, pp. 231–43.

Coleman, A. (1985) *Utopia on Trial: Vision and Reality in Planned Housing*. London: Hilary Shipman.

Connerly, C.E. and Marans, R.W. (1985) 'Comparing two global measures of perceived neighborhood quality', *Social Indicators Research*, **17**, pp. 29–47.

Cook. D.A.G. and Morgan, H.G. (1982) 'Families in high-rise flats', *British Medical Journal*, **284**, p. 846.

Cooper Marcus, C. and Sarkissian, W. (1986) *Housing as if People Mattered*. Berkeley, CA: University of California Press.

Corden, C. (1977) *Planned Cities: New Towns in Britain and America*. London: Sage.

Cox, V.C., Paulus, P.B. and McCain, G. (1984) 'Prison crowding research – the relevance for prison housing standards and a general approach regarding crowding phenomena', *American Psychologist*, **39**, 10, pp. 1148–60.

Craik, K.H. and Appleyard, D. (1980) 'Streets of San Francisco: Brunswick's lens model applied to urban inference and assessment', *Journal of Social Issues*, **36**, 3, pp. 72–85.

Creer, R.N., Gray, R.M. and Treshow, M. (1970) 'Differential responses to air pollution as an environmental health problem', *Journal of the Air Pollution Control Association*, **20**, pp. 814–8.

Cronbach, L.J. (1990) *Essential of Psychological Testing*, 5th edn., New York: Harper and Row.

Croog, S.H., Lipson, A. and Levine, S. (1972) 'Help patterns in severe illness: The roles of kin network, non-family resources, and institutions', *Journal of Marriage and Family Living*, **34**, pp. 32–41.

Crowell, B.A., George, L.K., Blazer, D. and Landerman, R. (1986) 'Psychosocial Risk Factors and Urban/Rural Differences in the Prevalance of Major Depression, *British Journal of Psychiatry*', **149**, p. 307.

Cunningham, M.R. (1979) 'Weather, mood, and helping behaviour: Quasi-experiments with the sunshine Samaritans', *Journal of Personality and Social Psychology*, **37**, pp. 1947–56.

Curwen, M. and Devis, T. (1988) 'Winter mortality, temperature and influenza: Has the relationship changed in recent years?' *Population Trends*, **54**, pp. 17–20.

Daiches, S. (1981) 'People in Distress: A Geographical Perspective on Psychological Well-being', *Research Paper 197*, Department of Geography, Univeristy of Chicago, Chicago.

Damer, S. (1976) 'Wine Alley: The sociology of a dreadful enclosure', in Wiles, P. (Ed.) *The Sociology of Crime and Delinquency in Britain*, **2**, London: Martin Robertson.

Darely, J.M. and Latané (1968) 'Bys Fander Intersection in Emergencies: Diffusion of Responsibility', *Journal of Personality and Social Psychology*, **8**, pp. 377–83.

Darke, J. (1984a) 'Architects and user requirements in public-sector housing: 1. Architects' assumptions about the users' *Environment and Planning B: Planning and Deisgn*, **11**, pp. 389–404.

Darke, J. (1984b) 'Architects and user requirements in public-sector housing: 2. The sources for architects' assumptions', *Environment and Planning B: Planning and Design*, **11**, pp. 405–16.

Darke, J.(1984c) 'Architects and user requirements in public-sector housing: 3. Towards an adequate understanding of user requirements in housing', *Environment and Planning B: Planning and Design*, **11**, pp. 417–33.

Davies, D.R. and Hockey, G.R.J. (1966) 'The effects of noise and doubling the signal frequency on individual differences in visual vigilance performance', *British Journal of Psychology*, **57**, pp. 381–9.

DEAN, K. and JAMES, H.(1984) 'Depression and schizophrenia in an English city', in Freeman, H. (Ed.) *Mental Health and the Environment*, London: Churchill Livingstone.

DEAN, G., WALSH, D., DOWNING, H. and SHELLEY, E. (1981) 'First admissions of native-born and immigrants to psychiatric hospitals in south-east England in 1976', *British Journal of Psychiatry*, **139**, pp. 506–12.

DEAN, L., PUGH, W. and GUNDERSON, E. (1975) 'The behavioural effects of crowding', *Environment and Behaviour*, **10**, pp. 419–31.

DEGROOT, I. (1967) 'Trends in public attitudes toward air pollution', *Journal of the Air Pollution Control Association*, **16**, pp. 245–7.

DoE (DEPARTMENT OF THE ENVIRONMENT) (1972) *The Estate Outside the Dwelling: Reactions of Residents to Aspects of Housing Layout*. Design Bulletin **25**, London: HMSO.

DoE (DEPARTMENT OF THE ENVIRONMENT) (1981a,b,c) *An Investigation of Difficult to Let Housing*, **1**, **2**, and **3**. Housing Development Directorate occasional papers 3/80, 4/80, 5/80. London: HMSO.

DoE (DEPARTMENT OF THE ENVIRONMENT) AND DoT (DEPARTMENT OF TRANSPORT) (1977) *Residential Roads and Footpaths: Layout Considerations*. Design Bulletin **32**. London: HMSO.

DEVLIN, K. and NASAR, J.L. (1989) 'The Beauty and the Beast: Some Preliminary Comparisons of "high" versus "popular" residential architecture and some public versus architect judgements of same', *Journal of Environmental Psychology*, **9**, pp. 333–44.

DIENER, E. (1984) 'Subjective well-being', *Psychology Bulletin*, **95**, pp. 542–75.

DILLING, H. (1980) 'Psychiatry and primary health services: Results in a field study', *Acta Psychiatrica Scandinavica*, **62**, pp. 15–22.

DOHRENWEND, B.P. and DOHRENWEND, B.S. (1969) *Social Status and Psychological Disorder: A Casual Inquiry*, New York: Wiley.

DOHRENWEND, B.P. and DOHRENWEND, B.S. (1974) 'Social and cultural influences on psychopathology', *Annual Review of Psychology*, **41**, pp. 417–52.

DOHRENWEND, B.P., SHROUT, P.E., EGRI, G. and MENDELSOHN, F.S. (1980) 'Nonspecific psychological distress and other dimensions of psychopathology', *Archives of General Psychiatry*, **37**, pp. 1229–36.

DOWNEY, G., SILVER, R.C. and WORTMAN, C.B. (1990) 'Reconsidering the attribution-adjustment relation following a major negative event: Coping with the loss of a child', *Journal of Personality and Social Psychology*, **59**, 5, pp. 925–40.

DOSTOEVSKY, F. (1865) *Crime and Punishment*, Oxford: Oxford University Press (1986).

DUBOS, R. (1965) *Man Adapting*, New Haven, CT: Yale University Press.

EATON, W.W. and LASRY, J.C. (1978) 'Mental health and occupational mobility in a group of immigrants', *Social Science and Medicine*, **12**, pp. 53–8.

EBBESEN, E.B., KLOS, G.L. and KONECNI, V.J. (1976) 'Spatial ecology: Its effects on the choice of friends and enemies', *Journal of Experimental Social Psychology*, **12**, pp. 503–18.

EDWARDS, J., BOOTH, A. and EDWARDS, P. (1982) 'Housing type, stress, and family relations', *Social Forces*, **61**, 1, pp. 241–57.

ENGELS, F. (1969) *The Condition of the Working Class in England*, Frogmore: Panther Books.

EPSTEIN, Y.M. (1982) 'Crowding stress and human behaviour', in Evans, G.W. (Ed.) *Environmental Stress*. Cambridge: Cambridge University Press.

EPSTEIN, Y.M. and BAUM, A. (1978) 'Crowding: Methods of Study', in Baum, A. and Epstein, Y. (Eds) *Human Response to Crowding*. Hillsdale, NJ: Erlbaum.

EPSTEIN, Y.A and KARLIN, R.A. (1975) 'Effects of acute experimental crowding', *Journal of Applied Social Psychology*, **5**, pp. 34–53.

ERON, L.E. and PETERSON, R.A. (1982) 'Abnormal behaviour: Social approaches', *Annual Review of Psychology*, **33**, pp. 231–64.

EVANS, G.W. (1978) 'Human spatial behaviour: The arousal model', in Baum, A. and Epstein, Y. (Eds) *Human Response to Crowding*, Hillsdale, NJ: Erlbaum.

EVANS, G.W. (Ed.) (1982) *Environmental Stress*. Cambridge: Cambridge University Press.

References

Evans, G.W. and Campbell, J.M. (1983) 'Psychological perspectives on air pollution and health', *Basic and Applied Social Psychology*, **4 2**, pp. 137–69.

Evans, G.W and Jacobs, S.V. (1982) 'Air pollution and human behaviour', in Evans, G.W. (Ed.) *Environmental Stress*. Cambridge: Cambridge University Press.

Evans, G.W. and Lepore, S.J. (1993) 'Household crowding and social support: A quasiexperimental analysis', *Journal of Personality and Social Psychology*, **65**, 2, pp. 308–16.

Evans, G.W., Colome, S.D. and Shearer, D.F. (1988) 'Psychological reactions to air pollution', *Environmental Research*, **45**, pp. 1–15.

Evans, G.W., Jacobs, S.V., Dooley, D. and Catalano, R. (1987) 'The interaction of stressful life events and chronic strains on community mental health', *American Journal of Community Psychology*, **15**, 1, pp. 23–34.

Evans, G.W., Palsane, M.N., Lepore, S.J. and Martin, J. (1989) 'Residential density and psychological health: The mediating effects of social support', *Journal of Personality and Social Psychology*, **57**, 6, pp. 994–99.

Fagence, M. (1977) *Citizen Participation in Planning*, New York: Pergamon Press.

Fanning, D.M. (1967) 'Families in flats', *British Medical Journal*, **4**, pp. 382–6.

Farahat, A.M. and Cebeci, M.N. (1982) 'A housing project – intentions, realities and alternatives', *Housing Science*, **6**, pp. 209–27.

Faris, R.E. and Dunham, H.W. (1939) *Mental Disorders in Urban Areas*, Chicago, IL: University of Chicago Press.

Fernando, S. (1984) 'Racism as a cause of depression', *International Journal of Social Psychiatry*, **30**, pp. 41–9.

Festinger, L., Schacter, S. and Back, K. (1950) *Social Pressures in Informal Groups: A Study of Human Factors in Housing*, New York, Harper Bros.

Finlay-Jones, R.A. and Burvill, P.W. (1977) 'The prevalence of minor psychiatric morbidity in the community', *Psychological Medicine*, **7**, pp. 474–89.

Firey, W. (1945) 'Sentiment and symbolism as ecological variables', *American Sociological Review X*, (reprint).

Fischer, C.S. (1982) *To Dwell Among Friends: Personal Networks in Town and City*, Chicago, IL: University of Chicago Press.

Fisher, J.D., Bell, P.A. and Baum, A. (1984) *Environmental Psychology*. New York: Holt, Rinehart and Winston.

Flaherty, J.A., Moises Gavira, F. and Pathak, D.S. (1983) 'The measurement of social support: the social support network inventory', *Comprehensive Psychiatry*, **24**, 6, pp. 521–9.

Flemming, R., Baum, A. and Singer, J.E. (1985) 'Social support and the physical environment', in Cohen, S., Syme, L. (Eds) *Social Support and Health*, New York, Academic Press.

Fombonne, E. (1991) 'The use of questionnaires in child psychiatry research: Measuring their performance and choosing an optimal cut-off', *Journal of Child Psychology and Psychiatry*, **32**, 4, pp. 677–93.

Ford, W.S. (1973) 'Interracial public housing in a border city: Another look at the contact hypothesis', *American Journal of Sociology*, **78**, pp. 1426–47.

Fordyce, M.W. (1985) 'The Psychap inventory: a multi-scale test to measure happiness and its concomitants', *Social Indicators Research*, **18**, pp. 1–33.

Forrester, D., Chatterton, M. and Pease, K. (1988) 'The Kirkholt burglary prevention project, Rochdale', *Crime Prevention Unit: Paper 13*. London: Home Office.

Fowler, E.P. (1987) 'Street management and city design', *Social Forces*, **66**, 2, pp. 365–89.

Fowler, F.J and Mangione, T.W. (1982) 'Neighborhood crime, fear and social control: A second look at the Hartford program', Washington, DC, GPO.

Francois, J. (1980) 'Aircraft noise, annoyance and personal characteristics', in Tobias, J.W., Jansen, G. and Ward, W.D. (Eds) *Noise as a Public Health Problem: Proceedings of the Third International Congress, ASHA Report No. 10*. Rockville, MD: American Speech-Language Hearing Assocation.

FRANK, J.D. (1973) *Persuasion and Healing*. Baltimore, MD: John Hopkins Press.

FRANK, K.A. (1983) 'Community by design', *Sociological Inquiry*, **53**, pp. 289–311.

FREEDMAN, J. (1975) *Crowding and Behavior*, San Francisco, CA: Freeman.

FREEDMAN, J. (1979) 'Reconciling apparent differences between the responses of humans and other animals to crowding', *Psychological Review*, **86**, 1, pp. 80–5.

FREEMAN, H.F.(1984a) 'The scientific background', in Freeman, H. (Ed.) *Mental Health and the Environment*, London: Churchill Livingstone.

FREEMAN, H.F. (1984b) 'Mental health and the environment: housing', in Freeman, H. (Ed.) *Mental Health and the Environment*, London: Churchill Livingstone.

FREEMAN, H.F. (1986) 'Environmental stress and psychiatric disorder', *Stress Medicine*, **2**, pp. 291–9.

FREEMAN, H.F. (1988) 'Psychiatric aspects of environmental stress', *International Journal of Mental Health*, **17**, 3, pp. 13–23.

FRERICHS, R.R., BEEMAN, B.L. and COULSON, A.H. (1980) 'Los Angeles Airport noise and mortality – fault analysis and public policy', *American Journal of Public Health*, **70**, pp. 357–62.

FRIED, M. (1963) 'Grieving for a lost home', in Duhl, L.J. (Ed.) *The Urban Condition*. New York: Basic Books.

FRY, A. (1987) *Safe Space: How to Survive in a Threatening World*. London: Dent.

FRYDMAN, M.I. (1981) 'Social support, life events and psychiatric symptoms: A study of direct, conditional and interaction effects', *Social Psychiatry*, **16**, pp. 69–78.

GABE, J. and WILLIAMS, P. (1987) 'Women, housing, and mental health', *International Journal of Health Services*, **17**, 4, pp. 667–79.

GALLE, O., GOVE, W. and MCPHERSON, M. (1972) 'Population density and pathology: What are the relations for man?' *Science*, **176**, pp. 23–30.

GANS, H.J. (1961) 'Planning and social life: Friendship and neighbour relations in suburban communities', *Journal of the American Institute of Planners*, **19**, pp. 134–40.

GANS, H.J. (1962) *The Urban Villagers: Group and Class in the Life of Italian-Americans*, Toronto, Canada: Macmillan.

GASKELL, S.M. (1987) *Model Housing: From the Great Exhibition to the Festival of Britain*. London: Mansell Publishing.

GATTONI, F. and TARNOPOLSKY, A. (1973) 'Aircraft noise and psychiatric morbidity', *Psychological Medicine*, **3**, pp. 516–20.

GELDER, M., GATH, D. and MAYOU, R. (1983) *Oxford Textbook of Psychiatry*. Oxford: Oxford University Press.

GELLER, D. (1980) 'Responses to urban stimuli: A balanced approach', *Journal of Social Issues*, **36**, pp. 86–100.

GENERAL HOUSEHOLD SURVEY (1980) **11**, London: HMSO.

GESTEN, E.L. and Jason, L.A. (1987) 'Social and community interventions', *Annual Review of Psychology*, **38**, pp. 477–60.

GIDDENS, A. (1990) *The Consequences of Modernity*. Cambridge: Polity.

GIGGS, J.A. (1973) 'The distribution of schizophrenics in Nottingham', *Transactions of the Institute of British Geographers*, **59**, pp. 55–76.

GILLIS, A.R. (1977) 'High-rise housing and psychological strain', *Journal of Health and Social Behaviour*, **18**, pp. 418–31.

GILLIS, A.R., RICHARD, M.A. and HAGAN, J. (1986) 'Ethnic susceptibility to crowding: An empirical analysis', *Environment and Behaviour*, **18**, 6, pp. 683–703.

GITTUS, E. (1976) *Flats, Families and the Under-fives*, London: Routledge and Kegan Paul.

GLADSTONE, F.J. (1978) 'Vandalism amongst adolescent schoolboys', in Clarke, R.V.G. (Ed.) *Tackling Vandalism. Home Office Research Study 47*, London: HMSO.

GLASS, D.C. and SINGER, J.E. (1972) *Urban Stress: Experiments on Noise and Social Stressors*. New York: Academic Press.

GOLDBERG, D. (1972) *The Detection of Psychiatric Illness by Questionnaire*, Oxford: Oxford University Press.

References

GOLDBERG, D. and BLACKWELL, B. (1970) 'Psychiatric illness in general practice. A detailed study using a new method of case identification', *British Medical Journal*, **2**, pp. 439–43.

GOLDBERG, D. and HUXLEY, P. (1980) *Mental Illness in the Community*, London: Tavistock Publications.

GOLDSMITH, J.R. (1968) 'Effects of air pollution on human health', in Stern, A.C. (Ed.) *Air Pollution*. New York: Academic Press.

GOODMAN, M. (1974) 'The enclosed environment', *Royal Society Health Journal*, **4**, pp. 165–75.

GORDEN, E.B. (1965) 'Mentally ill West Indian immigrants', *British Journal of Psychiatry*, **111**, pp. 877–87.

GORE, S. (1978) 'The effect of social support in moderating the health consequences of unemployment', *Journal of Health and Social Behaviour*, **19**, pp. 157–65.

GOTTESMAN, I.I. and SHIELDS, J. (1982) 'Schizophrenia: The epigenetic puzzle', Cambridge: Cambridge University Press.

GRANATI, A., ANGELEPI, F. and LENZI, R. (1959) 'L'influenza dei rumori sul sistema nervoso', *Folio Medica*, **42**, pp. 1313–25.

GRANDJEAN, E. (1974) *Sozio-psychologische untersuchungen vor den fluglarms*. Bern.

GREENBERG, S.W. and ROHE, W.M. (1984) 'Neighborhood design and crime: A test of two perspectives', *Journal of American Planning*, **50**, 1, pp. 48–61.

GREENBLATT, M., BECERRA, R.M. and SERAFETINIDES, E. (1982) 'Social networks and mental health: An overview', *American Journal of Psychiatry*, **139**, 8, pp. 977–84.

GUTMAN, R. (1966) 'Site planning and social behaviour', *Journal of Social Issues*, **22**, 4, pp. 103–15.

HACKNEY, J., LINN, W., KARUZA, S., BUCKLEY, R., LAW, D., BATES, D., HAZUCHA, M., PENGELLIS, L. and SILVERMAN, F. (1977) 'Effects of ozone exposure in Canadians and Southern Californians', *Archives of Environmental Health*, **32**, pp. 110–6.

HAHN, M. (1966) *California Life Goals Evaluation Schedules*. Palo Alto, CA: Western Psychological Services.

HALPERN, D.S. (1987) 'Architectural preference and mere exposure effects: The role of recognition in attitudinal enhancement by exposure', Unpublished BA research project.

HALPERN, D.S. (1990) 'Active citizenship and a healthy society', Extracts in: Report of the Commission on Citizenship, *Encouraging Citizenship*, London: HMSO.

HALPERN, D.S. (1991) 'Environmental criminology: A review of the evidence', Unpublished manuscript.

HALPERN, D.S. (1993) 'Minorities and mental health', *Social Science and Medicine*, **36**, 5, pp. 597–607.

HALPERN, D.S. and REID, J. (1992) 'Effect of unexpected demolition announcement on health of residents', *British Medical Journal*, **304**, pp. 1229–30.

HANNAY, D.R. (1984) 'Mental health and symptom referral in a city', in Freeman, H. (Ed.) *Mental Health and the Environment*, London: Churchill Livingstone.

HARE, E.N. and SHAW, G.K. (1965) *Mental Health on a New Housing Estate*, Maudsley Monograph 12, Oxford: Oxford University Press.

HARRIES, K.D. and STADLER, S.J. (1988) 'Heat and violence: New findings from Dallas field data', 1980–1981. *Journal of Applied Social Psychology*, **18**, pp. 129–38.

HARRISON, G., HOLTON, A., NEILSON, D., OWENS, D., BOOT, D. and COOPER, J. (1989) 'Severe mental disorder in Afro-Caribbean patients: Some social, demographic and service factors', *Psychological Medicine*, **19**, pp. 683–96.

HARTMAN, C. (1963) 'Social values and housing orientations', *Journal of Social Issues*, **19**, 2, pp. 155–68.

HEADEY, B., HOLMSTROM, E. and WEARING, A. (1984) 'Well-being and ill-being: Different dimensions?' *Social Indicators Research*, **14**, pp. 115–39.

HEDGES, A., BLABER, A. and MOSTYN, B. (1980) *Community Planning Project: Cunningham Road Improvement Scheme*, London: Social and Community Planning Research.

HERRIDGE, C.F. 'Aircraft noise and mental health', *Journal of Psychosomatic Research*, **18**, pp. 239–43.

HIGGINS, P.M. (1984) 'Stress at Thamesmead', in Freeman, H. (Ed.) *Mental Health and the Environment*, London: Churchill Livingstone.

HILLIER, B. and HANSON, J. (1984) *The Social Logic of Space*, Cambridge, Cambridge University Press.

HIRSCH, F. (1977) *Social Limits to Growth*, London: Routledge and Kegan Paul.

HOCKNEY, G.R.J. (1968) 'Effects of noise on human efficiency and some individual differences', *Journal of Sound and Vibration*, **20**, pp. 299–304.

HOLAHAN, C.J. (1976) 'Environmental effects on outdoor social behaviour in a low-income urban neighbourhood: A naturalistic investigation', *Journal of Applied Social Psychology*, **6**, 1, pp. 48–63.

HOLAHAN, C.J. and MOOS, R.H. (1981) 'Social support and psychological distress: A longitudinal analysis', *Journal of Abnormal Psychology*, **90**, 4, pp. 365–70.

HOLLANDER, E.P. (1981) *Principles and Methods of Social Psychology*, Oxford: Oxford University Press.

HOLMES, T.H. AND RAHE, R.H. (1967) 'The Social Readjustment Rating Scale', *Journal of Psychosomatic Research*, **11**, pp. 213–18.

HOMANS, G.C. (1954) 'The cash posters: A study of a group of working girls', *American Social Review*, **19**, pp. 724–33.

HOPPENFELD, M. (1971) 'The Columbia Process', in LEWIS, D. (Ed.) *The Growth of Cities*, Architect Yearbook 13, Letchworth, England: Garden City Press.

HUNTER, A. (1978) 'Symbols of incivility', Paper presented at the meeting of the American Society of Criminology, Dallas, TX: Cited by Taylor, R.B. (1987).

HUNTER, A. and BAUMER, T.L. (1982) 'Street traffic, social interaction, and fear of crime', *Sociological Inquiry*, **52**,2, pp. 122–31.

HUNTER, J. (1978) 'Defensible space in practice', *The Architects' Journal*, 11 October, pp. 675–77.

HUPPERT, F.A., ROTH, M. and GORE, M. (1987) 'Psychological factors', in *The Health and Style Survey*, London: Health Promotion Research Trust, pp. 51–8.

INEICHEN, B. (1979) 'High-rise living and mental stress', *Biology & Human Affairs*, **44**, pp. 81–5.

INEICHEN, B. and HOOPER, D. (1974) 'Wives' mental health and children's behaviour problems in contrasting residential areas', *Social Science and Medicine*, **8**, pp. 369–74.

INGHAM, J., RAWNSLEY, K. and HUGHES, D. (1972) 'Psychiatric disorder and its declaration in contrasting areas of South Wales' *Psychological Medicine*, **2**, pp. 281–92.

INNES, C.A. (1986) *Population Density in State Prisons*, Bureau of Justice Statistics Bulletin, No. NCJ–103204. Washington, DC: Bureau of Justice Statistics.

JACO, G. (1959) 'Mental health of the Spanish-American in Texas', in Opler, M.K. (Ed.) *Culture and Mental Health*, New York: Macmillan.

JACOBS, J. (1961) *The Death and Life of Great American Cities*, New York: Random House.

JACOBS, M. and STEVENSON, G. (1981) 'Health and housing: A historical examination of alternative perspectives', *International Journal of Health Services*, **1**, 1, pp. 105–22.

JEFFORDS, C.R. (1983) 'The situational relationship between age and fear of crime', *International Journal of Aging and Human Development*, **17**, 2, pp. 103–11.

JENKINS, L.M., TARNOPOLSKY, A., HAND, D.J. and BARKER, S.M. (1979) 'Comparison of three studies of aircraft noise and psychiatric hospital admissions conducted in the same area', *Psychological Medicine*, **9**, pp. 681–93.

JEPHCOTT, P. (1971) *Homes in High Flats*, Edinburgh: Oliver and Boyd.

JETER, I.K. (1976) 'Unidentified hearing impairment among psychiatric patients', *American Speech and Hearing Association*, **18**, pp. 843–5.

JONES, F.L. (1967) 'Ethnic concentration and assimilation: An Australian case study', *Forces*, **43**, 3, pp. 412–23.

References

JONES, P.N. (1979) 'Ethnic areas in British cities', in Herbert, D.T. and Smith, D.M. (Eds) *Social Problems and the City*, Oxford: Oxford University Press.

JONSSON, E. and SÖRENSEN, S. (1973) 'Adaptation to community noise – a case study', *Journal of Sound and Vibration*, **26**, pp. 571–5.

KAMMANN, R. and FLETT, R. (1983) 'Affectometer 2: A scale to measure current level of general happiness', *Australian Journal of Psychology*, **35**, pp. 259–65.

KANNER, A.D., COYNE, J.C., SCHAEFER, C. and LAZARUS, R.S. (1981) 'Comparison of two methods of stress measurement: Daily hassles and uplifts versus major life events', *Journal of Behavioural Medicine*, **4**, pp. 1–39.

KAPLAN, H.I. and SADOCK, B.J. (1988) *Synposis of Psychiatry*, 5th edition. Baltimore, MD: Williams and Williams.

KARLIN, R.A., EPSTEIN, Y. and AIELLO, J. (1978) 'Strategies for the investigation of crowding', in Esser, A. and Greenbie, B. (Eds) *Design for Communality and Privacy*, New York, Plenum.

KASL, S.V. (1974) 'Effects of housing on mental and physical health', *Man-Environment Systems*, **4**, pp. 207–26.

KASL, S.V. and HARBURG, E. (1975) 'Mental health and the environment: Some doubts and second thoughts', *Journal of Health and Social Behaviour*, **16**, pp. 268–82.

KASL, S.V. and Rosenfield, S. (1980) 'The residential environment and its impact on the mental health of the aged', in Birren, J.E. and Sloane, R.B. (Eds) *Handbook of Mental Health and Aging*, Englewood Cliffs, NJ: Prentice Hall.

KASL, S.V., WILL, J., WHITE, M. and MARCUSE, P. (1982) 'Quality of the residential environment and mental health', in Baum, A. and Singer, J.E. (Eds) *Advances in Environmental Psychology*, **4**, *Environment and Health*. Hillsdale, NJ: Lawrence Erlbaum Associates.

KEANE, C. (1991) 'Socioenvironmental determinants of community formation', *Environment and Behaviour*, **23**, 1, pp. 27–46.

KEATS, J. (1918) 'Endymion', in Bullett, G. (Ed.) *John Keats: Poems*, (1974) London: Dent.

KELLETT, J. (1989) 'Health and housing', *Journal of Psychometric Research*, **33**, 3, pp. 255–68.

KENDELL, R.E. (1975) *The Role of Diagnosis in Psychiatry*, Oxford: Blackwell.

KENNEDY, S., KIECOLT-GLASER, J. and GLASER, R. (1990) 'Social support, stress and the immune system', in Sarason, B., Sarason, I. and Pierce, G. (Eds) *Social Support: An Interactional View*, New York: Wiley.

KESSEL, W.I.N. (1960) 'Psychiatric morbidity in a London general practice', *British Journal of Preventative and Social Medicine*, **14**, pp. 16–22.

KESSLER, R., PRICE, R. and WORTMAN, C. (1985) 'Stress, social support, and coping processes' *Annual Review of Psychology*, **36**, pp. 531–72.

KLEIN, D. (1978) *Psychology of the Planned Community: The New Town Experience*, London: Human Sciences Press.

KLEIN, E. (1983) *Gender Politics: From Consciousness to Mass Politics*, Cambridge, MA: Harvard University Press.

KLEINER, R.J. and PARKER, S. (1970) 'Social-psychological aspects of migration and mental disorder in a Negro population', in Brody, E.B. (Ed.) *Behaviour in New Environments*, Beverley Hills, CA: Sage.

KLITZMAN, S. and STELLMAN, J.M. (1989) 'The impact of the physical environment on the psychological well-being of office workers', *Social Science and Medicine*, **29**, 6, pp. 733–42.

KNIPSCHILD, P. (1977) 'Medical effects of aircraft noise', *International Archives of Occupational and Environmental Health*, **40**, pp. 185–204.

KOBASA, S. (1979) 'Stressful life events, personality, and health: An inquiry into hardiness', *Journal of Personality and Social Psychology*, **37**, pp. 1–11.

KORTE, C., YPMA, A. and TOPPEN, C. (1975) 'Helpfulness in Dutch society as a function of urbanization and environmental input level', *Journal of Personality and Social*

Psychology, **32**, pp. 996–1003.

KRAUS, J. (1969) 'The relationship of psychiatric diagnosis, hospital admission rates, and size and age structure of immigrant groups', *Medical Journal of Australia*, **2**, pp. 91–5.

KRUPAT, E. (1985) *People in Cities*. Cambridge: Cambridge University Press.

KRUPINSKI, J. (1967) 'Sociological aspects of mental ill-health in migrants', *Social Science and Medicine*, **1**, pp. 267–81.

KRUPINSKI, J. (1984) 'Changing patterns of migration to Australia and their influence on the health of migrants', *Social Science and Medicine*, **18**, 11, pp. 927–37.

KUPER, L. (1953) *Living in Towns*, London: Cresset Press.

LEGRANGE, R.C. and FERRARO, K.F. (1989) 'Assessing age and gender differences in perceived risk and fear of crime', *Criminology*, **27**, 4, pp. 697–719.

LANGE, C. and JAMES, W. (1922) *The Emotions*, Baltimore: Williams and Wilkins.

LANGNER, T.S. (1962) 'A twenty-two item screening score of psychiatric symptoms indicating impairment', *Journal of Health and Social Behaviour*, **3**, pp. 269–76.

LARSEN, R.J., DIENER, E. and EMMONS, R.A. (1985) 'An evaluation of subjective well-being measures', *Soc. Indicators Res.*, **17**, pp. 1–17.

LAVE, L.B. and SESKIN, E.P. (1970) 'Air pollution and human health', *Science*, **169**, pp. 723–33.

LEFEBVRE, P. (1984) 'Hygiene mentale et grands ensembles en europe occidentale', *Societe Medico-Psychologique*. 21 Mars, pp. 527–42.

LEIGHTON, D., HARDING, J., MACKLIN, D., MacMILLAN, A. and LEIGHTON, A. (1963) *The Character of Danger: Stirling County Study*, **3**, New York: Basic Books.

LEPORE, S.J., EVANS, G.W. and SCHNEIDER, M.L. (1992) 'Role of control and social support in explaining the stress of hassles and crowding', *Environment and Behaviour*, **24**, 6, pp. 795–811.

LEVINE, R.V., MIYAKE, K. and LEE, M. (1989) 'Places rated revisited: psycho-social pathology in metropolitan areas. *Environment and Behaviour*, **21**, 5, pp. 531–53.

LEVY, L. and HERZOG, A.N. (1974) 'Effects of population density and crowding on health and social adaptation in the Netherlands', *Journal of Health and Social Behaviour*, **15**, pp. 228–40.

Levy, L. and ROWITZ, L (1973) *The Ecology of Mental Disorder*, New York: Behavioural Publications.

LEVY, R.L. (1983) 'Social support and compliance: A selective review and critique of treatment integrity and outcome measurement', *Social Science and Medicine*, **17**, 8, pp. 1329–38.

LEVY-LEBOYER, C. and NATUREL, V. (1991) 'Neighbourhood noise annoyance', *Journal of Environmental Psychology*, **11**, pp. 75–86.

LEWIS, D.A. and MAXFIELD, M.G. (1980) 'Fear in the neighborhood: An investigation of the impact of crime', *Journal of Research in Crime and Delinquency*, **17**, pp. 160–89.

LIN, N., DEAN, A. and ENSEL, W.M. (1981) 'Social support scales: A methodological note', *Schizophrenia Bulletin*, **7**, 1, pp. 73–89.

LITTLEWOOD, R. and LIPSEDGE, M. (1989) *Aliens and Alienists: Ethnic Minorities and Psychiatry* (2nd edition), London: Unwin Hyman.

LOWENTHAL, M.F. and HAVEN, C. (1968) 'Interaction and adaptation: Intimacy as a critical variable', *American Sociological Review*, **33**, pp. 20–30.

LOWRY, S. (1991) *Housing and Health*, London: *British Medical Journal*.

McDONALD, N. (1989) 'Jobs and their environment: The psychological impact of work in noise', *The Irish Journal of Psychology*, **10**,1, pp. 39–55.

MacDONALD, W.S. and ODEN, C.W. (1973) 'Effects of extreme crowding on the performance of five married couples during twelve weeks of intensive training', *Proceedings of the 81st Annual Convention of the American Psychological Association*, **8**, pp. 209–10.

McFARLANE, A.H., NEALE, K.A., NORMAN, G.R., ROY, R.G. and STREINER, D.L. (1981) 'Methodological issues in developing a scale to measure social support', *Schizophrenia Bulletin*, **7**, 1, pp. 90–100.

References

McGovern, D. and Cope, R.V. (1987) 'First psychiatric admission rates of first and second generation Afro-Caribbeans', *Social Psychiatry*, **22**, pp. 139–49.

McLean, E.K. and Tarnopolsky, A. (1977) 'Noise, discomfort and mental health', *Psychological Medicine*, **7**, pp. 19–62.

MacKenzie, D. and Goodstein, L.I. (1986) 'Stress and the control beliefs of prisoners: A test of the three models of control-limited environments', *Journal of Applied Social Psychology*, **16**, 3, pp. 209–28.

Maddi, S., Kobasa, S. and Hoover, M. (1979) 'An alienation test', *Journal of Humanistic Psychology*, **19**, pp. 73–6.

Magaziner, J. (1988) 'Living density and psychopathology: A re-examination of the negative model', *Psychological Medicine*, **18**, pp. 419–31.

Maguire, M. (1982) *Burglary in a Dwelling*, London: Heinemann.

Malpass, P. and Murie, A. (1987) *Housing Policy and Practice*, Second edn., MacMillan Education: Basingstoke.

Malzberg, B. (1964) *Mental Disease in Canada, 1950–1952: A Study of Comparative Incidence of Mental Disease among those of British and French Origin*, Albany: Research Foundation for Mental Hygiene.

Marañon, G. (1924) 'Contribution à l'etude de l'action emotive de l'adrenaline', *Revue Française d'Endocrinologie*, **2**, pp. 301–25.

Marshall, J. and Heslin, R. (1975) 'Boys and girls together: Sexual composition and the effect of density and group size on cohesiveness', *Journal of Personality and Social Psychology*, **31**, pp. 952–61.

Martin, C. (1990) 'Poor housing, unemployment and poverty: The effects on child health', *Radical Statistics Newsletter*, **44**.

Martin, F.M., Brotherston, J.H.F. and Chave, S.P.W. (1957) 'Incidence of neurosis in a new housing estate', *British Journal of Preventive Social Medicine*, **11**, pp. 196–202.

Maslach, C. (1979) 'Negative emotional biasing of unexplained arousal', *Journal of Personality and Social Psychology*, **37**, 6, pp. 953–69.

Massey, D.S. and Denton, N.A. (1988) 'Suburbanization and segregation in US metropolitan areas', *American Journal of Sociology*, **94**, 3, pp. 592–626.

Mathews, K.E. and Canon, L.K. (1975) 'Environmental noise level as a determinant of helping behaviour', *Journal of Personality and Social Psychology*, **32**, pp. 571–7.

Mavreas, V.G. and Bebbington, P.E. (1987) 'Psychiatric morbidity in London's Greek-Cypriot immigrant community', *Social Psychiatry*, **22**, pp. 150–9.

Maxfield, M.G. (1984) 'The limits of vulnerability in explaining fear of crime: A comparative neighborhood analysis', *Research in Crime and Delinquency*, **21**, 3, pp. 233–50.

Mayhew, P., Clarke, R.V.G., Burrows, J.N., Hough, J.M. and Winchester, S.W.C. (1979) 'Crime in public view', *Home Office Research Study 49*, London: HMSO.

Mayo, J.M. (1979) 'Effects of street forms on suburban neighbouring behavior', *Environment and Behaviour*, **11**, 3, pp. 375–97.

Meecham, W.C. and Smith, H.G. (1977) 'Effects of aircraft noise on mental hospital admissions', *British Journal of Audiology*, **II**, pp. 81–5.

Meltzer, H., Gill, B. and Petticrew (1994) 'The prevalance of psychiatric morbidity among adults aged 16–64, living in private households, in Great Britain', *OPCS Surveys of Psychiatric Morbidity in Great Britain*, Bulletin No. 1, London: Office of Population Censuses and Surveys.

Mendelsohn, R. and Orcutt, G. (1979) 'An empirical analysis of air pollution dose-response curves', *Journal of Environmental Economics and Management*, **6**, pp. 85–106.

Mercer, C. (1975) *Living in Cities*. Harmondsworth: Penguin.

Merton, R.K. (1949) 'Patterns of influence: A study of interpersonal influence and communication behaviour in a local community', in Lazaesfeld, P.F. and Stanton, F.N. (Eds) *Communications Research 1948–1949*, New York: Harper and Row.

MERTON, R.K. and KITT, A.S. (1950) 'Contributions to the theory of reference group behaviour', in Merton, R.K. and Lazarsfeld, P.F. (Eds) *Continuities in Social Research: Studies in the Scope and Method of the American Soldier*, Glencoe, IL: Free Press.

MEYER, R.G. and SALMON, P. (1984) *Abnormal Psychology*, London: Allyn and Bacon.

MILGRAM, S. (1970) 'The experience of living in cities', *Science*, **167**, pp. 1461–8.

MILGRAM, S. and SABINI, J. (1982) 'On maintaining urban norms: A field experiment in the subway', in Baum, A. and Singer, J.E. (Eds) *Advances in Environmental Psychology*, **4**, Hillsdale, NJ: Lawrence Erlbaum Associates.

MILLER, J.D. (1974) 'Effects of noise on people', *Journal of the Acoustical Society of America*, **56**, pp. 729–64.

MINSKY, M. (1987) *The Society of Mind*, London: Heinemann.

MINTZ, N.L. and SCHWARTZ, D.T. (1964) 'Urban ecology and psychosis: Community factors in the incidence of schizophrenia and manic-depression among Italians in Greater Boston', *International Journal of Social Psychiatry*, **10**, pp. 101–18.

MIROWSKY, J. and ROSS, C.E. (1989) *Social Causes of Psychological Distress*. New York: Aldine de Gruyter.

MITCHELL, R. (1971) 'Some social implications of high density housing', *American Sociology Review*, **36**, pp. 18–29.

MOLLER, C.B. (1968) *Architectural Environment and our Mental Health*, New York: Horizon.

MOORE, N.C. (1974) 'Psychiatric illness and living in flats', *British Journal of Psychiatry*, **125**, pp. 500–7.

MOORE, N.C. (1975) 'Social aspects of flat dwelling', *Public Health*, **89**, pp. 109–15.

MOORE, N.C. (1976) 'The personality and mental health of flat dwellers', *British Journal of Psychiatry*, **128**, pp. 259–61.

MOOS, W.S. (1964) The effects of "Foehn" weather on accident rates in the city of Zurich (Switzerland)', *Aerospace*, **35**, pp. 643–5.

MOREIRA, N.M. and BRYAN, M.E. (1972) 'Noise annoyance susceptibility', *Journal of Sound and Vibration*, **21**, pp. 449–62.

MORTON-WILLIAMS, J., HEDGES, B. and FERNANDO, E. (1978) *Road Traffic and the Environment*, London: Social and Community Planning Research.

MOSER, G. (1988) 'Urban stress and helping behaviour: Effects of environmental overload and noise on behaviour', *Journal of Environmental Psychology*, **8**, pp. 287–98.

MUECHER, H. and UNGEHEUER, H. (1961) 'Meteorological influence on reaction time, flicker fusion frequency, job accidents and use of medical treatment', *Perceptual and Motor Skills*, **12**, pp. 163–8.

MUELLER, D. (1980) 'Social networks: A promising direction for research on the relationship of the social environment to psychiatric disorder', *Social Science and Medicine*, **14**, (A), pp. 147–61.

MUHLIN, G.L. (1979) 'Mental hospitalization of the foreign-born and the role of cultural isolation', *International Journal of Social Psychiatry*, **25**, pp. 258–66.

MURPHY, H.B.M. and VEGA, G. (1982) 'Schizophrenia and religious affiliation in Northern Ireland', *Psychological Medicine*, **12**, pp. 595–605.

MYERS, D.G. (1990) *Social Psychology* (3rd edition). London: McGraw-Hill.

MYERS, K., HALE, C.S., MYKYTOWYCS, R. and HUGHES, R.L. (1971) 'Density space, sociability and health', in Esser, A.H. (Ed.) *Behaviour and Environment*, New York: Plenum.

NANDI, D.N., MUKHERJEE, S.P., BORAL, G.C., BANERJEE, C., GHOSH, A., SARKAR, S. and AJMANY, S. (1980) 'Socioeconomic status and mental morbidity in certain tribes and castes in India', *British Journal of Psychiatry*, **136**, pp. 73–85.

NEWCOMB, T.M. (1961) *The Acquaintance Process*, New York: Holt.

NEWMAN, O. (1973) *Defensible Space*, London: Architectural Press.

NEWMAN, O. (1981) *Community of Interest*, New York: Anchor Books.

NEWMAN, O. and FRANK, K. (1980) *Factors Influencing Crime and Instability in Urban Housing*

Developments, Washington, DC: GPO.

NEWMAN, O. and FRANK, K. (1982) 'The effects of building size on personal crime and fear of crime', *Population and Environment*, **5**, 4, pp. 203–20.

NYSTROM, S. and LINDEGARD, B. (1975) 'Predisposition for mental syndromes', *Acta Psychiatrica Scandinavica*, **51**, pp. 60–76.

ÖHRSTRÖM, E., BJÖRKMAN, M. and RYLANDER, R. (1988) 'Noise annoyance with regard to neurophysiological sensitivity, subjective noise sensitivity and personality variables', *Psychological Medicine*, **18**, pp. 605–13.

ORLEY, J. and WING, J. (1979) 'Psychiatric disorders in two African villages', *Archives of General Psychiatry*, **36**, pp. 513–20.

PAGE, R.A. (1977) 'Noise and helping behaviour', *Environment and Behaviour*, **9**, pp. 311–34.

PARKER, S. and KLEINER, R.J. (1966) *Mental Illness in the Urban Negro Community*, New York: The Free Press.

PARKER, J. (1985) 'Treating the town', Paper presented at conference, Health in towns: urban development, psycho-social disorders and mental health, 3–5 December, 1985.

PAYKEL, E. and DOWLATSHAHI, D. (1988) 'Life events and mental disorder', in Fisher, S. and Reason, J. (Eds) *Handbook of Life Stress, Cognition and Health*, Chichester: Wiley.

PEARLIN, L.I., LIEBERMAN, M.A., MENAGHAN, E.G. and MULLAN, J.T. (1981) 'The stress process', *Journal of Health and Social Behaviour*, **22**, pp. 337–56.

PENNEBAKER, J.W. and BRITTINGHAM, G.L. (1982) 'Environmental and sensory cues affecting the perception of physical symptoms', in Baum, A. and Singer, J. (Eds) *Advances in Environmental Psychology*, **4**, Hillsdale, NJ: Lawrence Erlbaum Associates.

PEREZ, M. (1988) 'Immune reactions and mental disorders', *Psychological Medicine*, **18**, pp. 11–3.

PERKINS, D.D., MEEKS, J.W. and TAYLOR, R.B. (1992) 'The physical environment of street blocks and resident', *Journal of Environmental Psychology*, **12**, pp. 21–34.

PHILLIPS, S. (1981) 'Network characteristics related to the well-being of normals: A comparative base', *Schizophrenia Bulletin*, **7**, pp. 117–24.

PIPE, R., BHAT, A., MATHEWS, B. and HAMPSTEAD, J. (1991) 'Section 136 and African/Afro-Caribbean minorities', *International Journal of Social Psychiatry*, **37**, 1, pp. 14–23.

POWER, A. (1984) *Local Housing Management: A Priority Estates Project Survey*, London: DoE.

POYNER, B. (1980) 'Street attacks and their environmental settings', The Tavistock Institute of Human Relations (unpublished); cited in Poyner, B. (1983) , Design Against Crime: Beyond Defensible Space, London: Butterworths.

POYNER, B. (1983) *Design Against Crime: Beyond Defensible Space*, London: Butterworths.

PRATT, G. and HANSON, S. (1988) 'Gender, class, and space', *Environment and Planning D: Society and Space*, **6**, pp. 15–35.

PRICE, C.A. (1977) 'The immigrants', in Davies, A.F., Encel, S. and Berry, M.J. (Eds) *Australian Society: A Sociological Introduction*, Melbourne: Longman Cheshire.

PRINCE OF WALES, HRH (1989) *A Vision of Britain: A Personal View of Architecture*, London: Doubleday.

PRINCE-EMBURY, S. and ROONEY, J.F. (1989) 'A comparison of residents who moved versus those who remained prior to restart of Three Mile Island', *Journal of Applied Social Psychology*, **19**, 11, pp. 959–75.

PUBLIC OPINION (1984) 'Need versus greed', (summary of Roper report), August/September: 25.

QUINTIN, D. (1988) 'Urbanism and child mental health', *Journal of Child Psychology Psychiatry*, **29**, 1, pp. 11–20

RABKIN, J.G. (1979) 'Ethnic density and psychiatric hospitalisation: Hazards of minority status', *American Journal of Psychiatry*, **136**, 12, pp. 1562–66.

RACK, P. (1982) *Race, Culture and Mental Disorder*, London: Tavistock Publications.

RAHAV, M., GOODMAN, A., POPPER, M. and LIN, S. (1986) 'Distribution of treated mental illness in the neighbourhoods of Jerusalem', *American Journal of Psychiatry*, **143**, 10, pp. 1249–55.

RAPOPORT, A. (1977) *Human Aspects of Urban Form: Towards a Man-environment Approach to Urban Form and Design*. New York: Pergamon Press.

RAPOPORT, A. (1982) 'The meaning of the built environment', Beverly Hills, CA: Sage.

RAVEN, J. (1967a) 'Sociological evidence on housing: 1. Space in the home', *Architectural Review*, July, pp. 68–74.

RAVEN, J. (1967b) 'Sociological evidence on housing: 2. the home environment', *Architectural Review*, September, pp. 236–40.

REEVES, F. (1983) *British Racial Discourse*. Cambridge: Cambridge University Press.

REPPETTO, T.A. (1974) *Residential Crime*, Cambridge, MA: Ballinger.

REYNOLDS, F. (1986) *The Problem Housing Estate*, Aldershot, Hants: Gower.

RICHARDS, C.B. and DOBYNS, H.F. (1957) 'Topography and culture: the case of the changing cage', *Human Organization*, **16**, pp. 16–20.

RICHMAN, N. (1974) 'The effects of housing on pre-school children and their mothers', *Developmental Medical Child Neurology*, **16**, pp. 53–8.

RICKELS, K. and DOWNING, R. (1967) 'Drug- and placebo-treated neurotic outpatients', *Archives of General Psychiatry*, **16**, pp. 369–72.

RIM, Y. (1975) 'Psychological test performance during climatic heat stress from desert winds', *International Journal of Biometeorology*, **19**, pp. 37–40.

ROBERTSON, A. (1989) *Sick Building Syndrome*, Granada Television.

ROBINS, L. and REGIER, D. (1991) *Psychiatric Disorders in America: The Epidemiological Catchment Area Study*, The Free Press.

ROBSON, P. (1989) 'Development of a new self-report questionnaire to measure self-esteem', *Psychological Medicine*, **19**, pp. 513–8.

RODIN, J., SOLOMON, S. and METCALF, J. (1978) 'Role of control in mediating perceptions of density', *Journal of Personality and Social Psychology*, **36**, pp. 989–99.

ROHE, W. (1985) 'Urban planning and mental health', *Prevention in Human Sciences*, **4**, pp. 79–110.

RONECK, D.W. (1981) 'Dangerous places: Crime and residential environment', *Social Forces*, **60**, 1, pp. 74–96.

ROSEN, S., BERGMAN, M., PLESTOR, D., EL-MOFTY, A. and SATTI, M. (1962) 'Presbycosis study of a relatively noise-free population in the Sudan', *Annuals of Ontology, Rhinology, and Laryngology*, **71**, pp. 727–43.

ROSENBERG, M. (1962) 'The dissonant religious context and emotional disturbance', *American Journal of Sociology*, **68**, 1, pp. 1–10.

ROSS, M., LAYTON, B., ERICKSON, B. and SCHOPLER, J. (1973) 'Affect, facial regard, and reactions to crowding', *Journal of Personal and Social Psychology*, **28**, pp. 69–76.

ROTTER, J., SEEMAN, M. and LIVERANT, S. (1962) 'Internal versus external locus of control: A major variable in behaviour therapy', in, Washburne, N. (Ed.) *Decisions, Values and Groups*. London: Pergamon.

ROTTON, J. and FREY, J. (1984) 'Psychological costs of air pollution: Atmospheric conditions, seasonal trends, and psychiatric emergencies', *Population and Environment*, **7**, 1, pp. 3–16.

ROYAL COMMISSION ON ENVIRONMENTAL POLLUTION (1995) *Transport and the Environment*, London: HMSO.

RUBACK, R.B., CARR, T.S. and HOPPER, C.H. (1986) 'Perceived control in prison: Its relation to reported crowding, stress, and symptoms', *Journal of Applied Social Psychology*, **16**, 5, pp. 375–86.

RUBACK, R.B. and INNES, C.A. (1988) 'The relevance and irrelevance of psychological research – the example of prison crowding', *American Psychologist*, **43**, 9, pp. 683–93.

RUBACK, R.B. and PANDEY, J. (1991) 'Crowding, perceived control, and relative power: An analysis of households in India', *Journal of Applied Social Psychology*, **21**, 4, pp. 315–44.

RUBACK, R.B. and PANDEY, J. (1992) 'Very hot and really crowded: Quasi-experimental

References

investigations of Indian "Tempos"', *Environment and Behaviour,* **24**, 4, pp. 527–54.

SAEGERT, S. (1980) 'The effect of residential density on low-income children', Presented at the annual meeting of the American Psychological Association, Montreal.

SAEGERT, S. and WINKEL, G.H. (1990) 'Environmental psychology', *Annual Review of Psychology,* **41**, pp. 441–77.

SALAME, P. and BADDELEY, A.D. (1982) 'Disruption of short-term memory by unattended speech: Implications for the structure of working memory', *Journal of Verbal Learning and Verbal Behaviour,* **21**, pp. 150–64.

SALK, J. and SALK, J. (1981) *World Population and Human Values,* New York: Harper.

SANUA, V.C. (1969) 'Immigration, migration and mental illness: A review of the literature with special emphasis on schizophrenia', in Brody, E.B. (Ed.) *Behaviour in New Environments,* Beverly Hills, CA: Sage.

SARASON, B.R., SARASON, I.G. and PIERCE, G.R. (1990) *Social Support: An Interactional View,* Chichester: Wiley.

SARASON, I., LEVINE, H., BASHAM, R. and SARASON, B. (1990) 'Assessing social support: The social support questionnaire', *Journal of Personality and Social Psychology,* **44**, 1, pp. 127–39.

SAUNDERS, P. (1989) 'A deep and natural desire?' Paper presented to the Sociology and Architecture Group, London: London School of Economics.

SCHACHTER, S. and SINGER, J.E. (1962) 'Cognitive, social and physiological determinants of emotional state', *Psychology Review,* **69**, pp. 379–99.

SCHMITT, R.C. (1966) 'Density, Health and Social Disorganization', *Planners,* **32**, pp. 38–40.

SCHWARZ, N. and CLORE, G.L. (1983) 'Mood, misattribution and judgments of well-being: Information and directive functions of affective states', *Journal of Personality and Social Psychology,* **45**, pp. 513–23.

SCOBIE, S. (1989) 'Geographical perspectives on the provision of psychiatric services: A review and bibliography', *Centre for Urban Policy Studies Working Paper 6.* School of Geography, University of Manchester.

SCOTT, J. (1988) 'Trend report: Social network analysis', *Sociology,* **22**, 1, pp. 109–27.

SELYE, H. (1978) *The Stress of Life,* New York: McGraw-Hill.

SEAMON, D. (1984) 'Emotional experience of the environment', *American Behavioural Scientist,* **27**, 6, pp. 757–70.

SELIGMAN, M.E.P. (1975) *Helplessness,* San Francisco, CA: Freeman.

SHAFFER, G.S. and ANDERSON, L.M. (1983) 'Perceptions of the security and attractiveness of urban parking lots', *Journal of Environmental Psychology,* **5**, pp. 311–23.

SHEETS, V.L. and MANZER, C.D. (1991) 'Affect, cognition, and urban vegetation: Some effects of adding trees along city streets', *Environment and Behaviour,* **23**, 3, pp. 285–304.

SHEPHERD, M., COOPER, B., BROWN, A.C. and KALTON, G.W. (1966) *Psychiatric Illness in General Practice,* London: Oxford University Press.

SHERROD, D.R. (1974) 'Crowding, perceived control and behavioural aftereffects', *Journal of Applied Social Psychology,* **4**, pp. 171–86.

SHORT, J.R. (1989) *The Humane City: Cities as if People Matter,* Oxford: Basil Blackwell.

SKOGAN, W.G. and MAXFIELD, M.G. (1981) *Coping with Crime: Individual and Neighborhood Reactions.* Beverly Hills, CA: Sage.

SMITH, A. (1976) *The Wealth of Nations.* (Abridged 1970 version, 1970) Harmondsworth: Penguin.

SMITH, A. (1991) 'A review of the non-auditory effects of noise on health', *Work and Stress,* **5**, 1, pp. 49–62.

SMITH, C. (1984) 'Geographical approaches to mental health', in Freeman, H.F. (Ed.) *Mental Health and the Environment,* London: Churchill Livingstone.

SMITH, S.J. (1988) 'Political interpretations of "racial segregation" in Britain', *Environment and Plan. D: Society and Space,* **6**, pp. 423–44.

SMITH, S. and HAYTHORN, W. (1972) 'Effects of compatability, crowding group size, and leadership seniority on stress, anxiety, hostility and annoyance in isolated groups', *Journal of Personality and Social Psychology*, **22**, pp. 67–79.

SNYDER, M., TANKE, E.D. and BERSCHEID, E. (1977) 'Social perception and interpersonal behaviour: On the self-fulfilling nature of social stereotypes', *Journal of Personality and Social Psychology*, **35**, pp. 656–66.

SNYDER, R.L. (1966) 'Fertility and reproductive performance of grouped male mice', in Benirschke, K. (Ed.) *Symposium on Comparative Aspects of Reproductive Behaviour*, Berlin: Springer Press.

SOCIAL and COMMUNITY PLANNING RESEARCH (1978) 'Road Traffic and the Environment, *ERSC Data Archive*, Study Number 992. University of Essex, Colchester.

SOMMERS, P. and MOOS, R. (1976) 'The weather and human behaviour', in Moos, R.H. (Ed.), *The Human Context: Environmental Determinants of Behaviour*, New York: Wiley.

SÖRENSEN, S. (1970) 'On the possibilities of changing the annoyance reaction to noise by changing the attitude to the source of annoyance', *Nordisk Hygienisk Tidskrift, Supplementum*, **1**, pp. 1–76.

SROLE, L., LANGER, T., MICHAEL, S.T., OPLER, M.D. and RENNIE, T. (1962) *Mental Health in the Metropolis: The Midtown Manhattan Study*. **1**. New York: McGraw-Hill.

STANSFELD, S., CLARK, C., JENKINS, L. and TARNOPOLSKY, A. (1985a) 'Sensitivity to noise in a community sample: 1. Measurement of psychiatric disorder and personality', *Psychological Medicine*, **15**, pp. 243–54.

STANSFELD, S., CLARK, C., TURPIN, G. and TARNOPOLSKY, A. (1985b) 'Sensitivity to noise in a community sample: 2. Measurement of psychophysiological indices', *Psychological Medicine*, **15**, pp. 255–63.

STOPES-ROE, M. and COCHRANE, R. (1990) 'Support networks of Asian and British families: Comparisons between ethnicities and between generations', *Special Behaviour*, **5**, pp. 71–85.

STORMS, M.D. and NISBETT, R.E. (1970) 'Insomnia and the attribution process', *Journal of Personality and Social Psychology*, **16**, 2, pp. 319–28.

STRAHILEVITZ, M., STRAHILEVITZ, A. and MILLER, J. (1979) 'Air pollutants and the admission rate of psychiatric patients', *American Journal of Psychiatry*, **132**, 2, pp. 205–7.

SUNDSTROM, E. (1986) *Work Places: The Psychology of the Physical Environment in Offices and Factories*, Cambridge: Cambridge University Press.

SUNDSTROM, E., TOWN, J.P., RICE, R.W., OSBORN, T.P. and BRILL, M. (1994) 'Office noise, satisfaction and performance', *Environment and Behaviour*, **26**, 2, pp. 195–222.

SWAN, J.A. (1970) 'Response to air pollution: A study of attitudes and coping strategies of high school youths', *Environment and Behaviour*, **2**, pp. 127–52.

TARNOPOLSKY, A. and CLARK, C. (1984) 'Environmental noise and mental health', in Freeman, H. (Ed.) *Mental Health and the Environment*, London: Churchill Livingstone.

TARNOPOLSKY, A. and MORTON-WILLIAMS, J. (1980) *Aircraft Noise and Prevalence of Psychiatric Disorders*. London: Social and Community Planning Research.

TARNOPOLSKY, A., WATKINS, G. and HAND, D.J. (1980) 'Aircraft noise and mental health: 1. Prevalence of individual symptoms', *Psychological Medicine*, **10**, 683–98.

TAYLOR, R.B. (1982) 'Neighborhood physical environment and stress', in Evans, G.W. (Ed.) *Environmental Stress*. Cambridge: Cambridge University Press.

TAYLOR, R.B. (1987) 'Toward an environmental psychology of disorder: Delinquency, crime, and fear of crime', in Skolols, D. and Altman, I. (Eds) *Handbook of Environmental Psychology*, **2**, 25, pp. 951–86.

TAYLOR, R.B.(1988) *Human Territorial Functioning*, Cambridge: Cambridge University Press.

TAYLOR, R.B. and HALE, M. (1986) 'Testing alternative models of fear of crime', *Journal of Criminal Law and Criminology*, **77**, 1, pp. 151–89.

TAYLOR, R.B., GOTTFREDSON, S.D. and BROWER, S. (1984) 'Block crime and fear: Defensible space, local social ties, and territorial functioning', *Journal of Research in Crime and Delinquency*, **21**, pp. 303–31.

TAYLOR, R.B., SHUMAKER, S.A. and GOTTFREDSON, S.D. (1985) 'Neighborhood-level links between physical features and local sentiments: Deterioration, fear of crime and confidence', *Journal of Architectural Planning and Research*, **2**, pp. 261–75.

TAYLOR, S. (1938) 'Suburban neurosis', *Lancet*, **I**, 759–61.

TAYLOR, S. and CHAVE, S. (1964) *Mental Health and Environment*, London: Longman.

TAYLOR, S.D. (1974) 'The geography and epidemiology of psychiatric disorders in Southampton', Unpublshed PhD thesis, University of Southampton.

TEWFIK, G.L. and OKASHA, A. (1965) 'Psychosis and immigration', *Postgraduate Medical Journal*, **41**, pp. 603–12.

TOPF, M. (1989) Sensitivity to noise – personal hardiness', *Environment and Behaviour*, **21**, 6, pp. 717–33.

TOWNSEND, P. (1979) *Poverty in the United Kingdom*, Harmondsworth: Penguin Books.

TURNER, J.C. (1984) 'Social identification and psychological group formation', in Tajfel, H. (Ed.) *The Social Dimension*, **2**, pp. 518–38. Cambridge: Cambridge University Press.

TYLER, T.R. (1980) 'Impact of directly and indirectly experienced events: The origin of crime-related judgements and behaviours', *Journal of Personality and Social Psychology*, **39**, 1, pp. 13–28.

UNGER, D.G. and WANDERSMAN, A. (1985) 'The importance of neighbours: The social, cognitive, and affective components of neighbouring', *American Journal of Community Psychology*, **13**, 2, pp. 139–69.

VALLET, M. and FRANCOIS, J. (1982) 'Evaluation physiologigue et psychologigue de l'avion sur le sommeil', *Travail Humain*, **45**, pp. 155–68.

VAN VLIET, W. (1983) 'Families in apartment buildings', *Environment and Behaviour*, **15**, pp. 211–34.

VENTURI, R. (1977) *Complexity and Contradiction in Architecture*, London: The Architectural Press.

VESLEY, D. (1985) 'Architecture and the conflict of representation', *A.A. Files*, **8**, pp. 21–38.

VRIT, A. and WINKEL, F.W. (1991) 'Characteristics of the built environment and fear of crime: A research note on interventions in unsafe locations', *Deviant Behaviour: An Interdisciplinary Journal*, **12**, pp. 203–215.

WALLER, I. and OKIHIRO, N. (1978) *Burglary: The Victim and the Public*, Toronto, Canada: University of Toronto Press.

WALMSLEY, D.J. (1988) *Urban Living*, Harlow: Longman.

WARD, C. (1973) *Vandalism*, London: The Architectural Press.

WATKINS, G., TARNOPOLSKY, A. and JENKINS, L.A. (1981) 'Aircraft noise and mental health: II. Use of medicines and health care services', *Psychological Medicine*, **11**, pp. 155–68.

WATTS, F. (1983) 'Socialization and social integration', in Watts, F.N. and Bennett, D.H. (Eds) *Theory and Practice of Psychiatric Rehabilitation*, Chichester: Wiley.

WEBB, S.D. (1984) 'Rural-urban differences in mental health', in Freeman, H.L. (Ed.) *Mental Health and the Environment*, London: Churchill Livingstone.

WECHSLER, H. and PUGH, T.F. (1967) 'Fit of individual and community characteristics and rates of psychiatric hospitalization', *American Journal of Sociology*, **73**, pp. 331–8.

WEDMORE, K. and FREEMAN, H. (1984) 'Social pathology and urban overgrowth', in Freeman, H. (Ed.) *Mental Illness and the Environment*, London: Churchill Livingstone.

WEIDEMANN, S. and ANDERSON, J.R. (1982) 'Residents' perceptions of satisfaction and safety', *Environment and Behaviour*, **14**, 6, pp. 695–724.

WEINSTEIN, N.P. (1978) 'Individual differences in relation to noise: A longitudinal study in a college dormitory', *Journal of Applied Psychology*, **63**, pp. 458–66.

WEISSMAN, N.M., MYERS, J.K. and HARDING, P.S. (1978) 'Psychiatric disorders in a US urban community: 1975/1976', *American Journal of Psychiatry*, **135**, pp. 459–62.

WELLS, B. (1965b) 'The psycho-social influence of building environments: Sociometric findings in large and small office spaces', *Building Science*, **1**, pp. 153–65.

WENER, R. and KEYS, C. (1988) 'The effects of changes in jail population densities on crowding, sick call, and spatial behaviour', *Journal of Applied Social Psychology*, **18**, 10, pp. 852–66.

WHITE, M., KASL, S.V., ZAHNER, G.E.P. and WILL, J.C. (1987) 'Perceived crime in the neighborhood and mental health of women and children', *Environment and Behaviour*, **19**, 5, pp. 588–613.

WICKER, A.W. (1979) *An Introduction to Ecological Psychology*, Cambridge: Cambridge University Press.

WILLMOTT, P. (1963) *The Evolution of a Community*, London: Routledge & Kegan Paul.

WILLMOTT, P. (1967) 'Social research and new communities', *Journal of the American Institute of Planners*, **33**, 6, pp. 387–98.

WILLMOTT, P. and COONEY, E. (1963) 'Community planning and sociological research: A problem of collaboration', *Journal of the American Insitute of Planners*, **29**, pp. 123–6.

WILNER, D.M., WALKLEY, R.P. and COOK, S.W. (1955) *Human Relations in Interracial Housing – A Study of the Contact Hypothesis*, Minneapolis, MN: University of Minnesota Press.

WILNER, D.M., WALKLEY, R.P., PINKERTON, T.C. and TAYBACK, M. (1962) *The Housing Environment and Family Life*, Baltimore, MD: John Hopkins University Press.

WILSON, S. (1978) 'Vandalism and defensible space on London housing estates', in Clarke, R.V.G. (Ed.) *Tackling Vandalism*, Home Office Research Study 47, London, HMSO.

WINCHESTER, S. and JACKSON, H. (1982) 'Residential burglary: The limits of prevention', *Home Office Research Study 74*, London: HMSO.

WINDLEY, P.G. and SCHEIDT, R.J. (1982) 'An ecological model of mental health among small-town rural elderly', *Journal of Gerontology*, **37**, pp. 235–42.

WING, J.K. (1974) 'Housing environments and mental health', in Parry, H.B. (Ed.) *Population and its Problems*, Oxford: Clarendon Press.

WING, J.K. (1976) 'Mental health in urban environments', in Harrison, G.A. and Gibson, J.B. (Eds) *Man in Urban Environments*, Oxford: Oxford University Press.

WINKEL, G.H. and HOLAHAN, C.J. (1985) 'The environmental psychology of the hospital: Is the cure worse than the illness?' in Wandersman, A. and Hess, R. (Eds) *Beyond the Individual: Environmental Approaches and Prevention*, London: Haworth.

WINNUBST, J., BUUNK, B. and MARCELISSEN, F. (1988) 'Social support and stress: Perspectives and processes', in Fisher, S. and Reason, J. (Eds) *Handbook of Life Stress, Cognition and Health*, Chichester: Wiley.

WIRTH, L. (1938) 'Urbanism as a way of life', *American Journal of Sociology*, **44**, 1–24.

YANCEY, W. (1971) 'Architecture, interaction, and social control: The case of a large-scale public housing project', *Environment and Behaviour*, **3**, pp. 3–21.

YOUNG, M. and WILLMOTT, P. (1957) *Family and Kinship in East London*, London: Routledge and Kegan Paul.

ZIGMOND, A.S. and SNAITH, R.P. (1983) 'The hospital anxiety and depression scale', *Acta Psychiatrica Scandinavica*, **67**, pp. 361–70.

ZUCKERMAN, M., SCHMITZ, M. and YOSHA, A. (1977) 'Effects of crowding in a student environment', *Journal of Applied Social Psychology*, **7**, 1, pp. 67–72.

Index

Page numbers in bold denote the first page of the chapter on that particular subject.